ABDOMINAL ULTRASOUND HOW, WHY AND WHEN

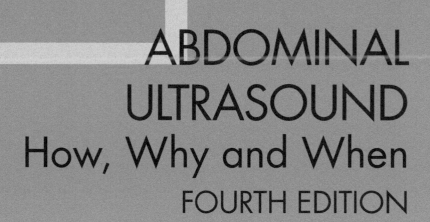

ABDOMINAL ULTRASOUND
How, Why and When
FOURTH EDITION

NICOLA J. DAVIDSON, BSc (Hons), MSc
Lead Sonographer
Worcestershire Acute NHS Trust
Worcester, UK

ELSEVIER

First edition 1999
Second edition 2004
Third edition 2011
Fourth edition 2023

Notices

Practitioners and researchers must always rely on their own experience and knowledge in evaluating and using any information, methods, compounds or experiments described herein. Because of rapid advances in the medical sciences, in particular, independent verification of diagnoses and drug dosages should be made. To the fullest extent of the law, no responsibility is assumed by Elsevier, authors, editors or contributors for any injury and/or damage to persons or property as a matter of products liability, negligence or otherwise, or from any use or operation of any methods, products, instructions, or ideas contained in the material herein.

ISBN 978-0-7020-8243-6

Content Strategist: Trinity Hutton; Poppy Garraway
Content Project Manager: Ayan Dhar

Printed in United Kingdom

Last digit is the print number: 9 8 7 6 5 4 3 2 1

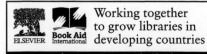

Working together
to grow libraries in
developing countries

www.elsevier.com • www.bookaid.org

CONTENTS

Contributors, vii

Preface, ix

1 **Optimizing the Diagnostic Information, 1**
Shivali Shah

2 **Ultrasound of the Liver, 21**
James R. Michael

3 **Ultrasound of the Gallbladder and Biliary Tree, 93**
James R. Michael

4 **Ultrasound of the Pancreas, 143**
Sharan Wadhwani

5 **Ultrasound of the Spleen and Lymphatic System, 167**
Nicola J. Davidson

6 **Ultrasound of the Renal Tract, 185**
Nicola J. Davidson

7 **Ultrasound of the Testes and Male Pelvis, 229**
Simon J. Freeman and Pamela C. Parker

8 **Ultrasound of the Retroperitoneum and Gastrointestinal Tract, 265**
Ruth Reeve and Catherine Kirkpatrick

9 **Ultrasound of the Pediatric Abdomen, 289**
Lorraine C. Walsh

10 **Ultrasound of the Acute Abdomen, 321**
Nicola J. Davidson

11 **Interventional Techniques, 333**
Sidi H. Rashid

Index, 347

Contributors are listed in order of the chapters:

Shivali Shah, BSc (Hons), MSc
Clinical Application Specialist, Philips, Scotland (UK)

James R. Michael, BSc, MSc
Senior Lecturer in Medical Ultrasound, Birmingham City University, Birmingham, UK

Sharan Wadhwani, MB Ch.B, BSc (Hons), MRCS, FRCR
Consultant Radiologist, Hepatobiliary and Pancreatic Imaging, Queen Elizabeth Hospital, University Hospitals Birmingham NHS Trust, Birmingham, UK

Simon J. Freeman, MBBS, MRCP, FRCR
Consultant Radiologist, University Hospitals Plymouth NHS Trust, Plymouth, UK

Pamela C. Parker, DCR (R), MSc
Consultant Sonographer, Ultrasound, Hull University Teaching Hospitals NHS Trust, Hull, UK

Ruth Reeve, BSc, MSc
Clinical Specialist Sonographer, Portsmouth Hospitals NHS Trust, Portsmouth, UK
Clinical Academic Research Fellow, School of Health Sciences, Faculty of Environmental and Life Science, University of Southampton, Southampton, UK

Catherine Kirkpatrick, BSc (Hons), MSc
Consultant Sonographer & Clinical Lead Ultrasound, United Lincolnshire Hospitals NHS Trust, Lincoln, UK

Lorraine C. Walsh, DMU, PG Dip, MEd
Consultant Sonographer, Birmingham Children's Hospital, Birmingham, UK

Sidi H. Rashid, MB BCh (Hons), FRCR
Consultant Vascular & Interventional Radiologist, Worcestershire Acute Hospitals NHS Trust, Worcester, UK

Ultrasound is widely used within imaging departments but is now also becoming a more common sight on hospital wards, in clinics, and in primary care. The relatively easy access to equipment has seen the use of ultrasound soar. While this can have a positive impact on patients in providing faster access to diagnostics, the use of ultrasound in untrained or inexperienced hands can result in confusion and ultimately misdiagnosis.

This book is intended to support those new to ultrasound to understand its uses and limitations and to provide a practical approach to scanning. This includes an explanation of technique, ultrasound features of common pathologies, and considerations on patient presentation and potential management. There are also plenty of tips which can help in those more difficult cases.

As ultrasound technology has improved, the range of conditions which can be diagnosed, monitored, and assessed has also extended. It would, therefore, be impossible to include every pathology that may be encountered, but this book is intended to guide the novice and act as a reference for the more experienced sonographer and those wanting to expand their ultrasound knowledge.

This edition has been produced as a collaborative effort by sonographers and radiologists who are passionate about ultrasound and have a wealth of knowledge and experience to share from their specialist areas. The author would also like to acknowledge Jane Bates for the work in previous editions, providing the fundamental core aspects of abdominal ultrasound which have been built upon in this fourth edition. Finally, thanks to the ultrasound team in Worcestershire who have supported training within our departments sharing valuable knowledge to trainees past, present, and future.

Nicola J. Davidson

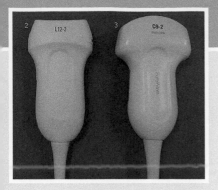

Optimizing the Diagnostic Information

Shivali Shah

CHAPTER OUTLINE

Introduction, 1
Technique, 1
Image Optimization, 2
The Use of Doppler, 6
Getting the Best out of Doppler, 8
Additional Imaging Technologies, 8
   Tissue Harmonic Imaging, 8
   Compound Imaging, 10
   Volume Ultrasound: 3D and 4D, 10
   Elastography: Transient and Shear
     Wave, 11
   Contrast-Enhanced Ultrasound (CEUS), 11
   Fusion Imaging, 11
   Needle Visualization, 12
Choosing a Machine, 12
   Image Quality, 13
   Machine Capabilities and Functions, 13

   Ergonomics, 14
   Upgradability and Maintenance, 14
Recording of Images, 14
Safety of Diagnostic Ultrasound, 15
Biological Effects of Ultrasound, 15
   Thermal Effects, 15
   Mechanical Effects, 16
Safety Indices (Thermal and Mechanical
   Indices), 16
Other Hazards, 16
The Safe Practice of Ultrasound, 17
Medicolegal issues, 17
Departmental Guidelines/Schemes of Work, 18
Quality Assurance, 18
   Equipment Tests, 18
References, 19

INTRODUCTION

With the ever-increasing demand for diagnostic and therapeutic radiological modalities, ultrasound remains a widely available, relatively cheap, safe imaging modality. However, it is operator-dependent to a greater degree than any other diagnostic imaging modality. The potential for variation in image acquisition, scanning techniques, and result interpretation is significant. Therefore, the only acceptable way to undertake diagnostic ultrasound is:
1. After appropriate training – practical and theoretical,
2. Preferably following an independent assessment by a qualified ultrasound practitioner (as not everyone can reach the desired standard),
3. By continually developing knowledge and technique with regular, relevant practice,
4. By employing audit of practice, preferably within a team setting, as prolonged isolated practice is more likely to result in poor standards of diagnosis.

TECHNIQUE

Ultrasound is devolving rapidly from radiology departments to other clinical environments, such as GP surgeries, hospital outpatient clinics, and theater environments. Pre-hospital and hospital emergency medicine practitioners also routinely employ point-of-care ultrasound in their practice. There is potential for ultrasound to be carried out by insufficiently trained personnel. A lack of understanding and/or appreciation by some has led to theoretical courses being considered "training." This notion is a gross underestimation of the reality and possibly one of the most disadvantageous legacies of this rapid proliferation of service provision.

Whatever the limitations of your equipment, a comprehensive and properly executed technique is essential. This is not just about acquiring images (unlike many other radiological imaging tests). It is about a comprehensive and confident evaluation of the organs (with representative images for audit and recording purposes). This can only be achieved with practical experience and reflective practice, close supervision, and continual feedback from qualified practitioners.

Knowing your limitations, knowing when you have not been able to execute a satisfactory scan, and being able to request assistance from expert practitioners, are some of the most valuable lessons you will learn.

Although the dynamic nature of the scan is a huge advantage over other forms of imaging, the potential for misdiagnosis is significant. The skilled operator continuously adjusts the technique to obtain the maximum diagnostic information. In any abdominal ultrasound survey, the operator assesses the limitations of the scan, and the level of confidence with which the pathologic condition can be excluded or confirmed.

IMAGE OPTIMIZATION

Ultrasound is a highly operator-dependent examination, and obtaining the best image quality is essential. Through training, the operator must learn the techniques by which their ultrasound machine's capabilities can be maximized. Misinterpretation can pose a significant risk to diagnoses and patient care.

It is imperative that the operator understands:

- Anatomy of the abdomen to obtain the most useful and relevant information by successfully navigating the viscera during an examination,
- The appearances on ultrasound of these anatomical structures, including a sound understanding of pathological processes, to enable image interpretation in the healthy and diseased states,
- The fundamentals of ultrasound, i.e., recognizing the advantages and disadvantages while scanning,
- Knowledge of the equipment being used, i.e., making the most of your machine (Box 1.1).

> ### BOX 1.1   Making the Most of Your Equipment
>
> 1. Use the highest frequency possible – try increasing the frequency when examining the pancreas or anterior gallbladder.
> 2. Use the lowest frame rate and highest line density possible. Restless or breathless patients will require a higher frame rate.
> 3. Use the smallest field practicable – sections through the liver require a relatively wide sector angle and a large depth of view, but when examining the common duct, for example, the field can be greatly reduced, thereby improving the resolution with no loss of frame rate.
> 4. Use the focal zone/range at the relevant, correct depth.
> 5. Use tissue harmonic imaging to increase the signal to noise ratio and reduce artifact.
> 6. Try different processing curves to highlight subtle abnormalities and increase contrast resolution.

Ultrasound manufacturers allow users to optimize and maximize image quality and enhance diagnostic information in numerous ways.

The essential controls:

2D gain: Controls the brightness of the image by amplifying all returning echoes in the image. Increasing and decreasing the gain will make the image brighter or darker, respectively. It is important to get this right as too low a gain will produce a dark/obscure image, and too high a gain will amplify mid-level echoes producing a very noisy image.

Focus: Usually presented as a zone or range. The placement of the focus is where the beam width is narrowest and most concentrated, improving the contrast and lateral resolution.[21] A large range or multiple foci will dramatically slow your frame rate (Fig. 1.1).

Depth: Controls your field of view. An increased depth will slow the frame rate, and because the echoes are taking longer to return, the image quality can deteriorate.

Zoom: Magnifies the region of interest. There are usually two types of zoom: Read Zoom, which allows the operator to instantly magnify an area of the image (however, the image can become very pixelated), and Write Zoom, which allows the user to select an area (via a box) and the machine will process and display

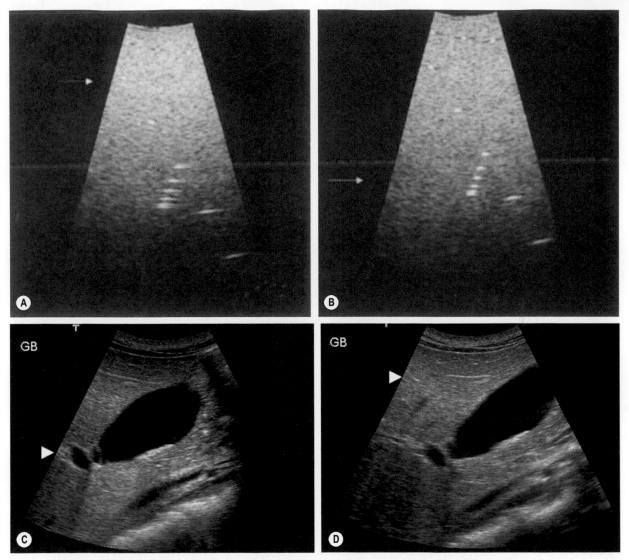

Fig. 1.1 The effect of focal zone placement. (A) With the focal zone in the near field, structures in the far-field are poorly resolved. (B) Correct focal zone placement improves both axial and lateral resolution of the wires. (C) The focal zone incorrectly set in the near field (arrowhead) makes it difficult to demonstrate small gallstones. (D) With the focal zone correctly set (arrowhead), the stones are resolved with a clear, diagnostic band of posterior shadowing.

only that area. The line density, frame rate, and image quality are superior when using the Write Zoom.[21]

Sector Width: The operator can alter the 2D size laterally. A smaller sector width will increase the lateral resolution.

Frequency: A high-frequency will give a higher resolution image. However, this will compromise penetration. Furthermore, vice versa, scanning a high body mass index patient may require the user to lower the frequency resulting in poorer resolution but better penetration (Fig. 1.2).

Dynamic range: Controls the amount of greyscale displayed on the image. It is the ratio between the largest and smallest displayed signal strength.[23] Operator-controlled, a high dynamic range will show a wider range of echoes; therefore, less contrast and a

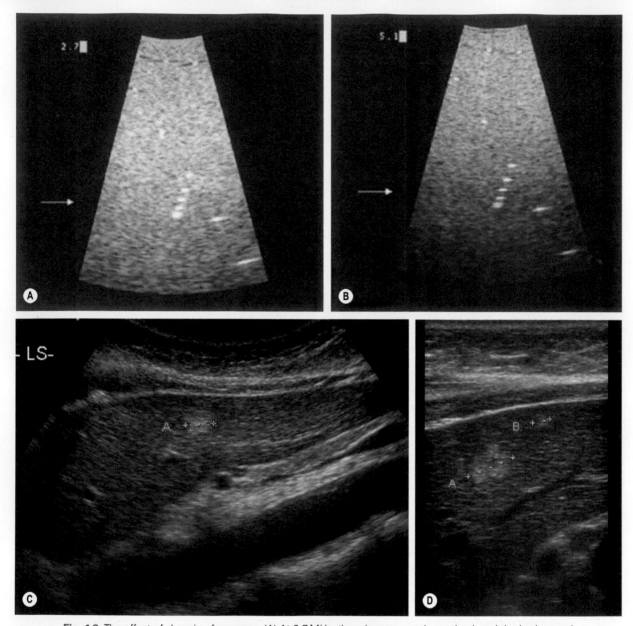

Fig. 1.2 The effect of changing frequency. (A) At 2.7 MHz, the wires are poorly resolved, and the background "texture" of the test object looks coarse. (B) The same transducer is switched to a resonant frequency of 5.1 MHz. Without changing any other settings, the six wires are now resolved, and the background texture appears finer. (C) A small nodule in the anterior portion of the left lobe of the liver was demonstrated with a 5.0 MHz transducer. (D) Using a higher frequency transducer, the nodule in (C) has improved detail, and a further small nodule (calipers B), not seen on the lower frequency, is detected near the anterior surface.

"softer image," and a low dynamic range with a narrow range/ratio will produce a more contrasted image.[21]

It is important not to suppress weak echoes by lowering the dynamic range by too much. Alternatively, a high dynamic range can create a noisy image.

Time gain compensation (TGC): Creates a more uniform image as the operator has control of tissue intensity at different depths.[23] The machine will automatically try to compensate for this at different depths; however, TGC is useful for looking at structures such as the bladder, gallbladder, or cysts where the posterior tissue signals are usually brighter and require adjusting.

Tissue Harmonic imaging and compound imaging are important controls (see Additional Imaging Technologies below) to optimize image quality. They are usually on/off controls.

Line Density: This may be achieved by either reducing the frame rate, reducing the sector angle, or depth of field (Fig. 1.3).

Regardless of the machine performance, a knowledgeable operator will optimize the above controls and get the best out of a machine. The operator is expected to know the limitations of the scan in terms of equipment

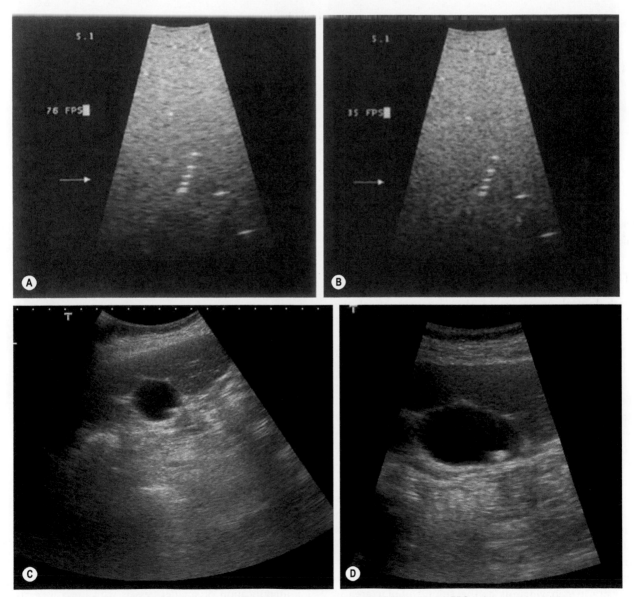

Fig. 1.3 The effect of line density. (A) Seventy-six frames per second (FPS). (B) 36 FPS – the resulting higher line density improves the image, making it sharper. (C) The gallbladder is displayed with a low line density, as the scanning area is large. (D) By reducing the field of view, the line density is increased, clarifying the small stone in the gallbladder.

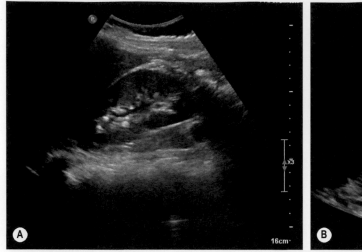
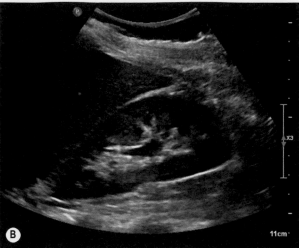

Fig. 1.4 The importance of using correct equipment settings: (A) Incorrect use of equipment settings makes it difficult to appreciate the structures in the right kidney. (B) By increasing the resonant frequency, decreasing the frame rate (increasing line density), and adjusting the focal zone, structures in the kidney are clarified.

capabilities, operator skills, clinical problems, and patient limitations and communicate them where necessary (Fig. 1.4).

THE USE OF DOPPLER

Pathological processes in the abdomen affect the hemodynamics of relevant organs, and the use of Doppler is an essential part of the diagnostic procedure. This is discussed in more detail in subsequent chapters.

Color Doppler is used to assess the patency and direction of flow of vessels in the abdomen, to establish the vascularity of masses or lesions, and to identify vascular flow disturbances such as stenoses. Flow information is color-coded (usually red toward and blue away from the transducer) and superimposed on the image. This gives the operator an immediate impression of a vascular "map" of the area (Fig. 1.5). This Doppler information is obtained simultaneously, often from a relatively large area of the image, sometimes at the expense of the grayscale image quality. The extra time taken to obtain the Doppler information for each line results in a reduction in frame rate and line density, which worsens as the color Doppler area is enlarged. Therefore, it is advisable to use a compact

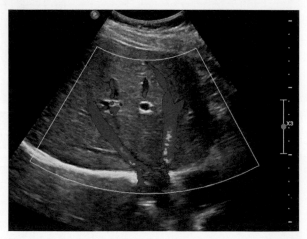

Fig. 1.5 Color Doppler of the hepatic vein confluence. Flow is colored blue to indicate a direction away from the transducer.

color "box" over the region of interest to maintain image quality.

Power Doppler also superimposes Doppler information on the grayscale image but without any directional information. It displays only the amount of energy (Fig. 1.6). It has the advantage of a stronger signal, allowing identification of smaller vessels with lower velocity flow than color Doppler. As it is less angle dependent than

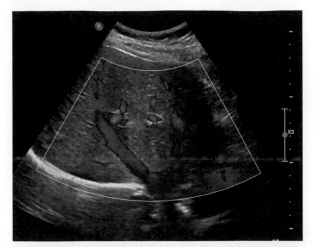

Fig. 1.6 Power Doppler of the hepatic vein confluence. Directional information is lost, but power Doppler can be superior to color in demonstrating low-velocity flow.

color Doppler, it is particularly useful for vessels that run perpendicular to the beam, such as the inferior vena cava. Recent advancements of Doppler include micro-sensitive color Doppler. This advanced Doppler algorithm is used to detect slow and weak blood flow, which normal color/power Doppler may not. The new ultra-sensitive Doppler removes clutter/noise from the ultrasound image, demonstrates low-velocity flow signals, and has improved the detection of microvessels (Fig. 1.7).[26]

Pulsed Doppler uses pulses of Doppler from individual elements or small groups of elements within the array. This allows the operator to select a specific vessel, which has been identified on the grayscale or color Doppler image, from which to obtain a spectrum. This gives further information regarding the flow envelope, variance, velocity, and downstream resistance of the blood flow (Fig. 1.8).

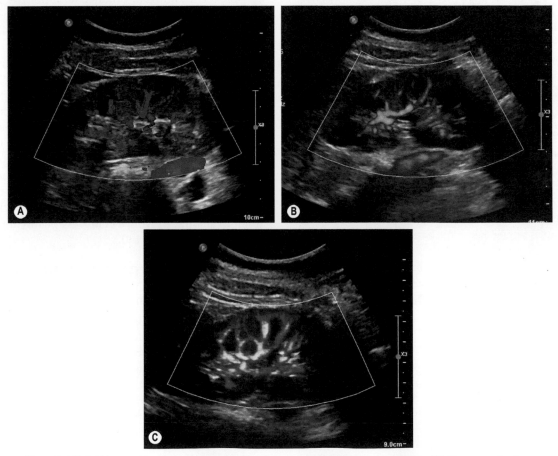

Fig. 1.7 (A) A kidney with color Doppler. (B) The same kidney with power Doppler. (C) The use of micro-sensitive Doppler to detect very slow flow. The vascularity of the kidney is more sensitive.

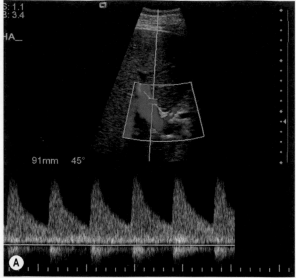

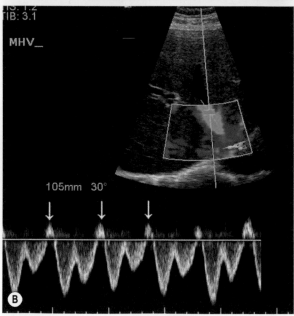

Fig. 1.8 Flow velocity waveforms. (A) Low-resistance flow toward the transducer from a normal hepatic artery. Good end-diastolic flow throughout the cycle with a "filled in" waveform indicating variance in flow. (B) In contrast, this hepatic vein trace with flow away from the transducer is triphasic, with a clear "envelope" consistent with less variance. The pulsatile nature of the flow incorporates brief flow toward the transducer (arrows) at the end of each cycle.

GETTING THE BEST OUT OF DOPPLER

Familiarity with Doppler controls is essential to avoid the pitfalls and increase confidence in the results. It is relatively straightforward to demonstrate flow in major vessels and to assess the relevant spectral waveform; most problems arise when trying to diagnose the *lack* of flow in a suspected thrombosed vessel and in displaying low-velocity flow in difficult-to-access vessels.

Doppler is known to produce false-positive results for vessel occlusion (Fig. 1.9), and the operator must avoid the pitfalls. It is essential that the Doppler settings are sensitive enough to detect the velocity of flow in the vessel (Box 1.2). This means that the angle of insonation to the direction of flow must be as close to 0 degrees as possible (i.e., the vessel must be flowing toward or away from the beam, not perpendicular to it), the pulse repetition frequency (PRF) must be set to detect slow flow, and the Doppler gain must be turned up sufficiently.

It is also possible to make mistakes if the settings are *too* sensitive, i.e., non-occlusive thrombus can be masked by too much color flow, and a very low PRF can result in aliasing – giving a confusing picture if the operator is unaware (Fig. 1.9).

ADDITIONAL IMAGING TECHNOLOGIES

Tissue Harmonic Imaging

Tissue harmonic imaging processes the harmonic frequency (usually twice the fundamental, transmitted frequency) by using pulse inversion. The reflected beam consists of the fundamental (transmitted) frequency together with diminishing amounts of harmonic frequencies. Using the harmonic has the effect of reducing artifact, improving spatial resolution, and consequently

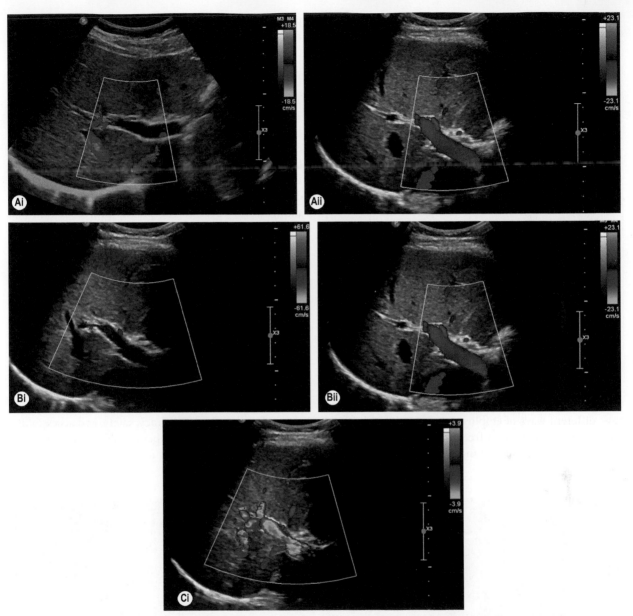

Fig. 1.9 (Ai) The portal vein appears to have no flow when it lies at 90 degrees to the beam – a possible misinterpretation for thrombosis. (Aii) When scanned intercostally, the vein is almost parallel to the beam, and flow is easily demonstrated. (Bi) Too high a PRF results in the false appearances of no flow in the left image. (Bii) Reducing the PRF demonstrates sufficient flow. (Ci) This portal vein looks blue because of a low PRF and aliasing, which could be mistaken for reversed flow. Increasing the PRF will correct any aliasing.

the conspicuity of structures.[1,2] Different manufacturers have different ways of employing this mode, and therefore, the results can differ from machine to machine. In some cases, the dynamic range may be reduced or the penetration impaired, so it is useful to be familiar with both fundamental and harmonic modes on your machine to get the best from the examination (Fig. 1.10).

Compound Imaging

There are two types of ultrasound compound imaging. The first, spatial compound imaging, insonates the tissues from several different angles. Theoretically, this enables the beam to be perpendicular to the various reflective surfaces for a greater proportion of the image, thus improving the definition around lesions and reducing artifact because of edge attenuation. It has been shown to improve the conspicuity of liver lesions and sharpen their margins.[3]

The second type of compound imaging uses several different transmission frequencies to achieve an optimum display of the tissues. With spatial compounding, the different angles of insonation may achieve better definition and improvement in clarity but also have the disadvantage of reducing or eliminating useful artifacts (such as posterior shadowing), which may assist the interpretation and diagnosis.[4]

Volume Ultrasound: 3D and 4D

Volume ultrasound has been used for many years because of its diagnostic accuracy, safety, and accessibility.

3D involves a large number of multiple 2D slices obtained, stored, and reconstructed to display as "volume"

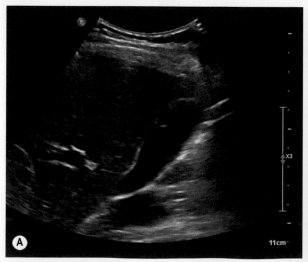
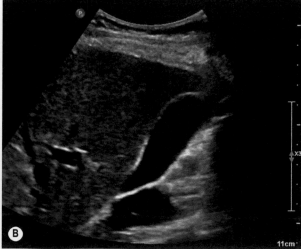

Fig. 1.10 The effect of tissue harmonic imaging: (A) A gallbladder without harmonics. (B) Tissue harmonic imaging was applied, which reduces artifact and clarifies the echogenicity.

information known as 3D. Consecutive 3D images are taken, repeated, and constructed to form a live 4D (three spatial dimensions plus motion) image.[22]

Depending on the transducer, the 3D/4D is captured either by a:

- Multi-element transducer being moved mechanically over a region,
- Electronic scanning, which has a matrix transducer array.

The acquisition of these volume datasets can help provide the operator with live information to better understand a structure/abnormality and eliminate movement artifacts (especially in the case of the matrix transducer). A further advantage is that such datasets may be examined and manipulated when the patient has left the department.[5,27]

Elastography: Transient and Shear Wave

Elastography is a common method used in abdominal organs to estimate the stiffness of tissue by means of compression.

In shear wave elastography, the ultrasound machine emits a push pulse, four times stronger than ultrasound, which generates shear waves in the body. The shear waves travel transversely through the tissue; additional detection pulses are generated to measure the propagation through the tissue. The wave speed measured is used to calculate the tissue stiffness. This is known as Acoustic Radiation Force Impulse technology. Shear waves that travel through tissue faster and generate high numbers are suggestive of increased tissue stiffness.

Another popular method includes "blind" transient elastography using a mechanical vibrating probe. This probe releases a very low frequency (approximately 50 Hz), which generates shear waves when transmitted through the tissues. The same principle applies where the probe detects these waves and displays a stiffness value from a single line of ultrasound. No 2D image is required.

Using the shear wave elastography function of the ultrasound machine is advantageous as the operator knows exactly where the pulse is transmitted, thereby avoiding potential miscalculations from cysts/vessels/ the gallbladder (where elastography cannot travel). Elastography has been shown to be a reliable, non-invasive method of estimating liver fibrosis and may avoid the need for some biopsy procedures.[6]

These specialist skills are best learned with a liver specialist who will set departmental protocols/guidelines of normal and abnormal values.

Contrast-Enhanced Ultrasound (CEUS)

CEUS is used to characterize lesions and to assess vasculature, and is often used as a second-line examination to assess pathologic conditions just after the initial ultrasound. A contrast agent made up of microbubbles is administered intravenously. These bubbles vibrate under beam interrogation producing a non-linear response. The asymmetric signal caused by this response is interpreted into the contrast image. Each lesion will have a behavior that is dependent on the "wash-in wash-out" time through the arterial, portal, and late phase. The pattern enables the operator to make a diagnosis without having to take a biopsy. Wash-in and wash-out characteristics for each tumor are individual. The reader is encouraged to undertake their own reading of this subject matter.

The natural breakdown of the microbubbles within minutes and its few adverse reactions are added benefits of CEUS, which also include non-ionizing imaging, easy accessibility, and reduction in the need for undertaking minimally invasive biopsies. However, it is also important to remember that CEUS cannot detect small lesions < 5 mm, it is often difficult to image subdiaphragmatic lesions, and confusion can occur when there are focal fatty areas.[25] Additionally, this technique is also limited by increased patient body habitus resulting from limited contrast penetration

It is important to perform CEUS with the assistance of a radiologist/liver specialist as expert guidance is often required.

Fusion Imaging

Fusion imaging is becoming more popular in the ultrasound world. Most commonly used in abdominal and prostate imaging, it can fuse multiple modalities (MRI/ CT/PET) to a multi-planar dynamic ultrasound scan. The process is enabled by combining previously acquired volumetric datasets to real-time ultrasound using electromagnetic tracking equipment.

Fusion imaging is a great tool to help the operator:

1. Find a lesion on ultrasound that has been seen on MRI/CT/PET. Often the operator struggles to find small, ambiguous lesions, unable to fully confirm on the ultrasound. Fusion helps identify the lesion on another modality and target the same area on ultrasound.

2. Find a lesion that has been seen on ultrasound but not on MRI/CT/PET. This can happen when non-contrast computed tomography (CT) examinations are performed and/or there is a small lesion. The operator can identify the target on ultrasound which automatically shows on the corresponding modality plane.

3. Re-examine a lesion under ultrasound. Ultrasound-to-ultrasound fusion can be performed to monitor and reassess a target.

4. Navigate a clear, safe path for an interventional examination.

A direct comparison of real-time ultrasound to existing datasets enables the operator to achieve confidence in the visualization and localization of structures/abnormalities. The ability to identify and set targets on historical datasets enables follow-up scans to be performed by ultrasound, thus reducing the requirement for serial CT scans.

Needle Visualization

When performing an interventional examination, the needle is often seen best using the in-plane approach. The in-plane technique enhances the needle better as it is perpendicular to the ultrasound beam. Often, there are instances when this is not possible, especially if an out-of-plane approach is necessary or even the need for a steeper angle.[24] Many manufacturers have created a software package to help overcome this issue (Fig. 1.11). Enabled software will steer the beam obliquely so it can perpendicularly reflect off the needle enhancing the whole length.

CHOOSING A MACHINE

The practitioner is confronted with a dizzying range of equipment, from a hand-held kit the size of a large mobile phone (usually relatively low cost) to high-end complex and expensive machines. Choosing the right machine for the job can be a daunting task.

As far as abdominal scanning is concerned, it is advisable to go for the *best grayscale image* you can possibly afford. Do not be tempted by lavish (expensive) functionality on a machine, which increases the price of equipment with an indifferent or inferior basic grayscale image.

Take careful stock of the range of examinations you expect your machine to perform. Future developments that may affect the type of machine you buy include:

- Increase in numbers of patients calculated from trends in previous years.
- Increase in range of possible applications – an impending peripheral vascular service, for example – or regional screening initiative.
- Clinical developments and changes in patient management may require more, or different, ultrasound techniques – for example, medical therapies which require ultrasound monitoring, surgical techniques which may require intraoperative scanning, availability of hospital beds, and introduction/expansion of hospital services.
- Impending political developments by government or hospital management, resulting in changes in the services provided, the funding, or the catchment area.

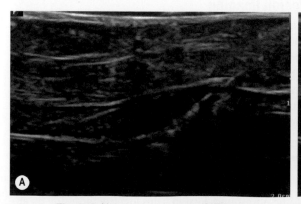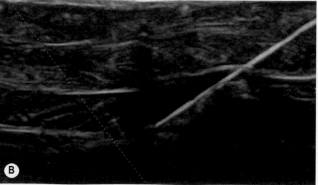

Fig. 1.11 Needle visualization. (A) The needle is entering from the top right-hand side corner of the image. It is very difficult to fully identify. (B) However, an algorithm with beam steering highlights the needle for the user.

- Other impending ultrasound developments – such as the use of CEUS, fusion imaging, needle visualization, ultrasound-guided therapies which may be required in the future.

The following points are useful to bear in mind when purchasing new equipment:

- Involve those who are regularly using ultrasound – the local radiology department, for example.
- The number/quantity of probes required and their ergonomic design (Fig. 1.12).

Consider the footprint, shape, and frequencies required: most modern transducers are broadband in design, enabling the operator to use a wide range of frequencies in one probe (Res/Gen/Pen mode). This is a potential advantage as it reduces the number of probes required for a general service. A curved array probe is suitable for most general abdominal applications, operating in the 2–6 MHz region. Additional higher frequency probes are useful for pediatrics and superficial structures. A small footprint is essential if neonatal and pediatric work is undertaken, and a 7–10 MHz frequency will probably be required. High-frequency probes are now available, ranging up to 35 MHz.

A biopsy attachment may be needed for invasive procedures. Depending on the range of work to be undertaken, linear probes, endoprobes, intraoperative probes, and other designs can be considered.

Image Quality

There are very few applications where this is not of paramount importance, and abdominal scanning requires the very best you can afford. A machine capable of producing a high-quality image is likely to remain operational for much longer (between five to seven years) than one capable of only poor quality, which will need replacement much sooner.

A poor quality image is a false economy in abdominal scanning (you are better compromising on functionality if funding is tight) as the compromises would impact the delivery of safe, high-quality patient care.

Machine Capabilities and Functions

The availability and ease of use of various functions differ from machine to machine. Some of the important issues to consider when buying a machine are:

- Ease of probe selection and switching process, simultaneous connection of several probes.
- Dynamic frequency capability.
- Dynamic focusing control, number, and pattern of focal zones/range.
- Functions such as beam steering, sector angle adjustment, zoom, frame rate adjustment, trackerball controls.
- TGC and power output controls.
- Cine facility – operation and size of memory.
- Programmable presets.
- Tissue harmonic and/or contrast harmonic imaging.
- Body marker and labeling functions.
- Measurement packages – operation and display.
- Color/power and spectral Doppler through all probes.
- Doppler sensitivity.
- Doppler controls – ease of use, programmable presets.
- Output displays.
- Report package option.

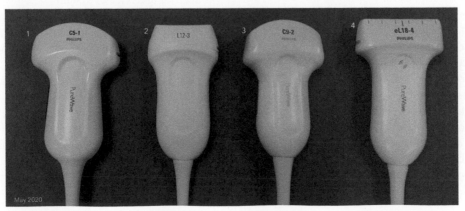

Fig. 1.12 Curved arrays (probes 1 and 3) suitable for abdominal scanning. Linear arrays (probes 2 and 4) are useful for superficial structures, e.g., gallbladder and anterior abdominal wall.

Ergonomics

The ultrasound machine must be usable by various operators in all the required situations. Work-related musculoskeletal disorders are a common cause of pain in sonographers, with some studies identifying that up to 90% of ultrasound practitioners experience pain. Careful consideration is not given to the scanning environment (see below). When choosing and setting up a scanning service, forethought should be given to the design of the ultrasound machine and the seating arrangements and examination couch. These should all be adjustable to facilitate the best scanning position for the operator. It is important for each practitioner to spend a few moments at the beginning of each examination optimizing the position of the equipment and patient to ensure a good posture can be achieved to reduce strain.[7]

TIP BOX

When scanning, the practitioner must consider their own posture to reduce the chance of injury. Points to consider include:-

- Ensure the position is not static – keep arm abduction to a minimum and try not to lean or twist.
- Reduce repetitive movements – if possible, perform a range of different scans.
- Do not grip the transducer tightly and review different types of grip to minimize the risk of injury.
- If your main role is to scan, ensure you have adequate breaks and incorporate stretching into your daily routine.

Other considerations are:

- System dimensions and steering. The requirement for the system to be portable – for example, ward or theater work – or mobile for transportation to remote clinics. Machines used regularly for mobile work should be robust and easy to move.
- Moveable (swivel and tilt) monitor and control panel, including height adjustment for different operators and situations.
- Keyboard design – to facilitate easy use of the required functions without stretching or twisting.

Handheld portable machines are an option that may be considered.

Upgradability and Maintenance

A machine that is potentially upgradable has a longer, more cost-effective life and will be supported by the manufacturer over a longer period of time. Consider:

- Future software upgrades – possible effects and costs.
- Other available options for the future; additional transducers or add-on facilities.
- Various maintenance contract options and costs are available, including options on the replacement of probes, which should be considered when purchasing new equipment.

RECORDING OF IMAGES

It is good practice for departments to have guidelines for taking and retaining images within individual schemes of work, outlining the minimum expected.[8]

The advantages of recording images are:

- They provide a record of the quality of the scan and how it has been conducted, the organs examined, the extent of the scan, the type and standard of equipment, the settings used, and other scanning factors that can be an invaluable tool in providing a medicolegal defense,
- They provide a valuable teaching aid,
- They help to ensure good governance within departments: promoting the use of good techniques, they can be used to ensure protocols are followed and provide an excellent audit tool,
- They can be used to obtain a second opinion on difficult or equivocal cases and provide a basis for discussion with clinical colleagues.

The disadvantages are:

- The cost of buying, operating, and maintaining the recording device or system,
- In some cases, the quality of images may not accurately reflect that of the image on the ultrasound monitor,
- Increased scanning time to accommodate the capturing of images,
- Storage and retrieval of images may be time and space-consuming,
- A hard copy may be mislaid or lost, but this can be mitigated by enforcement of strict patient confidentiality, data protection, and information governance policies and practices,
- If the examination has been *poorly* performed, the image may demonstrate that too!

The recording of images is encouraged. It allows for retrospective case review or clinical review, reduces the operator's vulnerability to litigation, and provides supporting evidence of the ultrasound diagnosis.[9] The operator must take responsibility for ensuring the scan has been performed to the required standard; any images produced for subsequent discussion are only *representative* of the examination and have been chosen by the operator as an appropriate selection.

Digital imaging networks (picture archiving and communications systems, or picture archiving and communication system) are convenient, quick, and relatively easy to use. The image quality is excellent, suffering little or no degradation in capture and subsequent retrieval, and the system can potentially be linked to a conventional imager should a hard copy be required.

Many systems now incorporate patient registration and reporting, further streamlining the ultrasound examination.

SAFETY OF DIAGNOSTIC ULTRASOUND

Within the field of clinical diagnostic ultrasound, it is currently accepted that there is insufficient evidence for any deleterious effects at diagnostic levels and that the benefits to patients outweigh the risks. As new techniques and technological developments come onto the market, new biophysical conditions may be introduced, which require evaluation with regard to safety,[10] and we cannot afford to become complacent about the possible effects. The situation remains under constant review.

Several international bodies continue to consider the safety of ultrasound in clinical use. The European Federation for Ultrasound in Medicine and Biology has confirmed the safety of diagnostic ultrasound and endorsed its "informed" use.[11] While the use of pulsed Doppler is considered inadvisable for the developing embryo during the first trimester, no such exceptions are highlighted for abdominal ultrasounds. The European Committee for Ultrasound Radiation Safety confirms that no deleterious effects have been proven in clinical medicine. It recommends, however, that equipment is used only when designed to national or international safety standards and that it is used only by competent and trained personnel. The World Federation for Ultrasound in Medicine and Biology confirms that the use of B-mode imaging is not contraindicated,[12] concluding that exposure levels and duration should be reduced to the minimum necessary to obtain the required diagnostic information.

The increase in the use of contrast agents in abdominal ultrasound has given rise to concern for safety, and while this is generally considered low risk, provided the appropriate contraindications are observed,[13,14] there is a theoretical risk of cavitation (see below). Once again, the requirement for proper training is emphasized.

Ultrasound intensities used in diagnostic ultrasound vary according to the mode of operation – pulsed Doppler usually has a higher level than B-mode scanning, which operates at lower intensities, although there may be overlap with color or power Doppler. The American Institute for Ultrasound in Medicine (AIUM) has suggested that ultrasound is safe below $100\,\mathrm{Wcm^{-2}}$.[15] This figure refers to the spatial peak temporal average intensity (I_{SPTA}).

However, the use of intensity as an indicator of safety is limited, particularly where Doppler is concerned, as Doppler intensities can be considerably greater than those in B-mode imaging. The United States Food and Drug Administration sets maximum intensity levels allowed for machine output, which differ according to the application.[16]

BIOLOGICAL EFFECTS OF ULTRASOUND

Harmful effects from ultrasound have been documented in laboratory conditions. These include *thermal effects* and *mechanical effects*.

Thermal Effects

During ultrasound scanning, these are demonstrated as a slight rise in temperature, particularly in close proximity to the transducer face. This local effect is usually of no significance, but the operator must be aware of the phenomenon. The most significant thermal effects occur at bone-tissue interfaces and are greater with pulsed Doppler. Increases in temperature of up to 5°C have been produced. Areas at particular risk are fetal bones and the interfaces in transcranial Doppler ultrasound scans.

Pulsed Doppler has a greater potential for heating than B-mode imaging as it involves greater temporal average intensities because of high PRF and because the beam is frequently held stationary over an area while obtaining the waveform. Color and power Doppler usually involve a greater degree of scanning and transducer movement, which involves a potentially lower heating potential than with pulsed Doppler. Care must be taken to limit the use of pulsed Doppler and not to hold the transducer stationary over one area for too long.

Mechanical Effects

Mechanical effects include cavitation and radiation pressure, which are caused by stresses in the tissues and depend on the amplitude of the ultrasound pulse. These effects are the greatest around gas-filled organs, such as lungs or bowel, and have, in laboratory conditions, caused small, surface blood vessels in the lungs to rupture.

Potentially, these effects could be a hazard when using contrast agents that contain microbubbles.

SAFETY INDICES (THERMAL AND MECHANICAL INDICES)

In order to inform users about the machine conditions which may potentially be harmful, mechanical and thermal indices are now displayed as an output display standard on all equipment manufactured after 1998. This makes the operator aware of the ultrasound conditions that may exceed the limits of safety and enables him/her to take avoiding action, such as reducing the power or restricting the scanning time in that area.

In simple terms, the mechanical index (MI) is related to amplitude and indicates how "big" an ultrasound pulse is, giving an indication of the chances of mechanical effects occurring. Therefore, it is particularly relevant in the abdomen when scanning gas-filled bowel or when using microbubble contrast agents. Gas bodies introduced by contrast agents increase the probability of cavitation.

The thermal index (TI) indicates the temperature rise that might occur within the ultrasound beam, aiming to estimate the reasonable worst-case temperature rise. The thermal index calculation alters, depending upon the application, giving rise to three indices: the soft tissue thermal index (TIS), the bone-at-focus index (TIB), and the bone-at-surface, or cranial index (TIC). The first of these is obviously most relevant for abdominal applications. In well-perfused tissue, such as the

liver and spleen, thermal effects are less likely because of the cooling effect of the blood flow. The display of safety indices is only a general indication of the possibility of biological hazards and cannot be translated directly into real heating or cavitation potential.[17]

These "safety indices" are limited in several ways. They require the user to be educated with respect to the implications of the values shown, and they do not take into account the duration of exposure, which is particularly important in assessing the risk of thermal damage. In addition, the TI does not take account of the patient's temperature, and it is logical to assume that increased caution is therefore required in scanning the febrile patient.

MI and TI are also unlikely to portray the optimum safety information during the use of contrast agents, in which, theoretically, heating effects and cavitation may be enhanced.[10]

OTHER HAZARDS

While most attention in the literature is focused on the possible biological effects of ultrasound, there are several other safety issues that are within the control of the operator:

- Electrical safety: All ultrasound machines should be subject to regular quality control and should be regularly checked for any signs of electrical hazards. Loose or damaged wiring, for example, is a common problem if machines are routinely used for mobile work. Visible damage to a transducer, such as a crack in the casing, should prompt its immediate withdrawal from service until a repair or replacement is affected.
- Microbiological safety: It is the responsibility of the sonographer to minimize the risks of cross-infection. Hospital-acquired infection is a serious and potentially life-threatening condition that must be minimized by careful infection control measures during and between scanning operations. Most manufacturers make recommendations regarding appropriate cleaning agents for transducers, which should be carefully followed. Sterile probe covers should be used in cases where there is an increased risk of infection, such as patients with open wounds, those on immunosuppression, or in a ward environment.
- "Operator" safety: By far the most serious hazard of all is that of the untrained or badly trained operator.

Misdiagnosis is a grave risk for those not aware of the pitfalls. Apart from the implications for the patient of subsequent incorrect management, the operator risks litigation which is difficult or impossible to defend if he/she has had inadequate training in ultrasound.

THE SAFE PRACTICE OF ULTRASOUND

It is fair to say that the safety of ultrasound is less of an issue in abdominal scanning than in obstetric or reproductive organ scanning. Nevertheless, it is still incumbent upon the operator to minimize the ultrasound dose to the patient in any practicable way.

The use of X-rays is governed by the *ALARA* principle – that of keeping the radiation dose as low as reasonably achievable. Although the risks associated with radiation are not present in the use of ultrasound, the general principle of keeping the acoustic exposure as low as possible is still good practice, and many people still refer to *ALARA* in the context of diagnostic ultrasound (Box 1.3).

MEDICOLEGAL ISSUES

Litigation in medical practice is increasing, and the field of ultrasound is no exception. The majority of cases involve, firstly, obstetric and, secondly, gynecological ultrasound. Nevertheless, it is prudent for the operator to be aware of the need to minimize the risks of successful litigation in all types of scanning procedures.

Patients have higher expectations of medical care than ever before, and ultrasound practitioners should be aware of the ways in which they can protect themselves medico-legally. The onus is upon the defendant to prove that he or she acted responsibly, and there are several helpful guidelines that should routinely be followed (Box 1.4).[13]

Depending on their profession, operators are constrained by codes of conduct of their respective colleges and/or Councils,[19] and there are many working with ultrasound who are unregulated. Delegation by senior medically qualified staff to non-medically qualified ultrasound practitioners is now accepted practice in the United Kingdom. It is incumbent upon the person delegating the scan (frequently a consultant radiologist) to ensure that the person to whom they delegate (practitioner or specialist registrar) is properly trained and skilled. The operator then becomes legally accountable for his/her professional actions. The same standard of care is expected from medically and non-medically qualified staff alike.[20] To avoid liability, a practitioner must comply with the Bolam test, in which they should be seen to act in accordance with practice accepted as proper by a responsible body of relevant medical people.

BOX 1.3 Steps for Minimizing the Ultrasound Dose

1. Ensure operators are properly trained, preferably on recognized training programs.
2. Minimize the output (or power) level. Use amplification of the received echoes to manipulate the image in preference to increasing the transmitted power.
3. Minimize the time taken to perform the exam.
4. Do not rest the transducer on the skin surface when not scanning.
5. Make sure the clinical indications for the scan are satisfactory and that a proper request has been received. Do not do unnecessary ultrasound examinations.
6. Be aware of the safety indices displayed on the ultrasound machine. Limit the use of pulsed Doppler to that necessary to contribute to the diagnosis.
7. Make the best use of your equipment – maximize the diagnostic information by manipulating the controls effectively.

BOX 1.4 Guidelines for Defensive Scanning (Adapted from Meire[18])

1. Ensure you are properly trained. Operators who have undergone approved training are less likely to make mistakes.
2. Act with professionalism and courtesy. Good communication skills go a long way to avoiding litigation.
3. Use written guidelines or schemes of work.
4. Ensure a proper request for the examination has been received.
5. A written report should be issued by the operator.
6. Record images to support your findings.
7. Clearly state any limitations of the scan which may affect the ability to make a diagnosis.
8. Ensure that the equipment you use is adequate for the job.

DEPARTMENTAL GUIDELINES/SCHEMES OF WORK

It is good and safe practice to use written guidelines for ultrasound examinations.[3] These serve several purposes:
- They may be used to support a defense against litigation (provided, of course, that the operator can prove they have followed such guidelines),
- They serve to impose and maintain a minimum standard, especially within departments that may have numerous operators of differing experience levels,
- They form a record of current practice.

Guidelines should ideally be:
- Written by and have input from those practicing ultrasound in the department (usually a combination of medically and non-medically qualified personnel), taking into account the requirements of referring clinicians, available equipment, and other local operational issues,
- Regularly reviewed and updated to take account of the latest literature and practices,
- Flexible – to allow the operator to tailor the scan to the patient's clinical presentation and individual requirements,
- Auditable – Audit of images is a way to ensure that protocols are being adhered to and to identify any issues with a practitioner's work.

The guidelines should be broad enough to allow operators to respond to different clinical situations in an appropriate way while ensuring that the highest possible standard of scan is always performed. In cases when it is simply not possible to adhere to departmental guidelines, the reasons should be stated on the report – for example, when the pancreas or appendix cannot be demonstrated because of body habitus or overlying bowel gas.

QUALITY ASSURANCE

The principles of quality assurance affect all aspects of the ultrasound service. These include staff issues (such as education and training, performance and continuing professional development), patient care, the work environment (including health and safety issues), and quality assurance of equipment. Unlike most other aspects of an ultrasound service, quality assurance checks on ultrasound equipment involve measurable and reproducible parameters.

Equipment Tests

After installation, a full range of tests and safety checks should be carried out and the results recorded. This establishes a baseline performance against which comparisons may later be made.

It is useful to record an image of a tissue-mimicking phantom with the relevant settings marked on it. Such images form a reference against which the machine's subsequent performance can be assessed and are especially useful if your machine seems to be performing poorly or the image seems to have deteriorated.

A regular testing regimen must then be set up to maintain quality and safety standards. This program can be set up in conjunction with the operators and the medical physics department, and relevant records should be kept. The use of a tissue-mimicking phantom enables the sonographer to perform certain tests in a reproducible and recordable manner (Fig. 1.13).

Checks should be carried out for all probes on the machine.

Suggested equipment checks include:
- Caliper accuracy,
- System sensitivity and penetration,
- Axial and lateral resolution,
- Slice thickness,
- Grayscale,
- Dead zone,
- Controls/functions,
- Imaging modes,
- Output power,
- Safety checks: electrical, mechanical, biological, and thermal, including a visual inspection of all probes and leads,
- Biopsy guide checks.

Some of these checks can be regularly carried out by users in the department, for example, caliper checks and biopsy guide checks. Others are more complex and are more appropriately undertaken by specialist medical physicists. All equipment should undergo regular servicing, and any interim faults should naturally be reported.

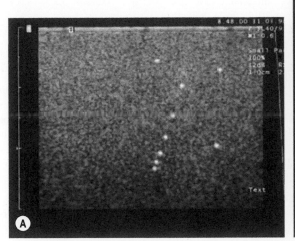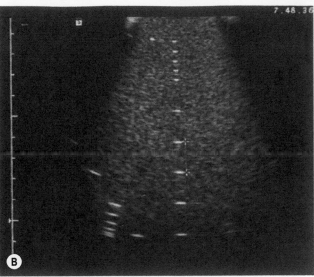

Fig. 1.13 Tissue-mimicking phantom. (A) When using a high-frequency linear array, cross-sections of the wires in the phantom are clearly demonstrated as small dots. (B) When using a curved array of a lower frequency, such as that used for abdominal scanning, the lateral resolution is seen to deteriorate in the far field as the beam diverges. The wires are displayed correctly in the near field but appear as short lines in the far field. Spacing of the wires is known, allowing caliper accuracy to be assessed.

REFERENCES

1. Desser TS, Jedrzejewicz MS, Bradley C. Native tissue harmonic imaging: basic principles and clinical applications. *Ultrasound Q.* 2000;16:40–48.
2. Choudhry S, Gorman B, Charboneau JW, et al. Comparison of tissue harmonic imaging with conventional US in abdominal disease. *Radiographics.* 2000;20:1127–1135.
3. Kim SH, Lee JM, Kim KG, et al. Comparison of fundamental sonography, tissue–harmonic sonography, fundamental compound sonography, and tissue–harmonic compound sonography for focal hepatic lesions. *Eur Radiol.* 2006;16:2444–2453.
4. Elliott S. A user guide to compound imaging. *Ultrasound.* 2005;13:112–117.
5. Elliott ST. Volume ultrasound: the next big thing? *Br J Radiol.* 2008;81:8–9.
6. Talwalkar JA, Kurtz DM, Schoenleber SJ, et al. Ultrasound–based transient elastography for the detection of hepatic fibrosis; systematic review and meta-analysis. *Clin Gastroenterol Hepatol.* 2007;5: 1214–1220.
7. Harrison G, Harris A. Work-related musculoskeletal disorders in ultrasound: Can you reduce risk? *Ultrasound.* 2015;23:224–230.
8. UKAS. *Guidelines for professional working practice.* London: UKAS; 1996.
9. BMUS. British Medical Ultrasound Society. Guidelines for the acquisition and retention of hard copy ultrasound images. *BMUS Bull.* 2000;8:2.
10. ter Haar G, Duck FA, eds. *The safe use of ultrasound in medical diagnosis.* London: BMUS/BIR; 2000.
11. EFSUMB. Clinical safety statement for diagnostic ultrasound. 2006. Available at: www.efsumb.org.
12. WFUMB. World federation for ultrasound in medicine and biology symposium on safety of ultrasound in medicine: conclusions and recommendations on thermal and non-thermal mechanisms for biological effects of ultrasound. Barnett SB, ed. *Ultrasound Med Biol.* 1998;24:1–55.
13. EFSUMB Study Group. Guidelines for the use of contrast agents in ultrasound. *Ultraschall Med.* 2004;25:249–256.
14. WFUMB. Safety symposium on ultrasound contrast agents: clinical applications and safety concerns. *Ultrasound Med Biol.* 2007;33:180–186.
15. American Institute for Ultrasound in Medicine (AIUM). Bioeffects considerations for the safety of diagnostic ultrasound. *J Ultrasound Med.* 1988;7.
16. Food and Drug Administration, United States Department of Health and Human Services. Information for manufacturers seeking marketing clearance of diagnostic ultrasound systems and transducers. Center for Devices and Radiological Health, Rockville, MD, 1997.
17. Duck FA. The meaning of thermal index (TI) and mechanical index (MI) values. *BMUS Bull.* 1997;5:36–40.

18. Meire HB, ed. Ultrasound-related litigation in obstetrics and gynecology: the need for defensive scanning. *Ultrasound Obstet Gynecol.* 1996;7:233–235.

19. Health Professions Council. Standards of conduct, performance and ethics. 2003. Available at: www.hpc-uk.org/publications/standards.

20. Dimond B. Red dots and radiographers' liability. *Health care risk report: clinical negligence.* 2000;10–13.

21. BMUS. British Medical Ultrasound Society. SCoR: Society and College of Radiographers. Guidelines for professional ultrasound practice. *revision.* 2019;4:70–81.

22. Elliott ST. Volume ultrasound: the next big thing? *Br J Radiol.* 2008;81:8–9.

23. Thoirs K. Physical and technical principles of sonography: a practical guide for non–sonographers. *Radiograph.* 2012;59:124–132.

24. Takatani J, Takeshima N, Okuda K, et al. Enhanced needle visualisation: advantages and indications of an ultrasound software package. *Anaesth Intensive Care.* 2012;40:856–860.

25. D'Onofrio M, Crosara S, De Robertis R, et al. Contrast-enhanced ultrasound of focal liver lesions. *Am J Roentgenol.* 2015;205:W56–W66.

26. Park AY, Kwon M, Woo OH, et al. A prospective study on the value of ultrasound microflow assessment to distinguish malignant from benign solid breast masses: association between ultrasound parameters and histologic microvessel densities. *Korean J Radiol.* 2019;20:759–772.

27. Wilson SR, Gupta C, Eliasziw M, et al. Volume imaging in the abdomen with ultrasound: how we do it. *Am J Roentgenol.* 2009;193:79–85.

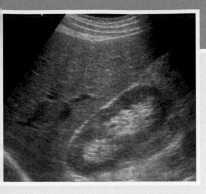

2

Ultrasound of the Liver

James R. Michael

CHAPTER OUTLINE

Introduction, 22
General Pointers on Upper Abdominal
  Technique, 23
The Liver, 23
  Normal Appearances, 23
  The Segments of the Liver, 29
  Hepatic Vasculature, 29
  Hemodynamics of the Liver, 31
  The Portal Venous System, 32
  The Hepatic Veins, 32
  The Hepatic Artery, 33
Pathology of the Liver and Portal Venous
  System, 35
  Focal Liver Lesions, 36
  The Mass Effect, 36
Benign Focal Liver Lesions, 36
  Simple Cysts, 36
  Complex Cysts, 37
  Polycystic Liver, 39
  Hydatid (Echinococcal) Cyst, 39
  Abscesses, 39
    Ultrasound Appearances, 40
    Clinical Features, 40
    Pyogenic Abscess, 40
    Amoebic Abscess, 40
    Candidiasis Abscess, 40
    Management of Hepatic Abscesses, 40
  Hematoma, 40
  Hemangioma, 42
  Focal Nodular Hyperplasia, 43
  Adenoma, 46
    Clinical Features, 46

Focal Fatty Change, 46
Focal Fatty Infiltration, 46
Focal Fatty Sparing, 48
Lipoma, 48
Granuloma, 48
Hepatic Calcification, 48
Malignant Focal Liver Lesions, 49
  Metastases, 49
    Ultrasound Appearances, 49
    Clinical Features and Management, 49
    Ultrasound of Other Relevant Areas, 52
  Hepatocellular Carcinoma (HCC), 52
  Cholangiocarcinoma, 56
Diffuse Liver Conditions, 56
  Fatty Infiltration (Steatosis), 56
  Non-Alcoholic Steatohepatitis, 57
  Cirrhosis, 57
    Ultrasound Appearances, 58
    Nodules in Cirrhosis, 58
    Hemodynamics in Cirrhosis, 61
    HCC in Cirrhosis, 61
    Hepatitis, 61
    Alcoholic Cirrhosis, 61
    Primary Biliary Cirrhosis (PBC), 61
    Secondary Biliary Cirrhosis, 62
    Other Causes, 62
    Clinical Features and Management, 62
    Portal Hypertension, 63
    Portal Vein Signs, 63
    Management, 68
  Hepatitis, 70
    Viral Hepatitis, 70

Other Causes of Acute Hepatitis, 70
Clinical Features, 70
Ultrasound Appearances, 70
Primary Sclerosing Cholangitis, 71
Budd-Chiari Syndrome, 71
Ultrasound Appearances, 72
Management, 73
Cystic Fibrosis, 73
Ultrasound Appearances, 73
Congestive Cardiac Disease, 73
HIV, 73
Liver Conditions in Pregnancy, 74
Acute Fatty Liver, 74
Hemolysis, Elevated Liver Enzymes, Low Platelet
Count (HELLP) Syndrome, 74
Liver Transplants, 75
Basic Doppler Principles, 76
Waveform Interpretation, 76
Acceleration Times (ms), 76
Resistive Index (RI) Values, 77
Preoperative Assessment, 78
Operative Procedure – Intraoperative
Ultrasound, 79
Postoperative Assessment, 79
Postoperative Ultrasound Appearances and
Complications, 80
Hepatic Artery, 80

Hepatic Artery Thrombosis (HAT), 80
Hepatic Artery Stenosis (HAS), 80
HA Pseudoaneurysm, 80
Portal Vein, 81
Portal Venous Complications, 81
IVC and Hepatic Veins, 83
Hepatic Venous and IVC Complication, 83
CBD, 84
Focal Lesions, 84
Post-Transplantation Malignancy, 84
Fluid Collections, 85
Rejection, 86
References, 86
**Appendix 2.1: LS Through the Right Lobe of the
Liver, 89**
**Appendix 2.2: LS Through the Inferior Vena
Cava, 89**
**Appendix 2.3: LS Through the Midline, Level of the
Aorta, 90**
**Appendix 2.4: Longitudinal, Oblique Section Along
the CBD, 90**
**Appendix 2.5: Transverse Oblique Section Through
the Hepatic Venous Confluence, 91**
**Appendix 2.6: TS Through the Level of the Porta
Hepatis, 91**
Appendix 2.7: TS at the Level of the Pancreas, 92

INTRODUCTION

Familiarity with normal anatomy and technical expertise in comprehensively examining an organ are essential. The latter can be obtained only by practice in a clinical environment under proper supervision (Box 2.1).

It is good practice, particularly on the patient's first attendance, to scan the whole of the upper abdomen, focusing particularly on the relevant areas and excluding or identifying any other significant pathologic condition. A full abdominal survey would usually include the liver, gallbladder, biliary tree, pancreas, spleen, kidneys, and retroperitoneal structures.[1] Apart from the fact that many pathological processes can affect multiple organs, several significant (but clinically occult) pathological processes are discovered incidentally, for example, renal carcinoma or aortic aneurysm.

BOX 2.1

Key points:
- Get properly trained before you attempt ultrasound diagnosis.
- Understand your limitations. Know when to ask for assistance and when to refer on.
- If you have not used your left hand throughout the scan, you have not performed an optimum examination.
- So, get properly trained – I cannot emphasize this too much!
- Have an independent practitioner assess your performance. If you do not feel ready to do this, you probably should not be scanning unsupervised.
- Audit your practice. Liaise with multidisciplinary teams/radiology department.

Thorough knowledge of anatomy is assumed at this stage, but diagrams of upper abdominal sectional anatomy are included in the appendices to this chapter for quick reference.

GENERAL POINTERS ON UPPER ABDOMINAL TECHNIQUE

Here are some general approaches help to get the best from the scanning examination and report:

- Scan systematically to ensure the whole of the upper abdomen has been thoroughly interrogated. The use of a worksheet indicating structures to be examined is helpful when learning.[1]
- Always scan any organ in at least two planes – preferably at right angles to each other. This reduces the risk of missing a pathologic condition and helps to differentiate an artifact from a true pathologic condition.
- Where possible, scan in at least two patient positions. It is surprising how the available ultrasound information can be enhanced by turning your patient decubitus or erect. Inaccessible organs flop into better view, and the bowel moves away from the area of interest.
- Use a combination of subcostal and intercostal scanning for all upper abdominal scanning. The different angles of insonation can reveal pathologic conditions and eliminate artifacts. Good technique is about finding a good acoustic window.
- Do not limit yourself to longitudinal and transverse sections. Use a variety of planes and angulations. Trace ducts and vessels along their courses. Use the transducer like a pair of eyes.
- Deep inspiration is useful in a proportion of patients, but not all. Sometimes it can make matters worse by filling the stomach with air and obscuring structures. An intercostal approach with the patient breathing gently often has far more success.
- Positioning patients supine, particularly if elderly or very ill, can make them breathless and uncomfortable. Raise the patient's head as much as necessary – a comfortable patient is much easier to scan.
- Images are a useful record of the scan and how it has been performed but do not make these your primary task. Scan first – sweeping smoothly from one aspect of the organ to the other in two planes, then take the relevant images to support your findings.
- Make the most of your equipment (see Chapter 1). Increase the confidence level of your scan by fully utilizing all the available facilities, using Doppler, tissue harmonics, changing transducers and frequencies, and manipulating the machine settings and processing options.
- Have a good understanding of blood testing and what pathologic conditions they might indicate (Table 2.2).

> **TIP BOX**
>
> Scan an organ in at least two planes, mapping the anatomy in your mind. As you scan, you should be building up an image of the organ in your head. It helps to have a good understanding of the anatomy you are imaging, especially regarding the "normal" appearances of the organ.

THE LIVER

Normal Appearances

The liver is a homogeneous, mid-gray organ on ultrasound. It has the same or slightly increased echogenicity compared to the cortex of the right kidney. Its outline is smooth, the inferior margin coming to a point anteriorly (Fig. 2.1). The liver is surrounded by a thin, hyperechoic capsule, which is difficult to see on ultrasound unless outlined by fluid (Fig. 2.2).

The smooth parenchyma is interrupted by vessels (see below) and ligaments (Figs. 2.3–2.15), and the liver itself provides an excellent acoustic window onto the various organs and great vessels situated in the upper abdomen.

The ligaments are hyperechoic, linear structures; the falciform ligament, which separates the anatomical left and right lobes, is situated at the superior margin of the liver and is best demonstrated when surrounded by ascitic fluid. It surrounds the left main portal vein (PV) and is known as the ligamentum teres as it descends toward the infero-anterior aspect of the liver

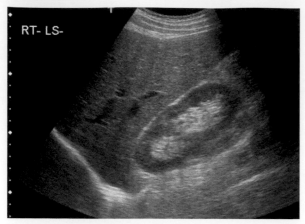

Fig. 2.1 Longitudinal section (LS) through the right lobe of the liver. The renal cortex is slightly less echogenic than the liver parenchyma.

(Figs. 2.9, 2.15). The ligamentum venosum separates the caudate lobe from the rest of the liver (Fig. 2.6).

The size of the liver is difficult to quantify, as there is such a large variation in shape between normal subjects. A measurement can be obtained in the midclavicular line measuring from the liver dome to the inferior margin, with a measurement up to 15 cm considered normal. However, direct measurements are notoriously inaccurate. Size is therefore usually assessed subjectively. Look particularly at the inferior margin of the right lobe, which should come to a point anterior to the lower pole of the right kidney (Fig. 2.1). A relatively common variant of this is the Reidel's lobe, an inferior elongation of segment V1 on the right. This is an extension of the right lobe over the lower pole of the

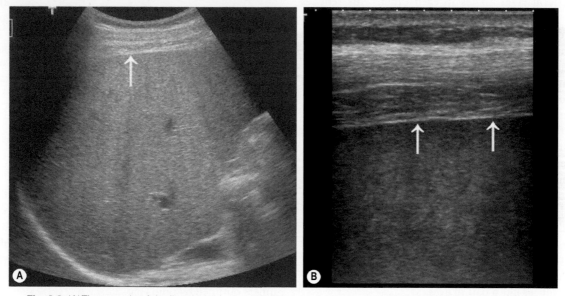

Fig. 2.2 (A) The capsule of the liver is a thin, hyperechoic layer seen anteriorly. (B) It is much better appreciated at higher frequencies (arrows) (7.5 MHz).

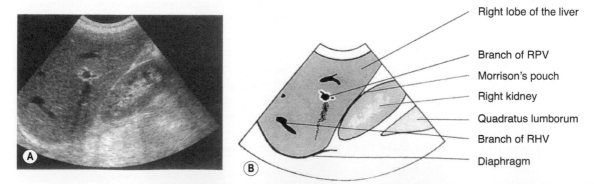

Right lobe of the liver

Branch of RPV

Morrison's pouch

Right kidney

Quadratus lumborum

Branch of RHV

Diaphragm

Fig. 2.3 LS through the right lobe of the liver and right kidney.

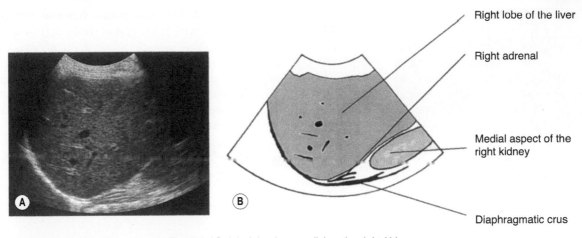

Right lobe of the liver

Right adrenal

Medial aspect of the right kidney

Diaphragmatic crus

Fig. 2.4 LS right lobe, just medial to the right kidney.

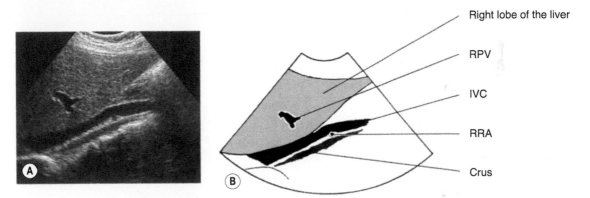

Right lobe of the liver

RPV

IVC

RRA

Crus

Fig. 2.5 LS through the right lobe, angled medially toward the inferior vena cava.

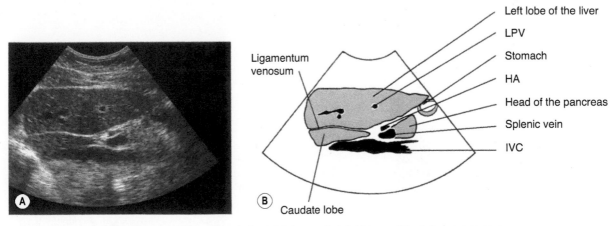

Ligamentum venosum

Left lobe of the liver

LPV

Stomach

HA

Head of the pancreas

Splenic vein

IVC

Caudate lobe

Fig. 2.6 LS midline, through the left lobe, angled right toward the inferior vena cava.

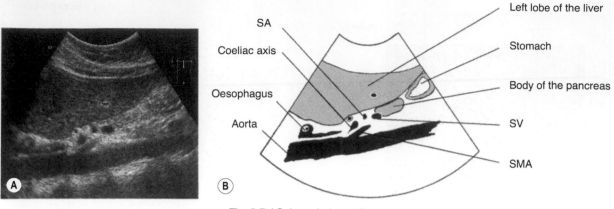

SA
Coeliac axis
Oesophagus
Aorta

Left lobe of the liver
Stomach
Body of the pancreas
SV
SMA

Fig. 2.7 LS through the midline.

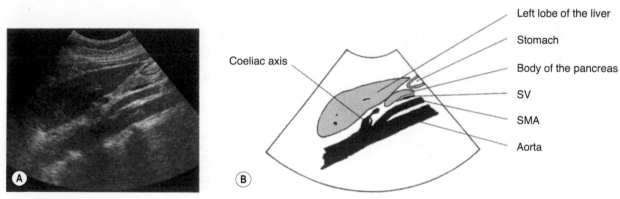

Coeliac axis

Left lobe of the liver
Stomach
Body of the pancreas
SV
SMA
Aorta

Fig. 2.8 LS just to the left of midline.

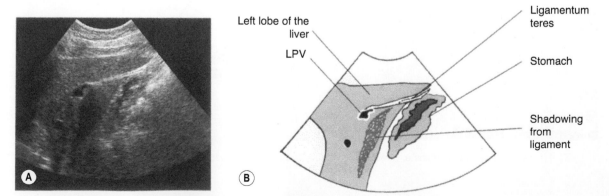

Left lobe of the liver
LPV

Ligamentum teres
Stomach
Shadowing from ligament

Fig. 2.9 LS, left lobe of the liver.

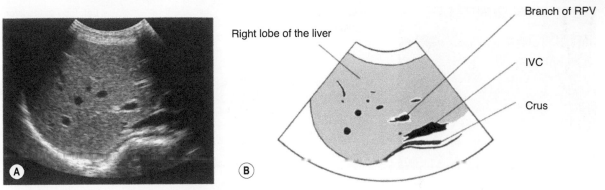

Fig. 2.10 TS through the liver, above the confluence of the hepatic veins.

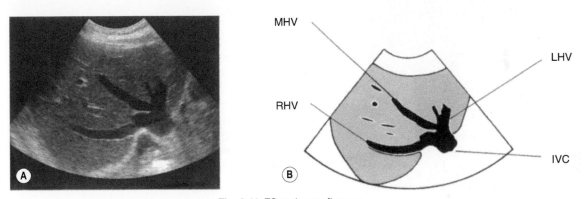

Fig. 2.11 TS at the confluence.

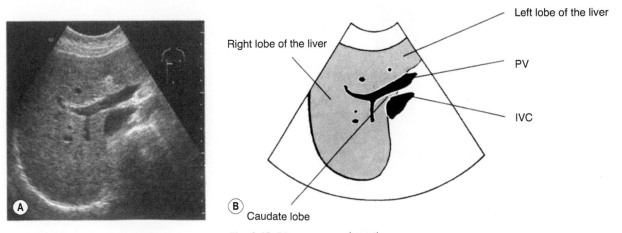

Fig. 2.12 TS at the porta hepatis.

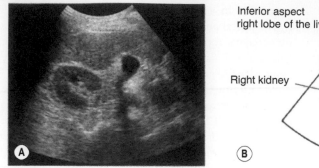

Inferior aspect
right lobe of the liver

Gallbladder

Right kidney

Shadowing
from the bowel

Fig. 2.13 TS through the right kidney.

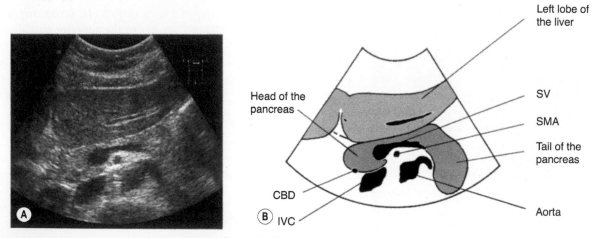

Left lobe of
the liver

Head of the
pancreas

SV

SMA

Tail of the
pancreas

CBD

IVC

Aorta

Fig. 2.14 TS at the epigastrium.

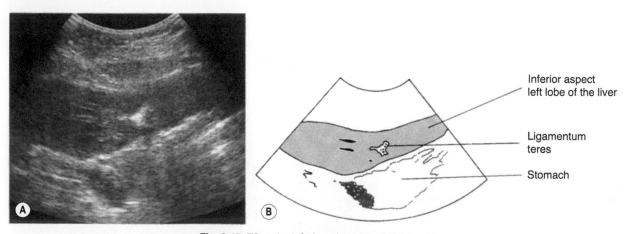

Inferior aspect
left lobe of the liver

Ligamentum
teres

Stomach

Fig. 2.15 TS at the inferior edge of the left lobe.

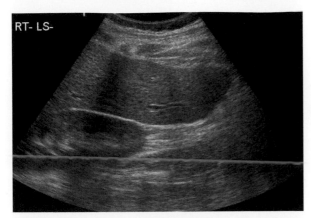

Fig. 2.16 LS through the right lobe, demonstrating a Reidel's lobe extending below the right kidney. (Compare with the normal liver in Fig. 2.1.)

kidney, with a rounded margin (Fig. 2.16) and is worth remembering as a possible cause of a palpable right upper quadrant "mass."

To distinguish mild enlargement from a Reidel's lobe, look at the left lobe – if this also looks bulky, with a rounded inferior edge, the liver is enlarged. A Reidel's lobe is often accompanied by a smaller, less accessible left lobe, with the overall liver volume remaining normal.

The Segments of the Liver

It is often sufficient to talk about the "right" or "left" lobes of the liver for the purposes of many diagnoses. However, when a focal lesion is identified, especially if it may be malignant, it is useful to locate it precisely in terms of the surgical segments. This allows subsequent correlation with other imaging, such as computed tomography (CT) or magnetic resonance imaging (MRI) and is invaluable in planning surgical procedures.

For example, planning for a radiofrequency ablation using US guidance would also want a prior scan of the known "focal lesion." Knowing segments can help locate subtle lesions between modalities, planning operations, and procedures efficiently and accurately to provide a high standard of care.

The segmental anatomy system, proposed by Couinaud in 1900,[2] divides the liver into eight segments, numbered in a clockwise direction. They are divided by the portal and hepatic veins, and the system is used by surgeons today when planning surgical procedures (Fig. 2.17). This system is also used when localizing lesions with CT and MRI.

Identifying the different segments on ultrasound requires the operator to form a mental three-dimensional (3D) image of the liver. The dynamic nature of ultrasound, together with the variation in planes of the scan, makes this more difficult to do than for CT or MRI. However, segmental localization of hepatic lesions by an experienced operator can be as accurate with ultrasound as with MRI.[3] Systematic scanning through the liver, in transverse section, identifies the main landmarks of the hepatic veins (Fig. 2.11), separating segments VII, VIII, IV, and II in the superior part of the liver. As the transducer is moved inferiorly, the portal vein appears, below which segments V and VI are located.

Hepatic Vasculature

The portal veins radiate from the porta hepatis, where the main portal vein (MPV) enters the liver (Fig. 2.18). The veins are encased by the hyperechoic, fibrous walls of the portal tracts, which make them stand out from the rest of the parenchyma. Also contained in the portal tracts are a branch of the hepatic artery (HA) and a biliary duct radicle. These latter vessels are too small to detect by ultrasound in the peripheral parts of the liver but can readily be demonstrated in the larger, proximal branches (Fig. 2.19).

At the porta, the HA generally crosses the anterior aspect of the portal vein, with the common duct anterior to this (Fig. 2.20). In a common variation, the artery lies anterior to the duct. Peripherally, the relationship between the vessels in the portal tracts is variable (Fig. 2.21).

The three main hepatic veins, left (LHV), middle (MHV), and right (RHV), can be traced into the inferior vena cava (IVC) at the superior margin of the liver (Fig. 2.11). Therefore, their course runs approximately perpendicular to the portal vessels – so a section of the liver with a longitudinal image of a hepatic vein is likely to contain a transverse section through a portal vein and vice versa. Unlike the portal tracts, the hepatic veins do

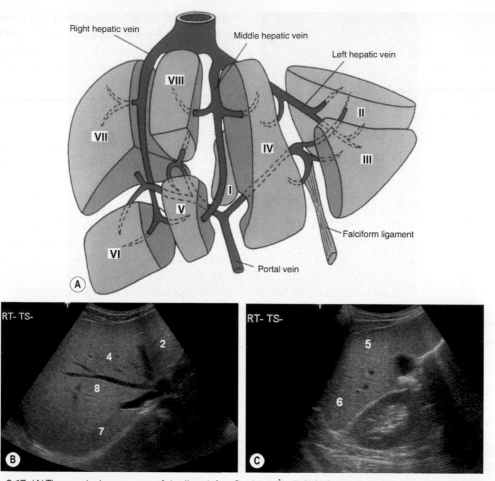

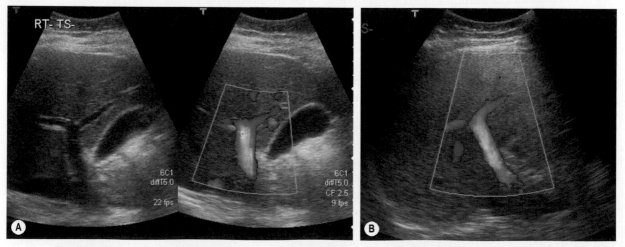

Fig. 2.17 (A) The surgical segments of the liver (after Couinaud[1]). (B & C) Segmental anatomy in TS of the liver.

Fig. 2.18 (A) The right and left branches of the portal vein. (B) Color Doppler demonstrates the main portal vein and left portal vein in red and the right portal vein in blue because of the relative direction of flow to the beam.

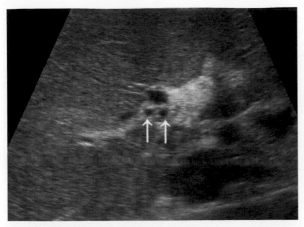

Fig. 2.19 The portal vein radicle is associated with a branch of the hepatic artery and a biliary duct (arrows) within the hyperechoic fibrous sheath.

operator. However, it may be a significant factor in planning and performing hepatic surgery, especially tumor resection, as the surgeon attempts to retain as much viable hepatic tissue as possible with intact venous outflow (Fig. 2.23).[4]

Hemodynamics of the Liver

Pulsed and color Doppler are important tools in understanding and diagnosing the extent of many disease processes. Doppler of the portal venous and hepatic vascular systems gives information on the patency, velocity, and direction of flow. The appearance of the various spectral waveforms relates to the downstream resistance of the vascular bed (see Chapter 1).

not have a fibrous sheath, and their walls are therefore less reflective. Maximum reflectivity of the vessel walls occurs with the beam perpendicular (Fig. 2.22).

The anatomy of the hepatic venous confluence varies. In most cases, the single, main RHV flows directly into the IVC, and the middle and left have a common trunk. In 15%–35% of patients, the LHV and MHV are separate. This usually has no significance to the

TIP BOX

Doppler should always be used in conjunction with the real-time image and in the context of the patient's presenting symptoms. Used in isolation, it can be highly misleading. Familiarity with the normal Doppler spectra is integral to the upper abdominal ultrasound scan.

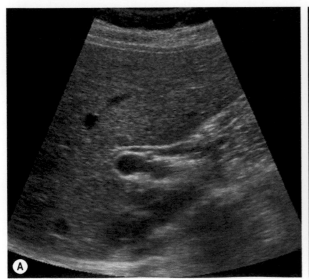

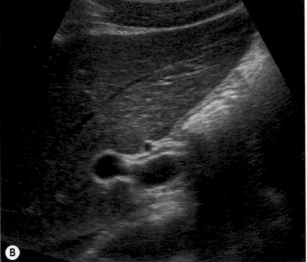

Fig. 2.20 (A) The porta hepatis. (B) A variant with the hepatic artery anterior to the duct.

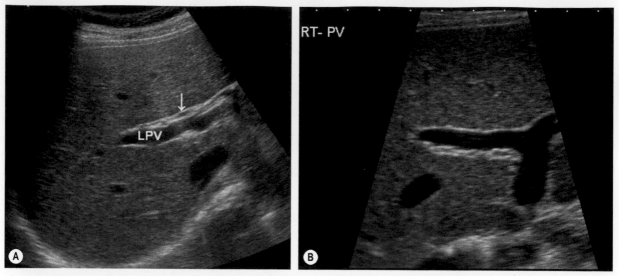

Fig. 2.21 The relationship of the biliary duct to the portal vein varies as the vessels become more peripheral. In (A), the duct (arrow) lies anterior to the left portal vein. In (B), the duct is posterior to the right portal vein.

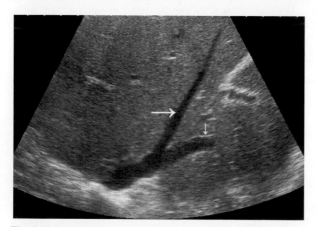

Fig. 2.22 Hepatic vein walls are less prominent than portal vein tract walls (large arrow). When the beam is perpendicular to the wall, as in this branch of the left hepatic vein (small arrow), it is reflective.

The Portal Venous System

Color Doppler is used to identify blood flow in the splenic and portal veins (Figs. 2.24, 2.25). The direction of flow is normally hepatopetal, i.e., toward the liver. The main, right, and left portal branches can best be imaged by using a right oblique approach through the ribs so that the course of the vessel is roughly toward the transducer, maintaining an angle of less than 60 degrees with the beam for the best Doppler signal.

The normal portal vein diameter is highly variable but does not usually exceed 16 mm in a resting state on quiet respiration. The diameter increases with deep inspiration and in response to food and posture changes. An increased diameter may also be associated with portal hypertension in chronic liver disease. An absence of postprandial increase in diameter is also a sign of portal hypertension.

The normal portal vein waveform is monophasic (Fig. 2.26) with gentle undulations, which are because of respiratory modulation and cardiac activity. This characteristic is a sign of the normal, flexible nature of the liver and may be lost in some fibrotic diseases.

The mean portal vein velocity is normally between 12 cm/s and 20 cm/s, but the normal range is wide. (A low-velocity is associated with portal hypertension. High velocities are unusual but can be because of anastomotic stenosis in transplant patients.)

The Hepatic Veins

The hepatic veins drain the liver into the IVC, which leads into the right atrium. Two factors shape the hepatic venous spectrum; the flexible nature of the normal liver, which can expand easily to accommodate blood flow, and the close proximity of the right atrium, which causes a brief "kick" of blood back into the liver during atrial systole (Fig. 2.27). This causes the spectrum to be triphasic.

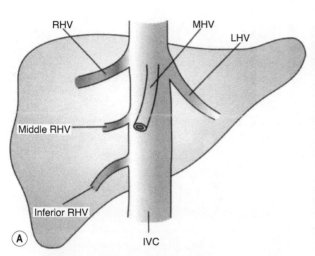

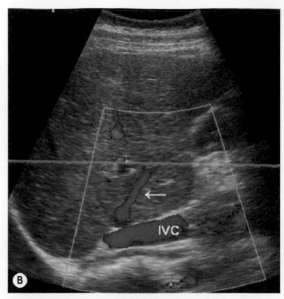

Fig. 2.23 (A) Configuration of the hepatic venous system. (B) Inferior middle hepatic vein (arrow) draining into the inferior vena cava.

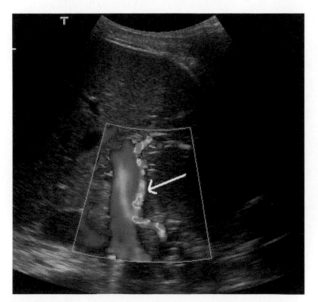

Fig. 2.24 Main portal vein at the porta hepatis demonstrating hepatopetal flow. The higher velocity hepatic artery lies adjacent to the main portal vein (arrow).

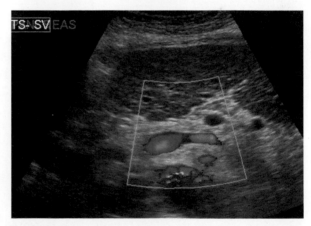

Fig. 2.25 TS through the epigastrium demonstrating the normal splenic vein with flow toward the liver. Note the change from red to blue as the vessel curves away from the transducer.

The veins can be seen on color Doppler to be predominantly blue with a brief red flash during atrial contraction.

Various factors cause alterations to this waveform – heart conditions, liver diseases, and extrahepatic conditions which compress the liver, such as ascites. Abnormalities of the hepatic vein waveform are therefore highly unspecific and should be taken in context with the clinical picture. As you might expect, the pulsatile nature of the spectrum decreases toward the periphery of the liver, remote from the IVC.

The Hepatic Artery

The main HA arises from the coeliac axis and carries oxygenated blood to the liver from the aorta. Its origin

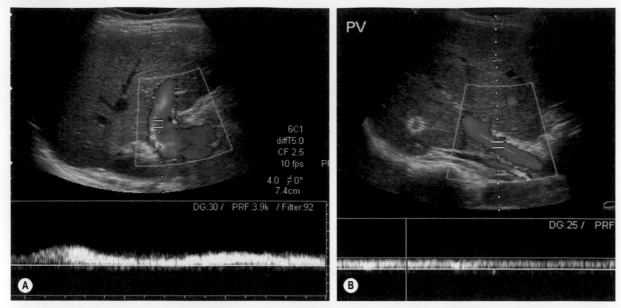

Fig. 2.26 Normal portal vein waveform. (A) Respiratory modulations are evident. (B) Portal vein velocity can be measured by using the angle corrector line in the spectral sampling box to indicate the direction of flow.

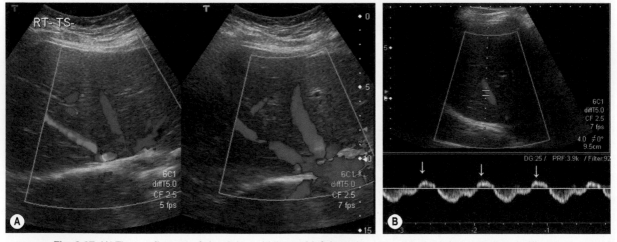

Fig. 2.27 (A) The confluence of the right, middle, and left hepatic veins with the inferior vena cava. Flow is predominantly hepatofugal – indicated by the blue color in the left-hand image, but briefly reverses under the influence of atrial systole – indicated in red in the right-hand image. (B) This is demonstrated by the normal triphasic waveform. Atrial systole appears as hepatopetal flow (arrows).

makes it a pulsatile vessel, and the relatively low resistance of the hepatic vascular bed means that there is continuous forward flow throughout the cardiac cycle (Fig. 2.28). The HA may be elusive on color Doppler in a normal subject because of its small diameter and

tortuous course. Use the MPV as a marker, scanning from the right intercostal space to maintain a low angle with the vessel. The HA is just anterior to this and of a higher velocity (i.e., it has a paler color of red on the color map, see Fig. 2.24).

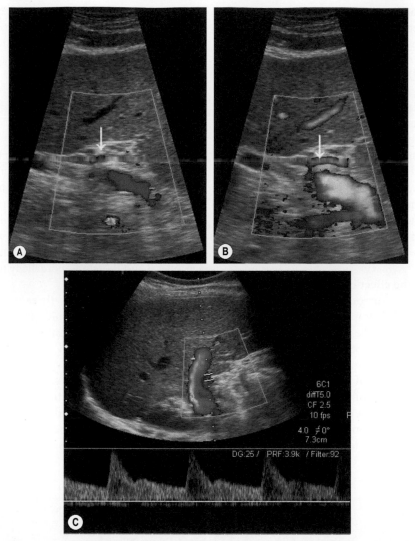

Fig. 2.28 (A) The hepatic artery may be difficult to locate with color Doppler, especially if the vessel is perpendicular to the beam. (B) Power Doppler is less angle-dependent and demonstrates the artery (arrow). (C) The normal hepatic artery waveform demonstrates a relatively high-velocity systolic peak with good forward end-diastolic flow.

PATHOLOGY OF THE LIVER AND PORTAL VENOUS SYSTEM

Ultrasound is frequently the first-line of investigation for suspected liver pathologic conditions, and the decision to proceed to secondary investigative procedures, such as further radiology or histology, is determined by the findings of the initial ultrasound scan. It is used in diagnosing, staging, and monitoring liver disorders. However, ultrasound has a much greater role than that of a first-line exclusion test and serves as a reliable tool for more focused, complex examinations. Developing technology and techniques now result in improved diagnostic accuracy and are increasingly obviating the need for further radiology. Ultrasound is used to both diagnose and treat conditions using ultrasound-guided invasive procedures.

Intraoperative and laparoscopic ultrasound, using high-frequency, direct contact techniques, set the standard for liver imaging in many cases.

Focal Liver Lesions

Focal liver lesions are common and once seen, require accurate characterization. For example, in some cases, such as simple cysts, the ultrasound appearances are pathognomonic, requiring no further investigation. In other cases, contrast-enhanced ultrasound (CEUS) provides a rapid and definitive diagnosis, obviating the need for further investigation or follow-up. In other cases, ultrasound appropriately directs the patient's further management (such as further radiological imaging for staging, characterization, or biopsy).

The Mass Effect

This term describes the effect of a focal mass, whether benign or malignant, on surrounding structures and is a useful diagnostic tool. It implies the lesions displacing or invasive nature, i.e., the displacement of vessels and/or invasion or distortion of adjacent structures and tissues because of the increasing bulk of a lesion. This effect differentiates a true mass from an infiltrative process such as steatosis or an artifact.

Masses that are large and/or closely adjacent to a vessel demonstrate the effect more readily. Of course, the mass effect does not differentiate benign from malignant masses or help in any way to characterize the mass. It is particularly useful when the mass is isoechoic compared with the normal liver (Fig. 2.29). In such cases, the effect of the mass on adjacent structures may be the main clue to its presence.

BENIGN FOCAL LIVER LESIONS

Simple Cysts

One of the most frequently seen liver lesions, the simple cyst, is either congenital (from abnormal development of a biliary radicle) or acquired (from trauma or previous infection). It is asymptomatic unless large enough to cause a mass effect compressing and displacing adjacent structures and is usually an incidental finding during the ultrasound scan. Frequently, small cysts are peripheral and therefore more likely to be missed on ultrasound than CT.

The simple cyst has three acoustic properties, which are pathognomonic: it is anechoic, has a well-defined smooth capsule, and exhibits posterior enhancement (increased through-transmission of sound) (Fig. 2.30). Although theoretically, it is possible to confuse a simple cyst with a choledochal cyst, the latter's connection to the biliary tree is usually demonstrable on ultrasound. A radioisotope hepatobiliary iminodiacetic acid scan will confirm the biliary connection if doubt exists.

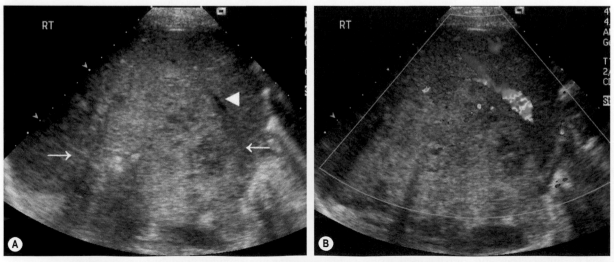

Fig. 2.29 The mass effect. (A) A large isoechoic lesion (arrows) displaces the middle hepatic vein (arrowhead). (B) Color flow of the same case.

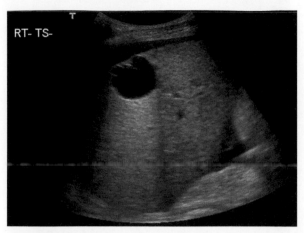

Fig. 2.30 Typical liver cyst demonstrating a band of posterior enhancement, smooth capsule, and fine septum. Note the ascites.

Complex Cysts

Some cysts may contain a thin septum, which is not a significant finding. Occasionally hemorrhage or infection may occur in a simple cyst, giving rise to low-level, fine echoes within it (Fig. 2.31). Such cysts are usually treated conservatively, although the larger ones may be monitored with ultrasound, particularly if symptomatic. Percutaneous aspiration of larger cysts under ultrasound guidance may afford temporary decompression but is rarely performed, as they invariably recur, and there is a risk of infection. Laparoscopic fenestration (deroofing), where part of the cyst wall is removed, allowing

drainage, provides a more permanent solution to large, symptomatic cysts (Table 2.3).

A rare cause of a cystic lesion in the liver is the cystadenoma, a benign epithelial tumor that may appear uni- or multilocular. These have a pre-malignant potential, rarely progressing to form a cystadenocarcinoma. Close monitoring with ultrasound will demonstrate a gradual increase in size, changes in the appearances of the wall of the cyst, such as thickening or papillary projections, and internal echoes in some cases, which may indicate malignant change. Cystic malignant liver lesions are uncommon, and the majority represent necrotic metastases, but it is extremely important to recognize suspicious malignant features such as solid nodules or thickened walls and septations (Fig. 2.32). A diagnostic aspiration may be performed under ultrasound guidance, and the fluid may contain elevated levels of carcinoembryonic antigen if malignant.[2] Cystadenomas are usually surgically re-moved because of their malignant potential (Fig. 2.33).

Rarely, cystic lesions in the liver may be because of other causes. These include pancreatic pseudocyst (within an interlobular fissure) in patients with acute pancreatitis or mucin-filled metastatic deposits in primary ovarian cancer. An arteriovenous (AV) malformation, a rare finding in the liver, may look like a septated cystic lesion. However, Doppler will demonstrate flow throughout the structure.

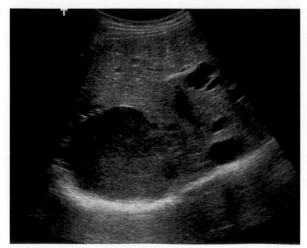

Fig. 2.31 Large, infected hepatic cyst containing low-level echoes.

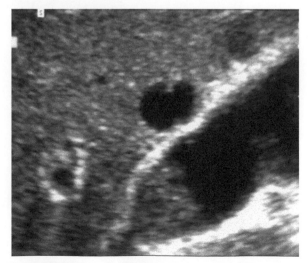

Fig. 2.32 Small cyst adjacent to the gallbladder containing a nodule. This was a mucinous metastasis from ovarian carcinoma.

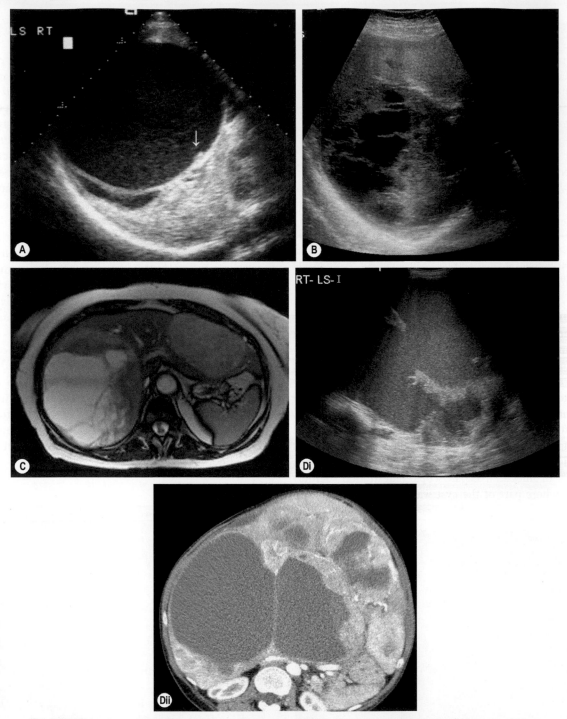

Fig. 2.33 (A) Large cystadenoma containing echoes and a septum. The cyst was large enough to cause obstructive jaundice as the patient's presenting symptom. The diagnosis was made by ultrasound-guided aspiration. A small nodule is present (arrow), which raises the suspicion for malignancy, and the cyst subsequently developed into a cystadenocarcinoma. (B) A cystadenocarcinoma in a young woman presenting with altered liver function tests, demonstrating the complex nature of the mass. (C) Magnetic resonance imaging of the case in (B). (Di) A rare primary neuroendocrine tumor of the liver, demonstrating a large complex, mainly cystic lesion, diagnosed with ultrasound-guided biopsy. (Dii) Computed tomography is valuable in indicating the extent of the disease.

Polycystic Liver

There is a fine dividing line between a liver that contains multiple simple cysts and polycystic liver disease. The latter usually occurs with polycystic kidneys, a common autosomal dominant condition readily recognizable on ultrasound (see Chapter 6), but rarely may affect the liver alone, sparing the kidneys (Fig. 2.34). The appearances are of multiple, often septated cysts of varying sizes throughout the liver. The cumulative enhancement behind the numerous cysts imparts a highly irregular echogenicity to the liver texture and may make it extremely difficult to pick up other focal lesions which may be present.

The polycystic liver is usually asymptomatic but easily palpable, and if the kidneys are also affected, the abdomen can look very distended. As with cysts in the kidneys, hemorrhage or infection in a cyst can cause localized pain. Treatment of the cysts by drainage is not successful, and in rare cases, hepatic transplantation offers the only viable option in patients with intractable symptoms.

Hydatid (Echinococcal) Cyst

Hydatid disease comes from a parasite, Echinococcus granulosus, which is endemic in the Middle East and sheep-farming areas but rare in the United Kingdom. The worm lives in the alimentary tract of infected dogs, which excrete the eggs. These may then be ingested by cattle or sheep and subsequently complete their lifecycle in a human. The parasite spreads via the bloodstream to the liver, where it lodges, causing an inflammatory reaction. The resulting cyst can be slow-growing and asymptomatic, and they may be single or multiple, depending on the degree of infestation.

Ultrasound may demonstrate a spectrum of appearances, from cystic through to solid, and the diagnosis can be made by looking carefully at the wall and contents; the hydatid cyst has two layers to its capsule, which may appear thickened, separated, or detached on ultrasound. Daughter cysts may arise from the inner capsule, the honeycomb or cartwheel appearance (Fig. 2.35), and the cyst may contain floating membranes and fine sand or debris. A calcified rind around a cyst is usually associated with an old, inactive hydatid lesion.

The diagnosis of hydatid, as opposed to a simple cyst, is important, as any attempted aspiration may spread the parasite further by seeding along the needle track if the operator is unaware of the diagnosis. Hydatids may be treated successfully using percutaneous ultrasound-guided aspiration with sclerotherapy, although surgical resection is necessary for some cases.

Abscesses

Liver abscesses result from bacterial, fungal, or parasitic infection. The most common are pyogenic abscesses secondary to an abdominal infection, for example, cholangitis (via the biliary tree), diverticulitis, or appendicitis (via the portal vein). Diabetic patients and those with compromised immune response are particularly prone to such infections.

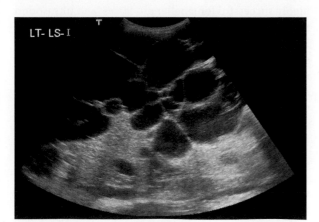

Fig. 2.34 Multiple cysts enlarging the left lobe of the liver in autosomal dominant polycystic kidney disease.

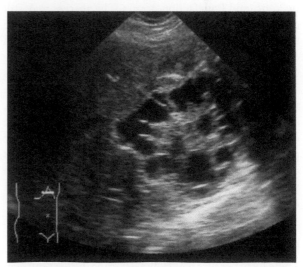

Fig. 2.35 Hydatid cyst demonstrating surrounding daughter cysts.

Ultrasound Appearances

Liver abscesses can vary in appearance dependent on cause, location and age of abscess. Initially, on ultrasound the abscess will appear as an ill-defined mass with a solid, hypoechoic appearance and in the early stages vascularity may appear increased with colour Doppler.

In time, the abscess will have a more cystic appearance as it liquifies. Solid components may still be visible, with or without signs of necrosis, air may also be seen. Once treatment begins the vascularity will decrease and often become more peripheral.

Clinical Features

Patients present with fever and nocturnal sweats, often accompanied by right upper quadrant pain and vomiting. Abnormal liver function tests (LFTs) and anemia can also be present. A raised white cell count and erythrocyte sedimentation rate are features.

The clinical history helps the sonographer establish the nature of the focal lesion and the abscess cause. Abscesses of any type may be solitary or multiple. Since the ultrasound appearances of abscesses can be similar to those of necrotic tumors or hematoma, the clinical picture is particularly important in establishing the diagnosis. Ultrasound appearances of hepatic abscesses may display a spectrum of acoustic features. Their internal appearances vary considerably; in the very early stages, there is a zone of infected, edematous liver tissue, which appears on ultrasound as a hypoechoic, solid focal lesion. As the infection develops, the liver tissue becomes necrotic, and liquefaction occurs. The abscess may still appear full of homogeneous echoes from pus and can be mistaken for a solid lesion, but as it progresses, the fluid content may become apparent, usually with considerable debris within it. Because they are fluid-filled, abscesses demonstrate posterior enhancement (Fig. 2.36A). The margins of an abscess are irregular, often ill-defined, and frequently thickened. The inflammatory capsule of the abscess may demonstrate vascularity on color or power Doppler, but this is not invariable and depends on equipment sensitivity and size of the lesion. Infection with gas-forming organisms may account for the presence of gas within some liver abscesses (Fig. 2.36B).

There are three main types of abscesses.

Pyogenic Abscess

These form because of infection entering the liver through the portal venous system. Most commonly, appendiceal or diverticular abscesses are responsible, but intrahepatic abscesses are also seen in immunosuppressed patients and following postoperative infection. Pyogenic abscesses are frequently multiple, and the patient must be closely monitored after diagnosis to prevent rapid spread. They are still considered a lethal problem, which has increased in recent years because of increasingly aggressive surgical approaches to many abdominal neoplasms.

Amoebic Abscess

This is a parasitic infection that is rare in the United Kingdom but found frequently in parts of Africa, India, and the southern parts of the United States. Increasing worldwide travel means a more frequent recognition of such lesions with ultrasound,[5] and suspicion should be raised when the patient has visited these countries. It is usually contracted by drinking contaminated water and infects the colon, ulcerating the wall and subsequently being transported to the liver via the portal venous system. About 25% of infected patients form hepatic abscesses, and the infection may spread to other sites in the abdomen. Following initial ultrasound, CT is necessary to identify extrahepatic disease.

Candidiasis Abscess

This is a fungal infection that may be seen in immunosuppressed patients. It is a rare cause of abscess formation and is usually bloodborne. The resulting abscesses are likely to be small but multiple on presentation.

Management of Hepatic Abscesses

An ultrasound-guided aspiration to obtain pus for culture is useful for identifying the responsible organism. Aspiration combined with antibiotic therapy is usually highly successful for smaller abscesses, and ultrasound is used to monitor the resolution of the abscesses in the liver. Ultrasound-guided drainage is used for large lesions, and surgical removal is rarely required. Further radiology may be indicated to establish the underlying cause and extent of infection, e.g., barium enema or CT, particularly if an amoebic infection is suspected.

Hematoma

A hematoma results from trauma (usually, therefore, via the emergency department), but the trauma may also be iatrogenic, e.g., following a biopsy procedure (hence the value of using ultrasound guidance to avoid major vessels in the liver) or surgery. The liver hematoma may have similar acoustic appearances to those of an abscess but does not share the same clinical features or history (Fig. 2.37A).

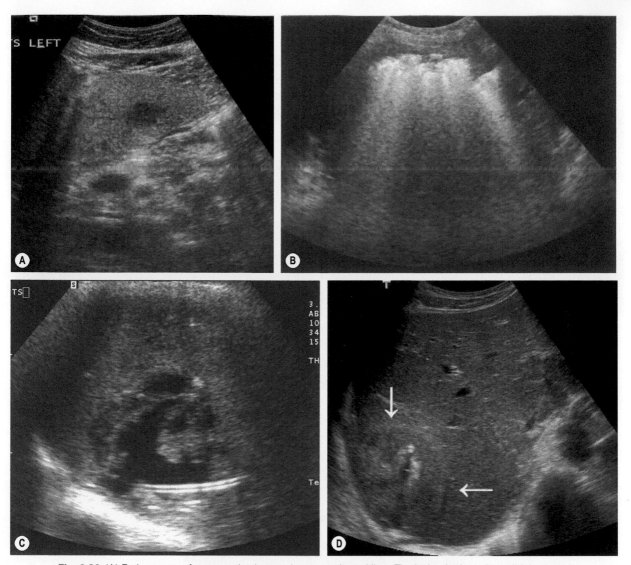

Fig. 2.36 (A) Early stages of a pyogenic abscess in a transplanted liver. The lesion looks quite solid, but note the posterior enhancement. (B) The gas contained within this large abscess in the right lobe of the liver obscures the full extent of the lesion. (Large abscesses like this, which contain gas, may mimic the acoustic appearances of normal bowel.) (C) A percutaneous drain was put into a liver abscess under ultrasound guidance. (D) A resolving abscess (arrows) demonstrates calcification, with no liquefied content.

Continued

The acoustic appearances depend upon the timing. A fresh hematoma may appear liquid and hypoechoic but rapidly becomes more solid looking and hyperechoic as the blood clots. As it resolves, the hematoma liquefies and may contain fibrin strands. It will invariably demonstrate a band of posterior enhancement and has irregular, ill-defined walls in the early stages. Later on, it may encapsulate, leaving a permanent cystic space in the liver, and the capsule may calcify. Injury to the more peripheral regions may cause a subcapsular hematoma which demonstrates the same acoustic properties. The hematoma outlines the surface of the liver, and the capsule can be seen surrounding it. This may cause a palpable enlarged liver (Fig. 2.37B).

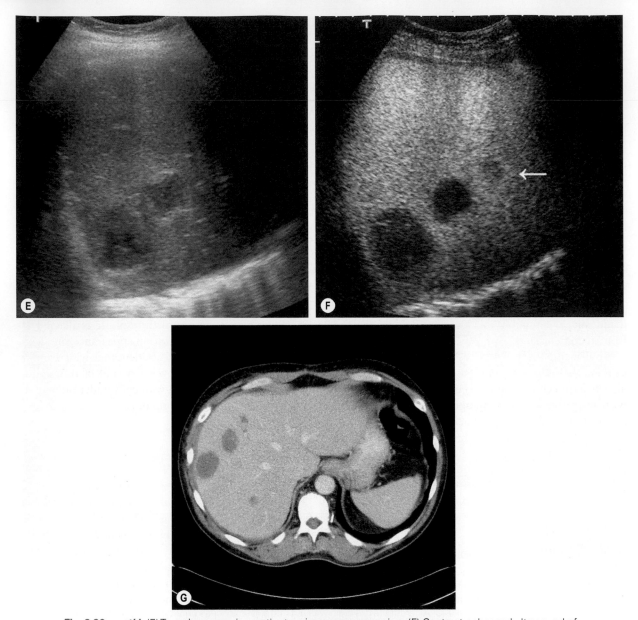

Fig. 2.36, cont'd (E) Two abscesses in a patient on immunosuppression. (F) Contrast-enhanced ultrasound of the case in E demonstrates a third smaller abscess (arrow) not visible pre-contrast. (G) Computed tomography confirms multiple abscesses.

Intervention is rarely necessary, and monitoring with ultrasound confirms eventual resolution. More serious hepatic ruptures, however, causing hemoperitoneum, may require surgery. CEUS is useful in demonstrating the extent of the injury and is particularly useful in the absence of a hemoperitoneum.

Hemangioma

This is the most common, solid benign tumor found in the liver. Hemangiomas are highly vascular, composed of a network of tiny blood vessels. They may be solitary or multiple. Most hemangiomas are small and found incidentally. They are rarely symptomatic but cause a

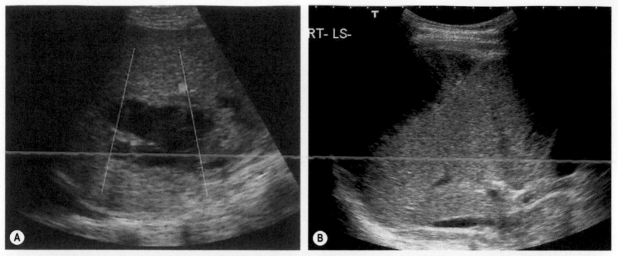

Fig. 2.37 (A) Intrahepatic hematoma following a road traffic accident with rib fractures. The lesion is relatively fresh and contains some low-level echoes. (B) A subphrenic hematoma displaces the liver inferiorly.

diagnostic dilemma, as they can be indistinguishable from liver metastases.

Their acoustic appearances vary; most are hyperechoic, well-defined rounded lesions, but they may also be hypoechoic or mixed echogenicity. In patients with fatty livers, the hemangioma frequently looks hypoechoic relative to the background of the hyperechoic hepatic parenchyma. Larger ones can demonstrate a spectrum of reflectivity depending on their composition and may demonstrate pools of blood and central areas of degeneration. They frequently exhibit slightly increased through-transmission, with posterior enhancement, particularly if large. This is probably because of the increased blood content compared with the surrounding liver parenchyma (Fig. 2.38).

As with many lesions, color or power Doppler is too insensitive to pick up the slow flow in hemangiomas or assist with lesion characterization. Microbubble contrast agents demonstrate a peripheral, globular enhancement with gradual centripetal filling to become isoechoic with the background liver in the sinusoidal phase.[6] CEUS frequently provides a definitive diagnosis at the time of scanning, reassuring the patient and obviating the need for further imaging of follow-up (Fig. 2.38).

When found in children, hemangiomas tend to be large and produce symptoms. These masses produce shunting of blood from the aorta via the main HA and in extreme cases, present with resulting cardiac failure. They are often heterogeneous in appearance, and larger vessels within them may be identified with Doppler. Although many regress over a period of time, others may have to be embolized with coils under radiological guidance to control the symptoms.

Focal Nodular Hyperplasia

Focal nodular hyperplasia (FNH) is the second most common solid, benign liver tumor. It is made up of a hyperplastic proliferation of liver cells with hepatocytes, Kupffer cells, and biliary and fibrous elements. It is most commonly found in young women and is usually discovered by chance, being asymptomatic. Its ultrasound characteristics vary, from hypo-, iso-, to hyperechoic compared with background liver (Fig. 2.39), and it may be multifocal. As with hemangioma, it presents a diagnostic dilemma when found on CT or ultrasound, as its characteristics vary. As with hemangioma, CEUS is extremely helpful in characterizing incidental FNH, as it usually displays rapid arterial stellate filling, followed by centripetal enhancement with contrast uptake isoechoic with background liver in the sinusoidal phase.[7] It may, however, be difficult to differentiate from the rarer adenoma, which also exhibits rapid arterialization on CEUS. There is also some early research into using microflow imaging, and early studies show that the microvessel patterns can differentiate between FNH and other pathologies.

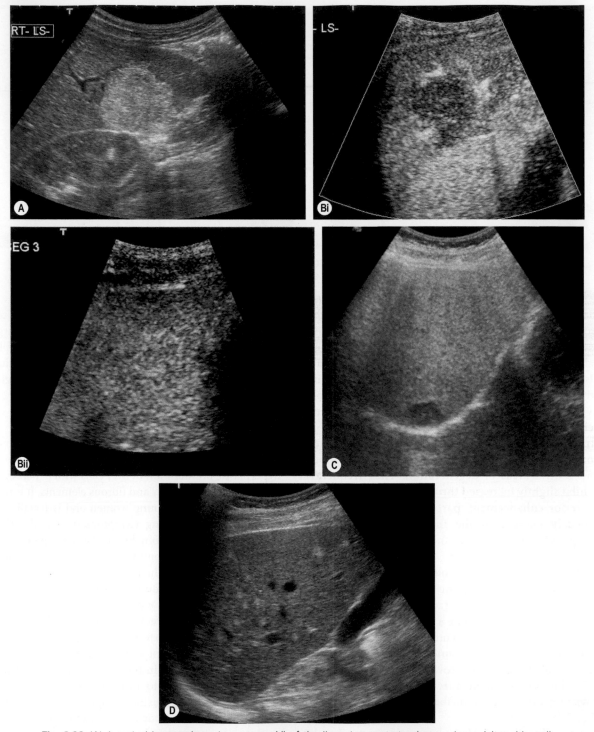

Fig. 2.38 (A) A typical hemangioma in segment VI of the liver demonstrates hyperechogenicity with well-defined borders. (Bi) Administration of contrast demonstrates characteristic peripheral nodular enhancement in the arterial phase. (Bii) The lesion gradually takes up the contrast to become isoechoic with background liver in the sinusoidal contrast phase confirming a benign hemangioma. (C) An atypical hemangioma appears hypoechoic on a background of fatty liver. Contrast-enhanced ultrasound confirmed its benign nature. (D) Multiple tiny hemangiomas throughout the liver.

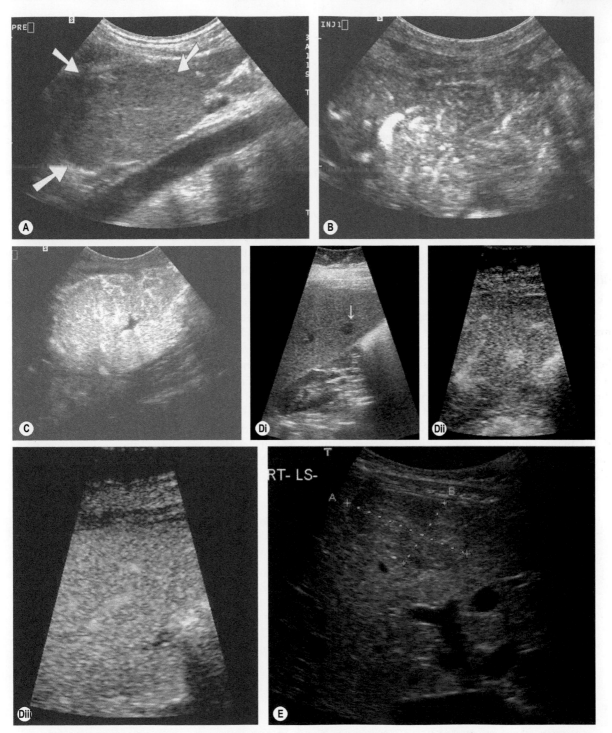

Fig. 2.39 Focal nodular hyperplasia (FNH): (A) In the left lobe (arrows). These are frequently almost isoechoic with normal liver tissue. (B) Following administration of microbubble contrast agent, FNH displays a "spoked-wheel" pattern of vascular enhancement during the early arterial phase. (C) The same lesion seconds later, showing a central scar. (Di) A tiny FNH (arrow) (Dii) blushes rapidly in the arterial phase of contrast administration and (Diii) becomes isoechoic with background liver in the sinusoidal phase. (E) Another example of an FNH, almost isoechoic with background liver.

Management of this benign mass is usually conservative, but surgical resection may be necessary for larger lesions.

Adenoma

The hepatic adenoma is a benign focal lesion consisting of a cluster of atypical liver cells (Fig. 2.40). There may be pools of bile or focal areas of hemorrhage or necrosis within this. This gives rise to a heterogeneous, patchy echotexture. The smaller ones tend to be homogeneous with a smooth texture. Their lipid content causes a tendency to be hyperechoic, although usually less reflective than a hemangioma, and many have similar reflectivity to the surrounding liver parenchyma.

Clinical Features

There is a particularly strong association between hepatic adenoma and oral contraceptive use, so these masses tend to present in younger women. Adenomas are also associated with glycogen storage disease and hemochromatosis. They may cause pain, particularly if they hemorrhage, and may be palpable. If present during pregnancy, they can enlarge and rupture under the influence of estrogen. In rare cases, malignant transformation may occur, so surgical removal is the management of choice, although occasionally, some adenomas regress if the oral contraceptive is discontinued.

Focal Fatty Change

Not a lesion as such but included here because of its focal appearance. It may pose a diagnostic dilemma on initial ultrasound.

Focal Fatty Infiltration

Fatty infiltration of the liver is a common occurrence that may affect the whole or part of the liver. It is associated with obesity and alcoholism and can also occur in pregnancy, diabetes, and with certain drugs. The deposition of fat confined to certain focal areas of the liver is related to the blood supply to that area. Fatty infiltration increases the reflectivity of the parenchyma, making it hyperechoic. This can simulate a focal mass, such as metastasis. Unlike a focal lesion, however, it does not display any mass effect, and the course of related vessels remains constant. It tends to have a characteristic straight-edged shape, rectangular or ovoid, corresponding to the region of local blood supply (Fig. 2.41). Foci of fatty change may be multiple or may affect isolated liver segments. The most common sites are in segment IV around the porta, in the caudate lobe (segment I), and in the posterior area of the left lobe (segment III).

CEUS is useful and accurate in differentiating focal fatty change from a true lesion, as the contrast uptake is identical to the background liver, and the contrast convincingly demonstrates the lack of mass effect (Fig. 2.41D). This technique usually obviates the need for further imaging in focal fatty change.

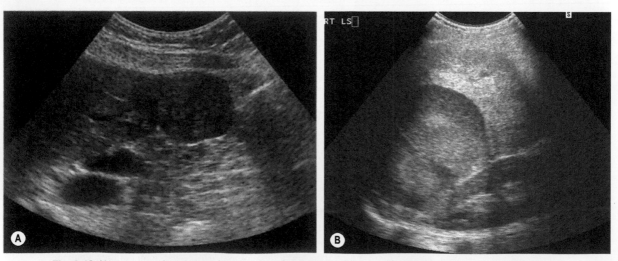

Fig. 2.40 (A) Adenoma in segment V of the liver in a young woman on the contraceptive pill. (B) An unusual example of cystic degeneration in a large adenoma.

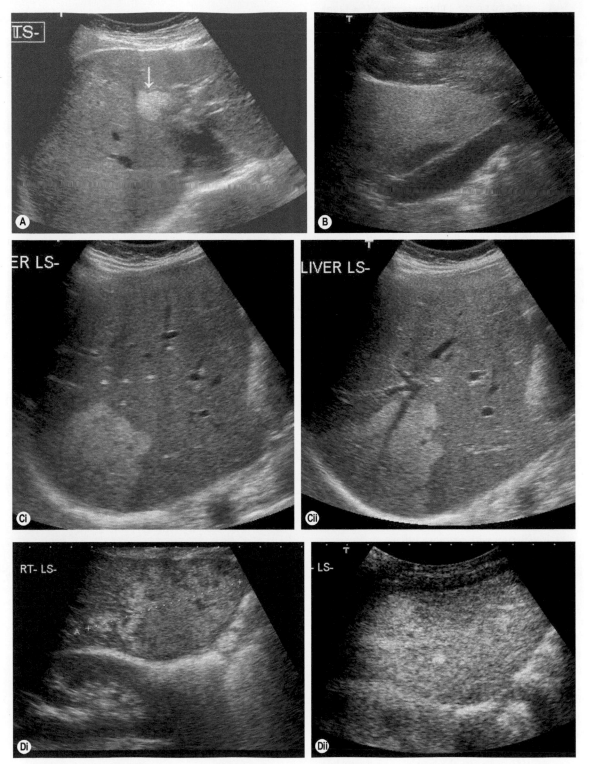

Fig. 2.41 (A) Focal fatty change (arrow) can mimic a focal lesion. (B) Focal fatty sparing in a characteristic position just anterior to the gallbladder. (Ci) Focal fatty change in the right lobe of the liver demonstrates a hepatic vein passing through it, (Cii) with no mass effect. (Di) An irregular focal lesion in segment VI in a patient with cirrhosis is suspicious for hepatocellular carcinoma. (Dii) Contrast-enhanced ultrasound demonstrates normal contrast take up in the arterial, portal, and sinusoidal phases, with no mass seen, confirming focal fatty change.

Focal Fatty Sparing

The reverse process may also occur, in which a diffusely fatty, hyperechogenic liver has an area that has been spared from fat deposition because of its blood supply. This area is less reflective than the surrounding liver and may mimic a hypoechoic neoplastic lesion, but as with focal fatty infiltration, it has regular outlines and shape and no mass effect. The most common sites for fatty sparing are similar to those for focal fatty infiltration: segment IV just anterior to the portal vein or gallbladder (Fig. 2.41B), segment I (the caudate lobe), and around the gallbladder fossa. Unlike a true focal lesion, fatty change does not exhibit a mass effect, and normal, undisplaced vasculature can be demonstrated with color Doppler (in the larger areas) or contrast ultrasound (particularly useful for the smaller focal areas) in both focal fatty infiltration and fatty sparing.

Lipoma

The hepatic lipoma is a relatively rare, benign hepatic tumor which is very similar in nature and acoustic appearance to focal fatty change. It differs in that it is a discrete tumor of fatty deposition, rather than an infiltrative process and so can exert a mass effect on surrounding vessels if large. The fat content makes the lipoma hyperechoic compared to the surrounding liver tissue.

Granuloma

Granulomas are benign liver masses that are associated with chronic inflammatory liver diseases. They have a particular association with primary biliary cirrhosis, sarcoidosis, or tuberculosis. They may be multiple and small, in which case the liver often looks coarse and hyperechoic. More often, they are small discrete lesions that may be hypo- or isoechoic, sometimes with a hypoechoic rim like a target, or calcified with distal shadowing (Fig. 2.42). They can undergo central necrosis. Differential diagnoses include metastases or regenerating nodules, and their appearance on ultrasound is non-specific.

Hepatic Calcification

Calcification occurs in the liver because of some pathological processes and may be seen following infection or parasitic infestation. It may be focal, usually the endstage of a previous abscess, hematoma, or granuloma, which usually indicates that the lesion in question is no longer active. It may also be seen within some metastases.

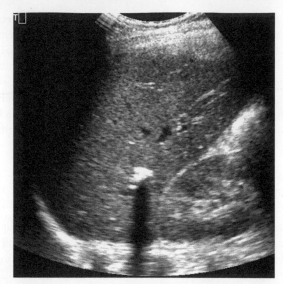

Fig. 2.42 A calcified granuloma demonstrates acoustic shadowing.

Calcification may also be linear in nature, following the course of the portal tracts. This can be associated with old tuberculosis or other previous parasitic infestations such as schistosomiasis (Fig. 2.43).[8] Occasionally, hepatic calcification is seen in children or in the fetus. This

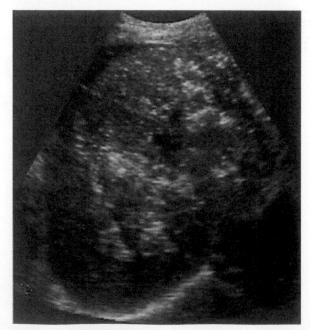

Fig. 2.43 Considerable deposits of calcification are seen in the liver in this patient with nephrotic syndrome.

is usually not a significant finding, but pre-natal infection should be excluded with toxoplasmosis, rubella cytomegalovirus, herpes simplex, and HIV (TORCH) screen. Calcification, which casts a strong and definite shadow, should be distinguished from air in the biliary tree, which casts a reverberative shadow and is usually associated with previous biliary interventions, such as endoscopic retrograde cholangiopancreatography (ERCP), sphincterotomy, or stent placement.

MALIGNANT FOCAL LIVER LESIONS

Metastases

The liver is one of the most common sites where malignant tumors metastasize. Secondary deposits are usually bloodborne, spreading to the liver via the portal venous system (e.g., in the case of gastrointestinal malignancies) or HA (e.g., lung or breast primaries) or spread via the lymphatic system. Some spread along the peritoneal surfaces, for example, ovarian carcinoma. This demonstrates an initial invasion of the subserosal surfaces of the liver (Fig. 2.44A), as opposed to the more central distribution seen with a hematogenous spread (Fig. 2.44B). The former peripheral pattern is more easily missed on ultrasound because small deposits are often obscured by near-field artifacts or rib shadows. It is therefore advisable for the operator to be aware of the possible pattern of spread when searching for liver metastases.

Ultrasound Appearances

The acoustic appearances of liver secondaries are extremely variable (Fig. 2.44). When compared with normal surrounding liver parenchyma, metastases may be hyperechoic, hypoechoic, isoechoic, or mixed pattern. It is not possible to characterize the primary source by the acoustic properties of the metastases. Metastases tend to be solid with ill-defined margins. Some metastases, particularly the larger ones, contain fluid because of central necrosis (Fig. 2.44E) or because they contain mucin, for example, from some ovarian primaries. Occasionally, calcification is seen within a deposit, causing distal acoustic shadowing, which may also develop following treatment with chemotherapy. For example, in some diseases, such as lymphoma, the metastases may be multiple but tiny, not immediately obvious to the operator as discrete focal lesions but as a coarse-textured liver (Fig. 2.44F). This type of appearance is non-specific and could be associated with several conditions, both benign and malignant.

Diagnosis of focal liver lesions, such as metastases, is made more difficult when the liver texture is diffusely abnormal or when there are dilated intrahepatic ducts because the altered transmission of sound through the liver masks small lesions. Other possible ultrasound features associated with metastases include a lobulated outline to the liver, hepatomegaly, and ascites.

If the finding of liver metastases is unexpected or the primary has not been identified, it is useful to complete a full examination to search for a possible primary carcinoma and to identify other sites of carcinomatous spread. Lymphadenopathy (particularly in the para-aortic, para-caval, and portal regions) may be demonstrated on ultrasound, and invasion of adjacent blood vessels and disease in other extrahepatic sites including spleen, kidneys, omentum, and peritoneum. CT is the usual next step to identify a possible primary site and stage the disease, in particular demonstrating extrahepatic disease that is often not seen on ultrasound.

Doppler is unhelpful in characterizing liver metastases, most of which appear poorly vascular or avascular. Fundamental non-contrast ultrasound lacks sensitivity in the diagnosis of liver metastases, as many lesions are either isoechoic or small (subcentimeter), rendering them almost invisible. The use of microbubble contrast agents radically improves the characterization and detection of metastatic deposits on ultrasound. The injection of a bolus of contrast agent when viewed using pulse-inversion demonstrates variable vascular phase enhancement in the arterial and portal phases, but the sinusoidal phase invariably lacks contrast uptake (Fig. 2.44G, H). This is a particularly useful technique as it increases the contrast resolution between metastasis and background liver, meaning that even subcentimeter lesions are reliably demonstrated. CEUS also increases the operator's confidence in the absence of metastases, particularly in cases with altered LFTs and prior history of malignancy (Fig. 2.44J). This is useful in obviating the need for further imaging in normal livers.

Clinical Features and Management

Many patients present with symptoms from their liver deposits, rather than the primary carcinoma. The demonstration of liver metastases on ultrasound may often prompt further radiological investigations for the primary. The symptoms of liver deposits may include non-obstructive jaundice, obstructive jaundice (which may occur if a large mass is present at the porta),

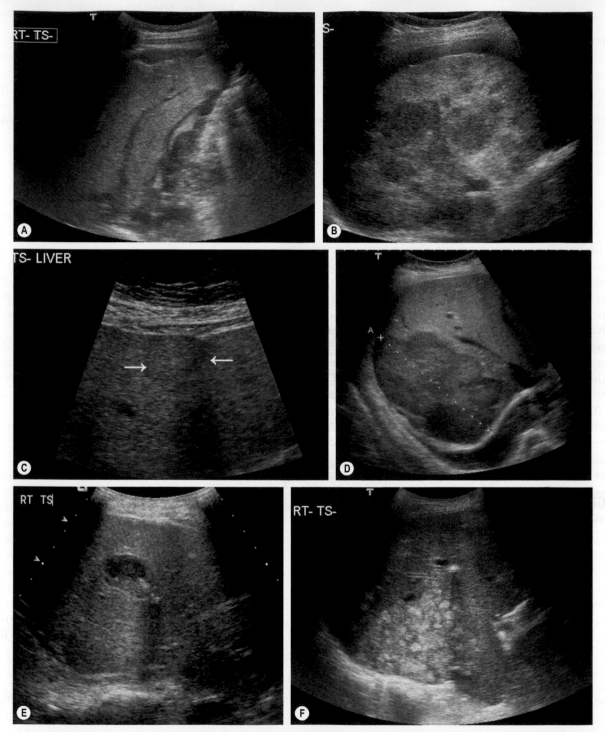

Fig. 2.44 Examples of liver metastases: (A) Peripheral, hypoechoic secondary deposits because of peritoneal spread from a primary ovarian carcinoma. (B) Bloodborne metastases from bowel carcinoma are distributed throughout the liver. (C) Solitary isoechoic metastasis was confirmed on magnetic resonance imaging. Isoechoic metastases are easy to miss, and the use of CEUS is invaluable in demonstrating them. (D) Large hyperechoic metastasis occupying segment VII of the right lobe. Note also the right pleural effusion. (E) A necrotic metastasis, demonstrating posterior acoustic enhancement. (F) Calcified metastases from breast carcinoma.

Continued

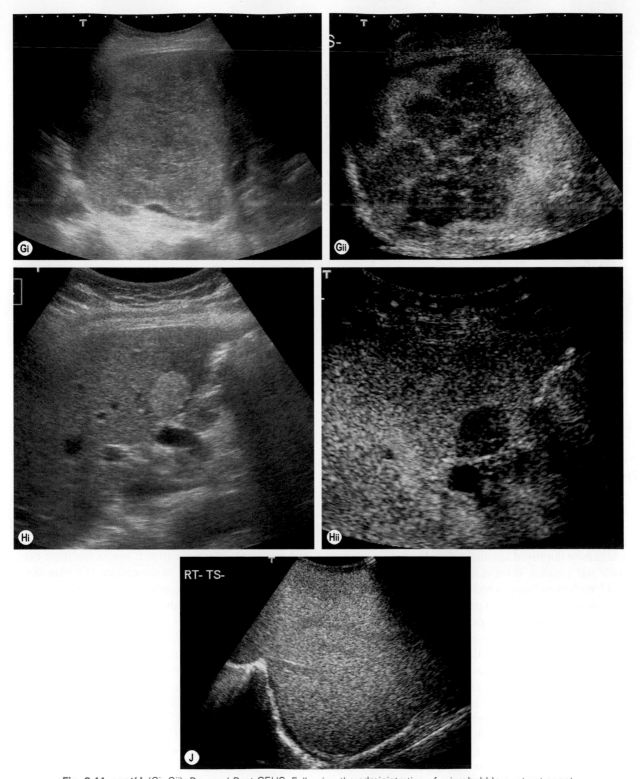

Fig. 2.44, cont'd (Gi, Gii), Pre- and Post CEUS. Following the administration of microbubble contrast agent, numerous metastases are discovered. These appear hypoechoic in the late portal venous phase, with no contrast uptake. (Hi, Hii) Pre- and Post CEUS of a solitary metastasis in a patient who has undergone surgery for bowel carcinoma. (J) Normal CEUS in a patient at risk of liver metastases. Contrast take up is homogeneous throughout the liver in the sinusoidal phase with no evidence of lesions. CEUS greatly increases the confidence in a negative scan.

TABLE 2.1	**Common Causes of Jaundice**
Non-Obstructive	
Unconjugated hyperbilirubinemia	Hemolysis
	Hematoma
	Gilbert's disease
Mixed hyperbilirubinemia	Hepatitis
	Alcoholic liver disease
	Cirrhosis of all types
	Multiple liver metastases
	Drug-induced liver disease
Obstructive	
Conjugated hyperbilirubinemia	Stones in the biliary duct
	Carcinoma of the duct, head of the pancreas, or ampulla
	Acute pancreatitis
	Other masses which compress the
	CBD (e.g., lymph node mass)
	Biliary atresia

BOX 2.2

Always:
- Take an oral history from the patient if possible – do not rely on the requested information.
- Obtain the results of any previous investigations, including previous radiology.
- Consider the possibility of multiple causes.

hepatomegaly, right-sided pain, increasing abdominal girth from ascites, and altered LFTs (Table 2.1). An ultrasound-guided biopsy may be useful in diagnosing the primary and complements further imaging such as X-rays and contrast bowel studies. Accurate staging of the disease is performed with CT, MRI, and/or PET-CT,[9] which have improved sensitivity for identifying extrahepatic and systemic disease, such as peritoneal deposits and lymphadenopathy, which can more accurately measure the adjacent spread of primary disease.

The prognosis for most patients with liver metastases has traditionally been poor, particularly if multiple, and depends to a large extent on the origin of the primary carcinoma. A regime of surgical debulking (removal of the primary carcinoma, adjacent invaded viscera, lymphadenopathy) together with chemotherapy can slow down the progress of the disease. Increasingly, however, there are treatment options that result in increased, good quality survival and, in some cases, a cure. This makes it important that secondary disease is diagnosed early and accurately to offer patients a significant chance of survival.

In an increasing number of cases, particularly those with metastases from a colorectal primary, which are less aggressive and grow more slowly, long-term survival is achieved by surgically resecting both the primary bowel lesion and then the liver deposits. The smaller and fewer the liver deposits, the better the prognosis. The success of this treatment means that tumors previously considered inoperable are now potentially curable. In such cases, it is particularly useful to localize the lesions using the segmental liver anatomy prior to surgery. Intraoperative ultrasound (IOUS) is then used to confirm the preoperative appearances and examine the tumor margins to plan the line of resection (Fig. 2.45).

Other treatment methods include chemoembolization and radiofrequency, microwave, or laser ablation, often under ultrasound guidance.[10] The success of these options depends on the number and size of the lesions and the nature of the primary. Currently, these methods are considered palliative rather than curative and are an option for patients who are unsuitable candidates for hepatic resection.

Ultrasound of Other Relevant Areas

In suspected or confirmed malignancy, the examination of the abdomen may usefully include all the sites likely to be affected. While the liver is one of the most common sites for the spread of the disease, it is also useful to examine the adrenals, spleen, and kidneys and look for lymphadenopathy in the para-aortic, para-caval, and portal regions.

If ascites are present, deposits may sometimes be demonstrated on the peritoneal or omental surfaces in patients with late-stage disease. These malignant plaques may also afford a useful site for ultrasound-guided biopsy to diagnose and palliatively treat the disease.

Hepatocellular Carcinoma (HCC)

This primary carcinoma of the liver is particularly common in Africa and the Far East, and demographics show an increasing incidence in Europe and the United Kingdom, now being the fifth most common cancer worldwide. Most HCCs (over 80%) arise in diseased

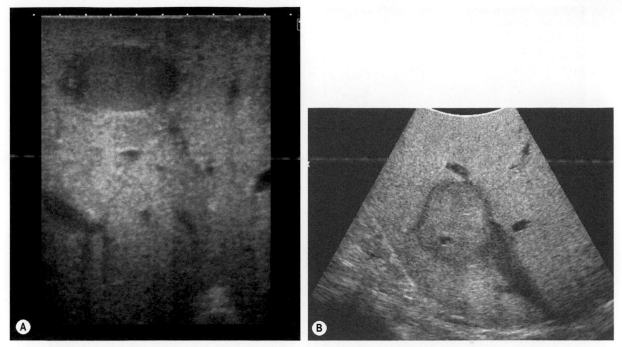

Fig. 2.45 (A) Intraoperative ultrasound scan demonstrates a small metastasis not identified on preoperative imaging. (B) Intraoperative ultrasound locates a metastasis prior to ultrasound-guided ablation.

livers, hence the strong association with alcoholic cirrhosis and hepatitis. One of the main reasons for ultrasound referral for assessment and surveillance in such patients is to exclude focal liver lesions, which could represent carcinoma. HCC is also associated with metabolic disorders and drug-related liver disease. Clinically, small tumors are asymptomatic but cause a raised serum alpha-fetoprotein (AFP). The relationship between cirrhosis and HCC prompts screening of such patients with AFP and ultrasound. The ultrasound appearances of HCC vary from hypo- to hyperechoic or mixed echogenicity lesions (Fig. 2.46). It is often particularly difficult, if not impossible, to locate small HCCs in a cirrhotic liver that is already coarse-textured and nodular. MRI may be useful in these cases[11,12] as it can differentiate HCC from other nodules, such as dysplastic nodules, which frequently occur in the cirrhotic liver. HCCs may be solitary or multifocal. The increase in such diseases as hepatitis C has caused the introduction of ultrasound/AFP screening programs in many centers. This has led to the more frequent detection of early, small HCCs, which can be indistinguishable on ultrasound from other regenerative liver nodules. Lesions of over 2 cm diameter in a cirrhotic liver have around a 90% chance of being malignant, and

CEUS can demonstrate tortuous feeding arteries, the tumor blush, and the hypoenhancement in the sinusoidal phase, which are characteristic of HCC (Fig. 2.46H).

CEUS appearances can be quite variable in HCC and should be interpreted with caution. The introduction of ultrasound screening, together with the improvement in image quality, has meant the discovery of ever smaller nodules. These frequently fail to demonstrate characteristic CEUS patterns, and MRI is the appropriate next imaging modality. The combination of MRI and CEUS when characteristic contrast patterns are present obviates the need for biopsy, an important consideration as it is associated with reduced survival in patients who subsequently receive a transplant. A biopsy may be performed to formulate a treatment plan in equivocal cases.

As with metastases, there is now a range of treatment options that can improve patient survival. Hepatic transplant is generally considered curative and traditionally offered in the absence of malignancy. However, patients with HCCs can still be considered for a transplant, provided the malignancy is limited, and their disease may be temporarily controlled using ultrasound-guided ablation if necessary.[13,14] In patients with advanced HCC, transcatheter arterial

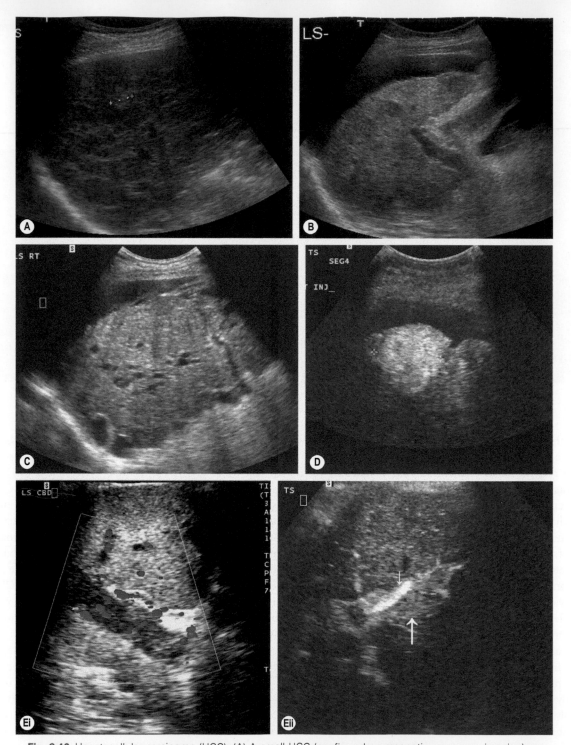

Fig. 2.46 Hepatocellular carcinoma (HCC): (A) A small HCC (confirmed on magnetic resonance imaging) on a background of cirrhosis. (B) Multifocal HCCs in a patient with cryptogenic cirrhosis. (C) A patient with chronic Budd-Chiari syndrome has a nodular liver with suspicion of a lesion near the anterior surface. (D) Administration of contrast in the same patient as (C) demonstrates increased uptake in the arterial phase, with hypoenhancement in the sinusoidal phase, helping to locate the lesion and characterize it as an HCC. (Ei) Tumor thrombus in the portal vein in a patient with multifocal HCC. (Eii) Contrast-enhanced ultrasound (EUS) of a case of invasive HCC; the portal vein (large arrow) shows contrast uptake because of tumor thrombus in the arterial phase. (HA, small arrow.)

Continued

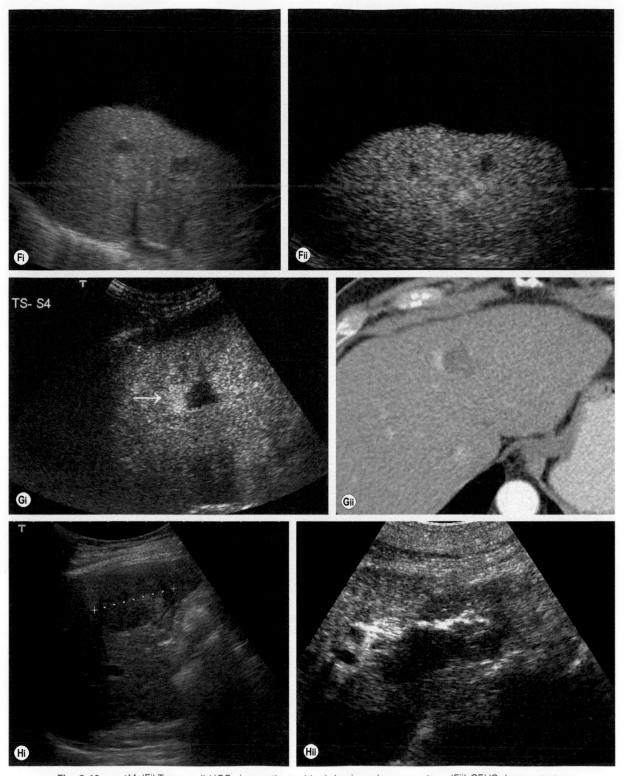

Fig. 2.46, cont'd (Fi) Two small HCCs in a patient with cirrhosis and gross ascites. (Fii) CEUS demonstrates typical hypoenhancement in the sinusoidal phase. (Gi) CEUS in an ablated HCC. The treated lesion is almost avascular, but a rim of tumor recurrence (arrow) is present around the lesion. (Gii) CT confirms tumor recurrence, and the lesion was re-ablated successfully.

Continued

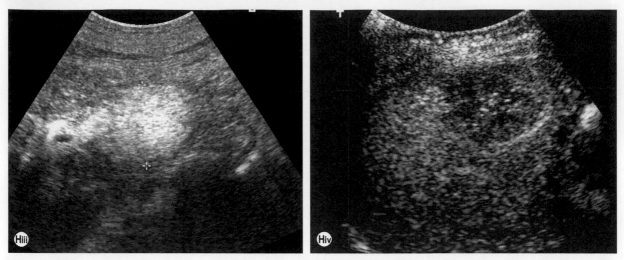

Fig. 2.46, cont'd (H) Typical CEUS of HCC: (Hi) pre-contrast lesion, (Hii) immediate post-injection shows a tortuous feeding artery followed by (Hiii) a blush of contrast uptake. (Hiv) Sinusoidal phase shows hypoenhancement.

chemoembolization (TACE) may slow the progress of the tumor, and high intensity focused ultrasound is a further technique that is promising in improving patient survival.[15]

Cholangiocarcinoma

This primary carcinoma of the bile ducts is discussed more fully in Chapter 3. Most commonly seen affecting the main biliary ducts, it also occurs in the intrahepatic biliary tree where it infiltrates the surrounding liver parenchyma, having the appearance of a solid mass. It may be solitary or multifocal, and a clue to its location is often the focal dilatation of ducts proximal to the obstructing mass. It has an association with sclerosing cholangitis and carries a relatively poor prognosis, as it tends to recur after transplantation (Table 2.4).

DIFFUSE LIVER CONDITIONS

Diseases that diffusely affect the liver may have non-specific ultrasound appearances. Suspicion is usually raised following altered LFTs (Table 2.2) and the diagnosis made histologically. Several diffuse liver conditions can cause hepatocellular (or non-obstructive) jaundice, which is associated with increased levels of unconjugated bile in the blood. Many of these can be demonstrated with ultrasound, while others cannot.

The main role of ultrasound in the jaundiced patient is to exclude any obstructive cause (by the presence or absence of biliary duct dilatation) and search for liver metastases or signs of a diffuse liver condition (Table 2.5).

Fatty Infiltration (Steatosis)

The process of accumulation of fat within the hepatic cells may be either focal (see above) or diffuse. Related to various conditions such as alcoholism, obesity, and diabetes, it is associated with any process which alters liver metabolism, and it is reversible in many circumstances. The acoustic properties of fat differ from those of normal liver tissue. The liver appears hyperechoic as the fat globules provide interfaces that are highly reflective. As the level of fat deposition increases, the level of echogenicity reaches that of the highly reflective portal tract walls. This has the effect of reducing the prominence of the portal tracts (Fig. 2.47) and making the liver appear smooth and homogeneous, with closely packed, fine echoes. The contrast between the liver and parenchyma of the right kidney is therefore increased (a particularly useful sign confirming that the correct gain settings have been used).

Hepatomegaly is also a feature, though not invariably. Finally, the attenuation of fat is greater than that of normal liver tissue; this has the effect of reduced penetration in the far-field rather as if the Time Gain

TABLE 2.2	Common Serum LFTs
Test	**Association with Increased Level**
Bilirubin	Obstructive or non-obstructive jaundice. (differentiation can be made between conjugated and unconjugated bilirubin)
Alkaline phosphatase (ALP) (liver enzyme)	Non-obstructive jaundice Metastases Other focal hepatic lesions
Alpha-fetoprotein	Hepatocellular carcinoma (HCC)
Prothrombin time	Malignancy Diffuse liver disease (often with portal hypertension)
Gamma-glutamyltransferase	Obstructive jaundice Alcoholic liver disease
Alanine aminotransferase (ALT)	Fatty liver
Aspartate aminotransferase (AST) (liver enzymes)	Obstructive or non-obstructive jaundice Hepatitis Viral infections Other organ failure (e.g., cardiac)
Protein (serum albumin)	Lack of protein is associated with numerous liver diseases. Low levels are associated with ascites, often because of portal hypertension

TABLE 2.3	Cystic Focal Liver Lesions Differential Diagnoses
SIMPLE CYST	Anechoic, thin capsule, posterior enhancement (may contain thin septae) Common finding, usually insignificant Consider polycystic disease if multiple (rarely an AV malformation may mimic a septated cyst; exclude by using color Doppler)
COMPLEX CYST	Thin capsule, internal echoes Hemorrhage or infection in a cyst Mucinous metastasis Cystadenoma Capsule thickened or complex, may also contain echoes Hydatid cyst Cystadenocarcinoma Intrahepatic pancreatic pseudocyst (rare)
SOLID/CYSTIC LESION	Irregular margin, internal echoes, debris/solid material Abscess Hematoma Necrotic metastasis Cavernous hemangioma

Compensation (TGC) paddles or slope control had been incorrectly set. In severe cases of infiltration, most of the sound is reflected back to the transducer in the first few centimeters, creating a highly reflective near-field band through which the sound cannot penetrate.

Fatty infiltration itself is not usually a significant finding; however, it often occurs in conjunction with other significant diffuse processes such as cirrhosis. Its increased attenuation reduces the ability of ultrasound to exclude other diseases or focal lesions, and therefore CT may be a useful adjunct. In cases of focal fatty change or sparing (see above), it may cause a diagnostic dilemma as it mimics a focal lesion. CEUS is useful in characterizing these areas (Fig. 2.47C).

Non-Alcoholic Steatohepatitis

Non-alcoholic steatohepatitis (NASH) or non-alcoholic fatty liver disease is when fat deposition in the hepatocytes is accompanied by inflammation and fibrosis in patients who consume little or no alcohol. In contrast to simple fatty liver, this process can cause irreversible damage leading to cirrhosis. Its incidence is increasing in developed countries, and it is strongly associated with obesity and diabetes.[16] It is an increasingly common reason for abnormal LFTs and referral for ultrasound (Fig. 2.47D).

Cirrhosis

Cirrhosis is a process associated with end-stage chronic liver disease (and not really a disease in itself). It can result from a wide range of pathological processes.

TABLE 2.4	**Common Solid Focal Liver Lesions: Differential Diagnoses**
BENIGN	**Hemangioma** Usually, hyperechoic. Common incidental finding **Focal nodular hyperplasia** Common, usually asymptomatic lesion, often in young women **Focal fatty change** No mass effect **Adenoma** Uncommon. Associated with the contraceptive pill **Granuloma** Associated with chronic inflammation/infection. May calcify **Regenerating nodules** Associated with cirrhosis. Multiple lesions **Abscess** May appear solid in the early stages. Look for posterior enhancement. Fever and pain **Infarct** Associated with HA thrombosis in liver transplant
MALIGNANT	**Metastasis** Wide spectrum of possible acoustic appearances **HCC** Associated with cirrhosis **Cholangiocarcinoma** Associated with cholestatic disease. Proximal biliary dilatation

TABLE 2.5	**Causes of Non-Obstructive (Medical) Jaundice**
Hemolysis	In which red cells are destroyed, releasing the hemoglobin (from which bilirubin is derived) into the surrounding tissue
Hematoma	Hemolytic process
Gilbert's disease	A defect in the hepatic uptake of bilirubin
Viral hepatitis, cirrhosis of all types, alcoholic or drug-induced liver disease	Destruction of the liver cells by these diseases prevents the mechanism of hepatic uptake and excretion of bilirubin. Both conjugated and unconjugated bilirubin are present
Abscess	Intrahepatic Malignancy Multiple and/or large lesions prevent the take up and excretion of bilirubin by the liver cells

Ultrasound Appearances

In cirrhosis, bands of fibrous tissue are laid down in the liver parenchyma between the hepatic lobules. This distorts and destroys the normal architecture of the liver, separating it into nodules. The process may be micronodular, which gives a generally coarse echotexture, or macronodular, in which discrete nodules of 1 cm and above can be distinguished on ultrasound (Fig. 2.48).

The hepatocellular damage which causes cirrhosis gives rise to hepatic fibrosis, a precursor of cirrhosis. The fibrosis itself may have very little effect on the ultrasound appearances of the liver, but when advanced, it is more highly reflective than normal liver tissue, giving the appearance of a bright liver often with a coarse texture.[11]

Unlike fatty change, which is potentially reversible, fibrosis results from irreversible damage to the liver cells.

The picture is further complicated by the association of fibrosis with fatty change, which also increases the echogenicity. However, the acoustic attenuation properties of fibrosis are similar to the normal liver so that the ultrasound beam can penetrate to the posterior areas using normal TGC settings. In contrast, fat increases both the echogenicity and the attenuation, preventing penetration to the far-field (Fig. 2.47).

The cirrhotic liver tends to shrink as the disease progresses. However, it may be normal in size or may undergo disproportionate changes within different lobes. In some patients, the right lobe shrinks, giving rise to relative hypertrophy of the caudate and/or left lobes, for example. This is likely to be because of the venous drainage of the different areas of the liver.

Nodules in Cirrhosis

The nodular nature of the cirrhotic liver may give rise to a diagnostic dilemma. Nodular regeneration is often present, in which the liver responds to the fibrosis and architectural disturbance with the nodular regrowth of hepatocytes, visible as lumps on the ultrasound scan.

Dysplastic nodules are composed of hepatocytes that have undergone a benign change. Low-grade nodules are non-malignant and usually small (subcentimeter) but slightly larger than the background cirrhotic nodules.

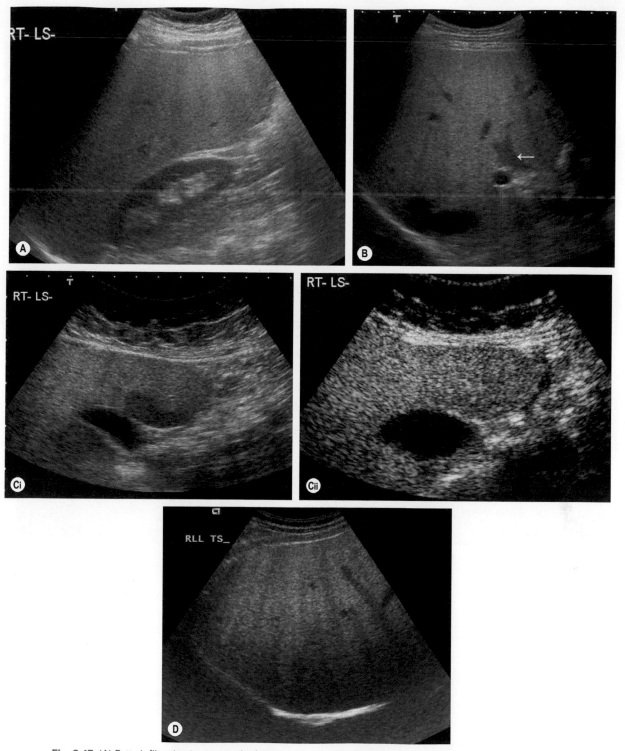

Fig. 2.47 (A) Fatty infiltration increases the hepatorenal contrast. The portal tracts are reduced in prominence, giving a more homogeneous appearance. Attenuation is increased so that it is more difficult to penetrate to the back of the liver. (B) Fatty liver with reduced portal tract prominence and a focal area of fatty sparing (arrow). (Ci) Fatty liver in a patient taking chemotherapy following resection for bowel carcinoma. The new finding of an area of fatty sparing anterior to the gallbladder needs definitive characterization. (Cii) CEUS demonstrates contrast take up identical to background liver throughout all phases, confirming fatty sparing. (D) Non-alcoholic steatohepatitis demonstrating a coarse-textured, fatty, and fibrotic liver.

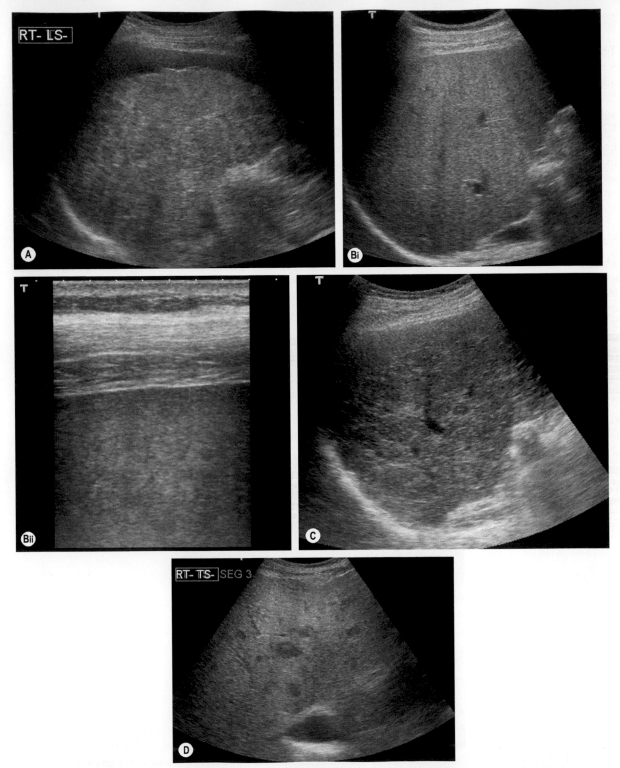

Fig. 2.48 (A) Micronodular cirrhosis in a patient with alcoholic liver disease. Ascites outlines the lobular anterior liver surface. (Bi) Micronodular cirrhosis in hepatitis C virus. (Bii) The nodular nature of the liver is better appreciated with a high-frequency probe. (C) Macronodular cirrhosis in a patient with primary biliary cirrhosis. Cirrhotic nodules are demonstrated throughout the peripheral hepatic substance with a lobulated liver outline. (D) Multiple dysplastic nodules in a patient with cirrhosis, confirmed on magnetic resonance imaging. (The differential diagnosis would be multifocal hepatocellular carcinoma.)

These nodules may progress into high-grade lesions, which have an increased arterial supply, are increasingly atypical of liver cells and are generally thought to be pre-malignant. Such nodules can be monitored with imaging and are at increased likelihood of undergoing malignant transformation to HCCs, although this process is not inevitable. The use of MRI with iron oxide is useful in characterizing nodules detected on ultrasound and identifying early malignant change. However, a nodule of 2 cm or more on ultrasound is almost certainly (over 90% chance) malignant and requires further staging.

Hemodynamics in Cirrhosis

The rigid nature of the diseased liver also causes hemodynamic changes, which can be demonstrated on color and spectral Doppler. Portal venous flow may also be compromised because of portal hypertension (see below), associated with numerous changes on ultrasound, including reduced velocity, reversed flow, or partial or total thrombosis. A compensatory increase in hepatic arterial flow to the liver may also be seen as a result of portal venous compromise in portal hypertension.

The normally triphasic hepatic venous waveform becomes flattened and monophasic because of increased hepatic resistance. This is a non-specific sign that occurs with numerous types of chronic liver disease or any condition, either intra- or extrahepatic, which compresses the venous flow, such as polycystic liver disease or the presence of ascites.[17] Its significance to the sonographer is that the monophasic hepatofugal flow may be mistaken for reversed portal venous flow if the operator is unaware.

HCC in Cirrhosis

Patients with cirrhosis are at increased risk of developing hepatocellular carcinoma, the detection of which may be particularly difficult in an already nodular liver. As there are treatment options for patients with cirrhosis and HCC, some of which are curative, if the malignancy is small, many institutions opt to screen cirrhotic patients with annual or six-monthly AFP and ultrasound.[18] This remains controversial, being more cost-effective in patients with hepatitis B cirrhosis than other causes of cirrhosis, and demonstrating doubtful overall cost-effectiveness in patients with normal levels of AFP.[19] Both CT and ultrasound have a low sensitivity for detecting small focal lesions in cirrhotic livers,[12] which continue to present a diagnostic challenge. However, improvements in ultrasound imaging

have enabled operators to identify smaller and more subtle nodules than previously possible. The use of ultrasound contrast agents may give a characteristic pattern, confirming HCC (Fig. 2.46),[20] but HCCs can be atypical, and the technique is less useful with subcentimeter lesions, such as dysplastic nodules. MRI using iron oxide is useful in characterizing small nodules and in detecting additional, small HCCs not identified on ultrasound.[21,22]

Hepatitis

Hepatitis B (HBV) and C (HCV) viruses are infections with a worldwide distribution. Transmission of infection is by exposure to bodily fluids, unsafe injection practices, blood transfusions, and mother-to-child infection, among other causes. Around 25% of cases will result in severe liver damage (depending on the age at diagnosis), and death from cirrhosis and/or HCC pose a massive health problem. It is estimated that 3% of the world's population is now infected with HCV,[23] which is now a leading factor in the development of HCC.[24]

Alcoholic Cirrhosis

The spectrum of alcoholic liver disease may take three forms: steatosis (alcoholic fatty liver), alcoholic hepatitis (often preceding cirrhosis), and finally, cirrhosis. The incidence of death from alcoholic cirrhosis continues to climb in the United Kingdom.

Alcoholic liver disease may be halted or reversed in the early stages in patients who discontinue alcohol intake, with subsequent nodular regeneration of hepatic tissue (Fig. 2.48D).

Primary Biliary Cirrhosis (PBC)

PBC is an autoimmune, progressive cholestatic liver disease that presents predominantly in middle-aged females. The term cirrhosis may be rather misleading for the early stages of this condition, which actually take the form of an inflammatory destruction of the intrahepatic bile ducts. These early stages of cholangitis are not, strictly speaking, cirrhotic. However, as the destruction progresses, bands of fibrosis form in the process of macronodular cirrhosis (Fig. 2.48C).

Treatment of PBC involves control of the associated symptoms of portal hypertension and pruritis, but its progression is inevitable. Liver transplantation now offers a successful therapeutic option for these patients, with a 70% survival at seven years.[25] Although the liver frequently looks normal on ultrasound in the early stages of the disease, lymphadenopathy can be demonstrated in up to 80% of PBC patients.[26]

Secondary Biliary Cirrhosis

Secondary biliary cirrhosis (SBC) occurs as a result of chronic biliary obstruction. Causes of SBC usually include benign strictures or chronic stone impaction in the common bile duct (CBD), causing progressive, gradual obstruction over a period of time. This causes ascending cholangitis and jaundice. The bile ducts may appear only mildly dilated on ultrasound. It is also a recognized sequel of biliary atresia in children.

Other Causes

Cirrhosis may be drug-induced, particularly in patients on long-term treatment or therapy, and may also result from prolonged exposure to some environmental toxins and to parasitic infections. It is associated with many other diseases, such as cystic fibrosis, human immunodeficiency virus (HIV), diabetes, ulcerative colitis, rheumatoid arthritis, NASH, Budd-Chiari disease, primary sclerosing cholangitis (PSC), or any long-term conditions, acquired or congenital, which can affect the liver.

Congenital forms of cirrhosis exist because of metabolic disorders: Wilson's disease (deposition of copper in the liver and kidneys), glycogen storage disease (inability to break down glycogen to glucose), hemochromatosis (deposition of iron in the liver and pancreas), and others. Liver congestion from heart failure can also lead to cirrhosis in severe, prolonged cases. Up to 10% of patients have cirrhosis from no recognizable cause. This is termed cryptogenic cirrhosis (Table 2.6).

Clinical Features and Management

Clinical presentation depends on the cause and may involve chronic symptoms or an acute episode. Pruritus, fatigue, and jaundice, with steatorrhea and deranged LFTs (raised alkaline phosphatase and serum bilirubin in PBC, raised alanine aminotransferase [ALT] and aspartate aminotransferase [AST] in alcoholic disease) are generally present by the later stages. This is followed by the symptoms of portal hypertension (see below), which is a poor prognostic feature associated with late-stage cirrhosis.

The process may be reversed in alcoholics who stop drinking. However, the prognosis of any cirrhotic condition is poor if malignancy is present. In severe cases, the management revolves around palliating the

TABLE 2.6	Summary of Possible Ultrasound Appearances in Cirrhosis
Normal Parenchyma	May appear normal, particularly in the early stages
Changes in texture	Coarse texture (micronodular)
Changes in reflectivity	Irregular nodular appearance (macronodular)
Changes in size and outline	Fibrosis increases the overall echogenicity (but not the attenuation)
Focal lesions	May be accompanied by fatty change, which increases both echogenicity and attenuation giving a hyper-reflective near-field with poor penetration to the posterior liver Small, shrunken liver Nodular, irregular surface outline Deep fissures Possible disproportionate hypertrophy of left or caudate lobes Increased incidence of HCC Regenerative or dysplastic nodules (low to high-grade)
Vascular	Signs of portal hypertension: Changes in portal vein velocity and direction Thrombosis (occlusive or non-occlusive) Varices and collaterals Increased hepatic arterial flow Flattened, monophasic hepatic venous flow on spectral Doppler (a non-specific finding)
Other signs	Ascites Splenomegaly Lymphadenopathy

symptoms of portal hypertension, as bleeding from varices is a major cause of morbidity and mortality.

The degree of fibrosis and severity of cirrhosis is currently usually established histologically by biopsy. This is an invasive technique with the potential for serious complications. However, these are minimized if the needle is guided into the liver under ultrasound control.

Elastography is currently being investigated as a possible non-invasive alternative to biopsy.[27] This technique transmits ultrasonic vibrations into the liver to measure its stiffness. The principle is that the more fibrotic the tissue, the stiffer it is and the faster the vibration is transmitted. Patients with cirrhosis are frequently monitored using six-monthly ultrasound and AFP in an attempt to diagnose HCC as early as possible. Liver transplant is now an established and highly successful treatment option for cirrhosis when the symptoms can no longer be controlled with drugs and may be considered curative in some patients.

Although the success of transplant is reduced in patients with malignancy, the presence of a modest burden of HCC is no longer a contraindication to transplant.[28] However, patients waiting for suitable transplant organs may have disease which progresses, making them unsuitable for transplantation when the opportunity occurs. Palliative measures such as percutaneous ablation or surgical resection can be employed to contain the effects of malignancy in a patient otherwise suitable for transplantation. Chemoembolization may benefit some patients with HCC and reasonably good liver function. In patients with advanced disease, palliation of symptoms, such as sclerotherapy of varices, ascitic drainage, or transjugular intrahepatic portosystemic shunt (TIPSS), may improve the quality of life.

Portal Hypertension

Portal hypertension occurs when the pressure in the portal venous system is raised. This may happen because of chronic liver disease, particularly in the cirrhotic stage when the nodular and fibrotic nature of the parenchyma impedes the flow of blood into the liver. It is significant because it causes numerous deleterious effects on the patient, many of which can be recognized on ultrasound (Table 2.6).

Raised portal venous pressure is associated with several complications. These are discussed below.

Portal Vein Signs

Portal vein flow is influenced by numerous factors, including prandial state, patient position, exercise, and cardiac output.[29] Its velocity varies considerably in both cirrhotic and healthy subjects, and it is essential to use color and spectral Doppler to investigate the portal flow properly.[30] The vein may appear dilated and tortuous, but not invariably.

Portal venous flow may be:

- Normal in direction (hepatopetal) and velocity.[31]
- Reduced in velocity (Fig. 2.49Ai),[32] 10 cm/s, although there is overlap with the normal range.
- Damped, in which there is a lack of normal respiratory variation of both the caliber and the waveform of the splenic and portal veins. The normal spectrum has a "wavy" characteristic, which may be lost.
- Reversed (hepatofugal) (Fig. 2.49B). This indicates serious liver disease. Interestingly, patients with hepatofugal PV flow are much less likely to suffer from bleeding varices, suggesting a type of protective mechanism here.
- "Balanced" in which both forward and reverse low-velocity flow is present in a condition that may precede imminent thrombosis or reversal (Fig. 2.49C).
- Thrombosed (Fig. 2.49D–F). Low-level echoes from the thrombus may be evident, but the vein may appear anechoic with fresh thrombus, as in the normal vein. The absence of power Doppler flow, provided the settings are appropriate, is a much better indicator for thrombosis than the gray-scale image. Although PV thrombosis most commonly results from portal hypertension in cirrhosis, there are many other causes, including inflammatory or malignant conditions which may surround, compress, or invade the portal and/or splenic veins (Table 2.7). Thrombosis may be occlusive or non-occlusive and may extend into the intrahepatic portal venous system. CEUS is useful in distinguishing a patent from a non-patent vein if technical difficulties limit the Doppler information (Fig. 2.49F).
- Hepatopetal main PV flow with hepatofugal peripheral flow may be a sign of HCC, requiring careful scanning to identify the lesion.
- Cavernous transformation. A network of collateral vessels may form around a thrombosed MPV at the porta, especially if the cause of thrombosis is because of extrahepatic causes (e.g., pancreatitis) rather than diseased liver. The appearance of cavernous transformation of the PV is quite striking (Fig. 2.50A), and color Doppler is particularly useful in its diagnosis.[33] Varices at the porta may be the cause of a false-negative ultrasound in the hunt for thrombosis (see below).

Technique is important in the diagnosis of portal vein thrombosis. False-positive results when the patent vein is

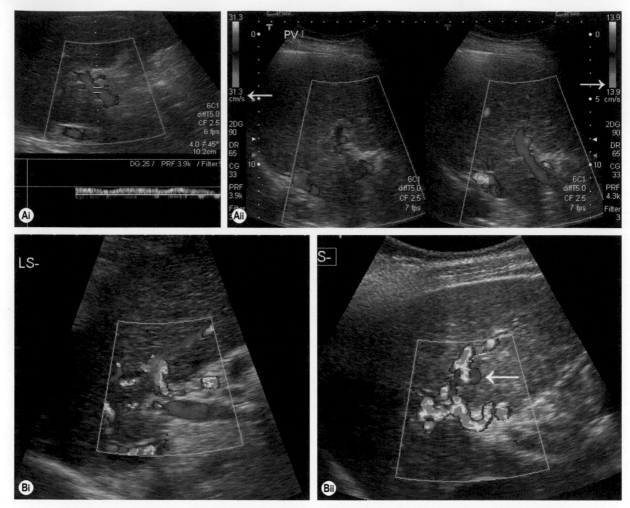

Fig. 2.49 The main portal vein in portal hypertension: (Ai) portal vein velocity is greatly reduced, at 3 cm/s. A low pulse repetition frequency (PRF) and increased color gain may be necessary to demonstrate this. (Aii) The left image shows a false-positive scan for portal vein thrombosis, as the PRF is high (arrow). The right-hand image demonstrates flow in a patent vein once the PRF is reduced. (Bi) Reversed portal vein flow in portal hypertension. (Bii) Compensatory, increased prominence of the hepatic arteries with reversed portal vein flow. The PRF is set to display the slow flow of the almost occluded portal vein (arrow), and so the high-velocity arterial flow demonstrates aliasing.

Continued

incorrectly diagnosed as thrombosed usually result from inadequate technique. The vein axis must be less than 60˘ to the transducer; an intercostal approach from the right lateral aspect is frequently most successful for this. Doppler sensitivity must be set to pick up low-velocity flow (a low scale or pulse repetition frequency (PRF)) and have the color gain correctly set. Ultrasound contrast is useful in identifying slow flow in a vessel that is technically difficult to scan. Contrast angiography with arterioportography is considered the gold standard for assessing portal vein patency, but this technique is time-consuming and invasive and has similar results to carefully performed ultrasound.[34]

False-negative results indicating that flow is present in a vein that is actually thrombosed are because of the detection of flow within a collateral vessel at the porta, which can be mistaken for the MPV.

Ascites is a transudate from the serosal surfaces of the gut, peritoneum, and liver. Small traces of ascites

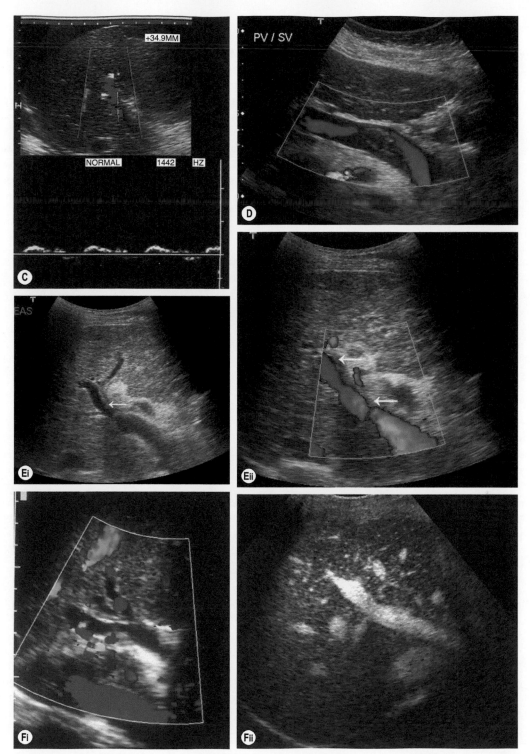

Fig. 2.49, cont'd (C) Balanced portal vein flow. Alternate forward and reverse low-velocity flow on the Doppler spectrum. The portal vein color Doppler alternates red and blue. (D) portal vein thrombosis. The portal vein is dilated and contains a non-occlusive thrombus. (Ei) The portal vein contains a rim of non-occlusive thrombus (arrow) on the anterior wall. (Eii) Color flow Doppler demonstrates a corresponding lack of flow. (F) Contrast-enhanced ultrasound may be useful in demonstrating low-velocity flow in the technically difficult portal vein; (Fi) false-positive for portal vein thrombosis, despite low PRF, because of an inadequate angle to display the Doppler shift. (Fii) Contrast demonstrates a patent portal vein.

TABLE 2.7	Causes of Portal Vein Thrombosis
Chronic liver disease	Especially when cirrhosis is present
Inflammatory	Pancreatitis; acute cholecystitis; necrotizing enterocolitis
Malignancy	Pancreatic tumor; gastric tumor
Coagulation disorders	May be associated with Budd-Chiari syndrome

may be missed if the correct technique, including focal zone placement, is not employed.

Splenomegaly is the result of back pressure in the portal and splenic veins. The spleen can enlarge to six times its normal size and extend both inferiorly and medially, making accurate measurement difficult.

Varices (Fig. 2.50), i.e., venous anastomoses flow from the high-pressure portal system to the lower pressure systemic circulation, which shunts the blood away from the portal system, have thinner walls than normal vessels, which makes them prone to bleeding.

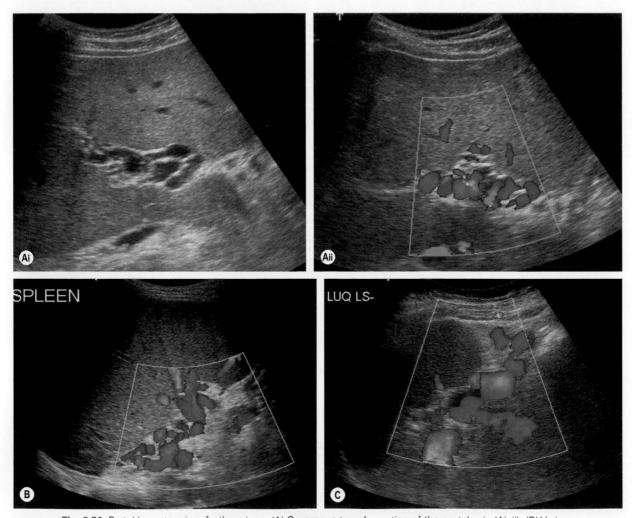

Fig. 2.50 Portal hypertension, further signs: (A) Cavernous transformation of the portal vein (Ai, ii). (B) Varices are demonstrated along the inferior border of the spleen. (C) Color Doppler demonstrates the tortuous vascular channel of a splenorenal shunt inferior to the spleen.

Continued

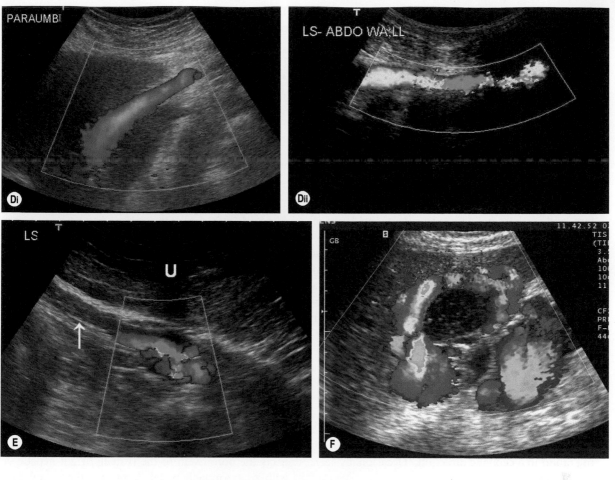

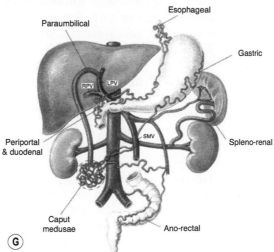

Fig. 2.50, cont'd (Di) Patent paraumbilical channel running along the ligamentum teres to the anterior abdominal wall in a patient with end-stage chronic liver disease and portal hypertension. (Dii) the vein is seen continuing inferiorly along the anterior abdominal wall. (E) A paraumbilical vein (arrow) culminates in a small caput-medusae just beneath the umbilicus (U). (F) Varices can be seen around the gallbladder wall in a case of hepatic fibrosis with portal hypertension. (G) Collaterals in portal hypertension.

The common sites are:

- Gastric and lower esophagus: esophageal varices are particularly prone to bleeding, and this is often the patient's presenting symptom. They are difficult to see on abdominal ultrasound because of the overlying stomach and are better demonstrated with endoscopic techniques. Left coronal scans may demonstrate tortuous vessels at the medial aspect of the upper pole of the spleen.
- Splenorenal: an anastomosis between the splenic and left renal veins, which is often seen on ultrasound as a large, tortuous vessel at the lower edge of the spleen (Fig. 2.50B–C). (These anastomoses are usually very efficient at redirecting the blood from the portal system, and so these patients have a lower incidence of gastric varices and, therefore, a better prognosis.)
- Peraumbilical: a substantial vessel can often be seen in the liver lying in the ligamentum teres (Fig. 2.50D–E) and running down the anterior abdominal wall to a knot of vessels at the umbilicus, the so-called "caput-medusae." (A patent paraumbilical channel of diameter 12 mm may occasionally be seen in normal patients.)
- Porta hepatis: varices around the MPV itself, especially if the latter is thrombosed (see below).
- Gallbladder wall: rarely, varices form around the gallbladder wall to bypass the MPV and feed into the intrahepatic portal branches (Fig. 2.50F).
- Coronary vein: a vessel may be seen arising from the portal vein near the superior mesenteric vein, directing blood in a cephalic direction. (Occasionally seen in normal patients.)
- The extent of portosystemic collaterals is usually underestimated on ultrasound. However, a systematic approach that investigates all the possible sites can demonstrate up to 90% of collaterals (Fig. 2.50G).[31,35]

The HA may be another ultrasound clue to compromised portal venous flow. The main HA may demonstrate increased flow velocity, especially if the portal vein is thrombosed. This is a compensatory mechanism to maintain the blood flow to the liver. The main HA may appear enlarged and more obvious than usual on ultrasound, and peripheral intrahepatic arterial flow (not readily demonstrated in a normal subject) may also become obvious (Fig. 2.51).

Management

The most pressing problem is often bleeding from varices, especially esophageal varices, and patients may present with melena or hematemesis. Management may involve medical means, endoscopic techniques (either injection sclerotherapy of esophageal varices or banding,

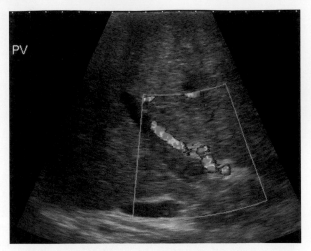

Fig. 2.51 A thrombosed portal vein. High-velocity compensatory arterial flow is seen anterior to the portal vein.

in which a ring is placed around the base of the varix causing thrombosis), compression using a Sengstaken tube with an inflated balloon, surgical, or the placement of a percutaneous TIPSS. These methods are relatively temporary and can relieve pressure in the portal venous system, controlling portal hypertensive complications to plan further management.

TIPSS is a percutaneous radiological intervention used to relieve the symptoms of portal hypertension, including bleeding varices and refractory ascites.[36] It connects the portal vein to the (usually) right hepatic vein with an expandable metal shunt. A catheter and guidewire are passed, under X-ray control, through the jugular vein to the IVC and into the hepatic vein. A pathway is then forged with a needle through the liver parenchyma to join the portal vein with the insertion of a shunt to keep the channel open. Portal venous blood then effectively bypasses the liver, flowing straight into the hepatic vein.

Ultrasound may be used to monitor stent patency (Fig. 2.52). Shunt stenosis or occlusion is a common problem, particularly in long-term shunts, which can be detected with routine post-procedure ultrasound screening and treated with reintervention. The most common site for stenosis is at the junction of the stent with the portal vein. The velocity of blood flow in the shunt should be between 100 cm/s and 200 cm/s, and this should be consistent throughout the stent. A variety of Doppler parameters can be used to detect the malfunction of the shunt.

A shunt velocity of less than 50 cm/s is a sign of stenosis,[37] but this has not been reproducible in all institutions,

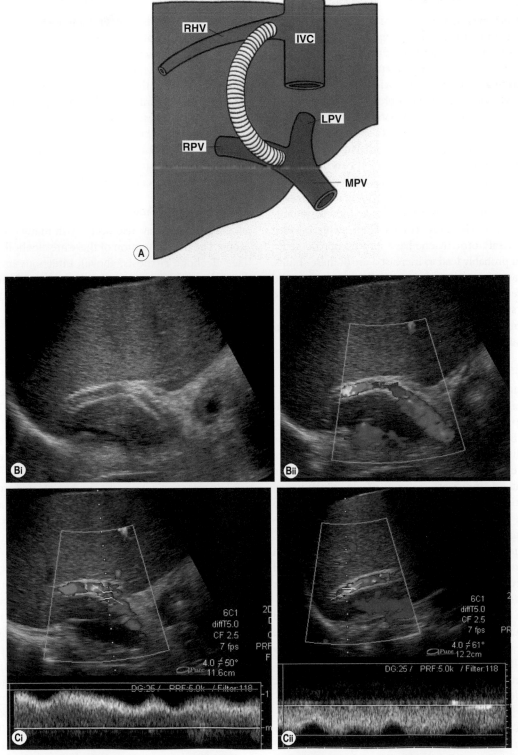

Fig. 2.52 (A) Transjugular intrahepatic portosystemic shunt (TIPSS). (Bi) TIPSS in a patient with severe portal hypertension. (Bii) Color Doppler demonstrates its patency, with a higher velocity in the hepatic venous end. (C) Flow is in the correct direction with the velocity measured at the portal vein end (Ci) and the hepatic venous end (Cii).

and other factors such as a change of 50 cm/s or more from the baseline scan, a localized elevation of velocity at the stenotic site (with an upper limit of normal of up to 220 cm/s), or an increase in the velocity gradient (as the stenotic stent exhibits an increased maximum velocity and a decreased minimum velocity) are also poor prognostic signs.[38]

TIPSS is regarded as a temporary measure but can considerably improve the patient's condition pending treatment of chronic liver disease relieving hemorrhage from varices, relieving intractable ascites and stabilizing liver function. Although the technique is highly successful in decompressing the portal circulation, it is associated with subsequent stent dysfunction and portosystemic encephalopathy. However, results from stents covered with polytetrafluoroethylene have shown improvements, which will probably lead to increased use of these shunts. It is increasingly used as a bridge to a liver transplant and is also used as an alternative to surgery in patients who are poor surgical risks, although the diversion of blood away from the liver can result in adversely affected liver function and eventual encephalopathy.[39]

Hepatitis

Viral Hepatitis

Acute viral hepatitis may be caused by one of several viruses, hepatitis A, B, C, D, or E. The viruses that cause hepatitis B, C, and D may also go on to chronic disease and predispose the liver to HCC in the later stages. Vaccines exist only for A and B.

Hepatitis A and E are transmitted via contaminated food or drink and are particularly prevalent in third world countries. Hepatitis B, C, and D are likely to be transmitted through transfusion or sexual contact. Hepatitis C is now a particular threat to the world population, with an incidence of up to 170 million people worldwide and rising,[40] representing a potentially major problem for world health resources in the future. This epidemic results from numerous factors, including the use of infected (unscreened) blood products, high-risk sexual activity, and skin penetration through injected drug use and body piercing. Infection with the HCV virus usually goes unnoticed until symptoms occur some years later. This time lag provides a potential opportunity for infection of further individuals in the meantime and contributes to uncertainty over the actual infection rate worldwide. It may take up to 20 years for patients to develop cirrhosis, and up to 30 years for the formation of HCC.[41]

Fulminant hepatitis, with complete liver failure, is a rare complication of acute hepatitis B. Most patients with acute hepatitis recover completely, but hepatitis B, C, and D may go on to develop into chronic hepatitis.

This has two forms:

Chronic persistent hepatitis is a mild form of inflammation limited to the portal tracts. It is usually of comparatively little clinical significance and does not show ultrasound changes.

Chronic active hepatitis is a more serious and aggressive form of the disease which causes diffuse, persistent inflammation. This may eventually lead to cirrhosis, which can be associated with HCC.

Other Causes of Acute Hepatitis

Acute hepatitis may also occur with many other conditions. The most common of these are alcoholic hepatitis (see alcoholic cirrhosis, above), infectious mononucleosis, herpes virus, and cytomegalovirus. Patients with AIDS and those who are immunosuppressed are also particularly prone to hepatitis.

Clinical Features

It may be asymptomatic (patients who have antibodies present but deny having had the disease must have had subclinical disease at one time). Other signs include lethargy, nausea, vomiting, and jaundice. The liver is enlarged and tender in the acute phase. In many cases, particularly HBV and HCV, there is a considerable time lag, often of years, before symptoms and diagnosis.

The presence of hepatitis can be detected from blood tests, but the degree of liver damage must be made histologically, ideally with an ultrasound-guided biopsy.

Ultrasound Appearances

The liver frequently appears normal on ultrasound. If ultrasound changes are present in the acute stage, the liver is slightly enlarged with diffusely hypoechoic parenchyma. The normally reflective portal tracts are accentuated in contrast (Fig. 2.53A). This "dark liver" appearance is non-specific and may also occur in leukemia, cardiac failure, AIDS, and other conditions.

The inflammation may start at the portal tracts working outwards into the surrounding parenchyma: so-called periportal hepatitis. In such cases, the portal tracts become less well-defined and hyperechoic. The gallbladder wall may also be thickened, and some patients demonstrate portal lymphadenopathy. If the disease progresses to the chronic stage, the liver may reduce in size, becoming nodular and coarse in appearance (Fig. 2.53).

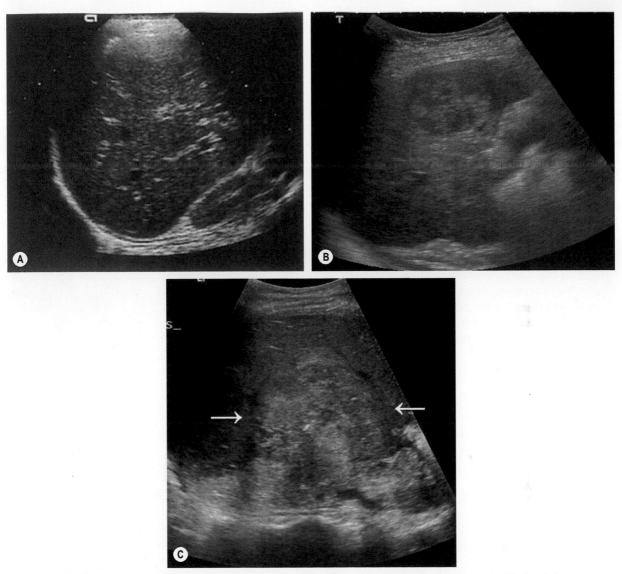

Fig. 2.53 (A) Subtle changes of edema in acute hepatitis; the liver is hypoechoic compared with the right kidney, mildly enlarged, and has prominent portal tracts. (B) Chronic hepatitis with cirrhosis, demonstrating a coarse-textured, nodular liver with a large hepatocellular carcinoma (HCC), later confirmed on magnetic resonance imaging. (C) Cirrhosis from hepatitis C, with a large, invasive HCC (arrows).

Primary Sclerosing Cholangitis

This is a primary disease of the biliary ducts, most frequently found in young men. Like PBC, it is a cholestatic disease. It is discussed more fully in Chapter 3 but is included here for reference as it may often result in a coarse liver texture, similar to that seen in some forms of cirrhosis, and is associated with the formation of cholangiocarcinoma.

Budd-Chiari Syndrome

Budd-Chiari is a relatively rare syndrome associated with partial or complete occlusion of the hepatic veins. There are numerous causes of hepatic vein occlusion, of which the main ones are:

• Congenital or acquired coagulation disorders, which may affect both the hepatic and portal veins, such as polycythemia or myeloproliferative disorder.

- Malignant primary or secondary liver tumor may invade the hepatic veins or may travel up the IVC (e.g., renal carcinoma) to occlude the hepatic vein confluence.
- Membranous web obstructing the IVC (surgically removable).
- Chronic infection or inflammatory diseases.

Ultrasound Appearances

In the acute stage, the liver may enlarge. As the condition progresses, compensatory hypertrophy of any "spared" segments usually occurs in the caudate lobe because the venous drainage from here is inferior to the main hepatic veins. The hepatic veins may be difficult or impossible to visualize (Fig. 2.54). Dilated serpiginous collateral veins may form to direct blood away from the liver, and in some cases, the portal venous flow reverses to achieve this. The spleen also progressively enlarges and, if the disease is long-standing, the liver becomes cirrhotic, acquiring a coarse texture.

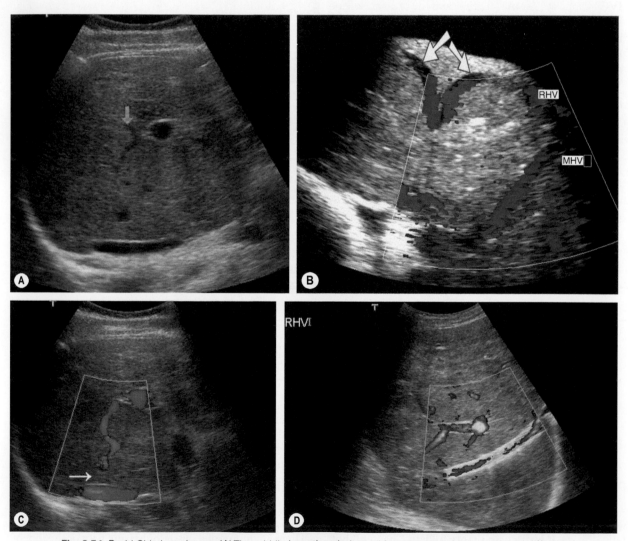

Fig. 2.54 Budd-Chiari syndrome. (A) The middle hepatic vein (arrow) is tortuous and strictured, and difficult to identify on ultrasound. (B) Large collaterals are seen (arrows) near the surface of the liver. (C) Thrombus, with lack of color flow, in the proximal right hepatic vein (RHV, arrow). Collateral vessels are present around the HV. (D) A patent stent in the RHV restores flow and reduces ascites.

Ascites may also be present, particularly if there is complete obstruction involving the IVC. The cause of IVC obstruction may be a web, which can occasionally be identified on ultrasound. If the cause is a coagulation disorder, the portal venous system may also be affected by thrombosis, causing portal hypertension.

Doppler is particularly helpful in diagnosing Budd-Chiari syndrome.[32] The hepatic veins and IVC may be totally or partially occluded; if partial, the waveforms may become flattened, losing their characteristic triphasic pattern. In some cases, flow may be reversed in the IVC hepatic and/or portal veins, and the presence of collateral vessels in the liver is another useful indicator on ultrasound.[42] Ultrasound may miss partial HV occlusion, but the use of contrast agents in suspected cases of Budd-Chiari syndrome may improve diagnostic accuracy.

Management

This depends upon the cause and severity of symptoms. Both medical and surgical treatments have mixed success. Transjugular intrahepatic porto-systemic shunts have been used in some centers as an alternative treatment with some success. Severe coagulative disorders resulting in decompensated cirrhosis may have to be transplanted, although there is a significant risk of recurrence. If the cause is an IVC web, this may be surgically removed. In some patients, palliative treatment with percutaneous stent placement in the hepatic veins can relieve the symptoms of ascites and varices.[43]

Cystic Fibrosis

Cystic fibrosis, one of the most common chromosomal abnormalities, has historically been associated with the pediatric population. However, increasing success in the management of this condition, particularly in specialist centers, has improved the current median survival to 40 years for a child born in the 1990s.[44]

Ultrasound Appearances

As the disease progresses into adulthood, signs of liver cirrhosis and portal hypertension may be demonstrated on ultrasound, although disease progression in the adult population tends to take a milder course than in the pediatric population (Fig. 2.55).[45] The liver may be steatotic, and fibrotic changes produce a coarse, hyperechoic appearance. Patients tend to be monitored regularly with ultrasound for disease progression and signs of portal hypertension. Splenomegaly, varices, ascites, and

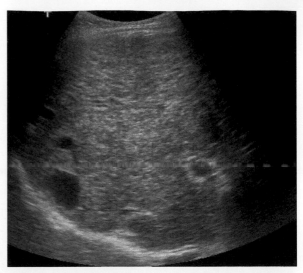

Fig. 2.55 Marked changes in the liver of an adult patient with cystic fibrosis.

possible portal vein thrombosis may be demonstrated (see above), although splenomegaly can be present without portal hypertension in this group. Changes in fibrosis can also be seen in the pancreas.

Congestive Cardiac Disease

Patients with cardiac failure frequently demonstrate dilated hepatic veins in the liver, sometimes with a dilated IVC. Although this may give the sonographer the overall impression of hypoechogenicity, because of the proliferation of large, anechoic vessels, the liver texture itself tends to be of either normal echogenicity or, in the later stages of failure, hyperechoic.

Mitral valve disease may cause altered waveforms in the hepatic veins. The usual triphasic flow becomes more pronounced, with a highly pulsatile waveform (Fig. 2.56A). The portal venous waveform may sometimes be altered in cases of tricuspid valve regurgitation. The normally monophasic flow may become bi-directional (Fig. 2.56B). This phenomenon, associated with congestive heart failure, also occurs in cirrhosis prior to portal vein thrombosis. However, the latter "balanced" flow is of very low-velocity while that because of tricuspid regurgitation is a higher velocity, more pulsatile waveform.

HIV

HIV is an increasing and significant health problem. Patients with HIV are frequently monitored with

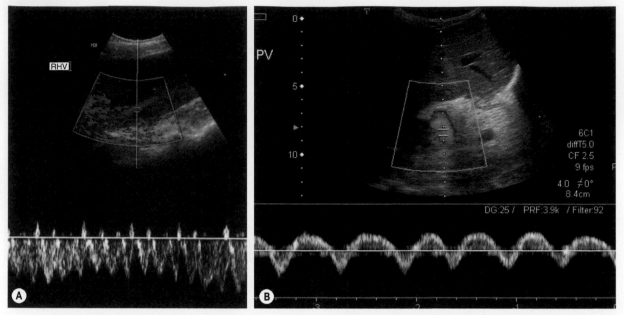

Fig. 2.56 (A) The waveform of the hepatic vein in a patient with mitral valve disease demonstrates increased pulsatility. (B) The portal vein has an abnormal, highly pulsatile flow waveform in a patient with tricuspid regurgitation. (This is quite distinct from the low-velocity "balanced flow" of portal hypertension.)

ultrasound, as they may display abdominal symptoms including fever and weight loss. A range of appearances may be present on ultrasound, including hepatomegaly and altered or coarse texture. Focal changes may occur in around 10% of patients with HIV, including lymphoma, sarcoma, tuberculous abscess, and HCC. Chronic liver damage over time may result in cirrhosis with associated nodules.[46]

Liver Conditions in Pregnancy

Acute Fatty Liver

This rare condition occurs in the third trimester of pregnancy. Acute fatty deposition in the liver tissue can cause abdominal pain, vomiting, and jaundice. The liver may appear sonographically normal or be diffusely hyperechoic, although focal areas of fatty deposition have also been reported. Acute fatty liver tends to resolve during the first month of the post-partum period but may, in rare cases, progress to cause liver failure (Table 2.8).

Hemolysis, Elevated Liver Enzymes, Low Platelet Count (HELLP) Syndrome

HELLP syndrome is a rare complication of pregnancy occurring in up to 20% of mothers with severe

TABLE 2.8	Causes of Changes in Liver Reflectivity
Increased echogenicity	Fatty infiltration (also increases attenuation) Fibrosis Cirrhosis Chronic hepatitis Cystic Fibrosis HIV
Decreased echogenicity	Acute hepatitis AIDS or HIV Leukemia Toxic Shock syndrome Can be normal, particularly in the young
Coarse or nodular texture	Cirrhosis – various causes Regenerating nodules Metastases/diffuse metastatic infiltration Chronic or granulomatous hepatitis PSC, PBC Diffuse infective process – e.g., with AIDS or immunosuppressed patients

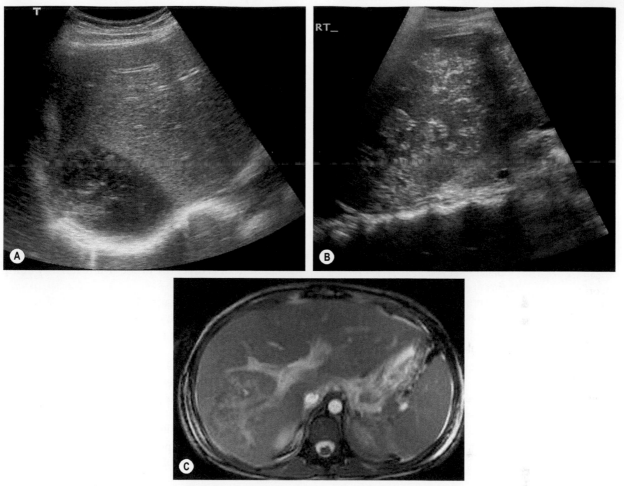

Fig. 2.57 (A) Spontaneous subcapsular hematoma in pregnancy in a patient with hemolysis, elevated liver enzymes, low platelet count (HELLP) syndrome. (B) Multiple areas of intrahepatic hemorrhage in HELLP. (C) Magnetic resonance imaging of the patient in (B).

pre-eclampsia.[47] Hemolytic anemia (H), elevated liver enzymes, and low platelet count cause abdominal pain, nausea, and fever. Its complications may include multiple areas of spontaneous hemorrhage (either subcapsular hematoma or intraparenchymal bleeding), infarction, or necrosis within the liver, which can be identified with ultrasound or MRI scanning (Fig. 2.57). The recognition and prompt diagnosis of acute fatty liver and HELLP syndrome reduce maternal morbidity by enabling emergency cesarean section to be performed (Table 2.8).

LIVER TRANSPLANTS

Liver transplants are performed for a large number of conditions (see Table 2.9) and is considered a curative treatment in many cases. Ultrasound assessment is a common examination performed both pre and post transplant. It is important that the operator is aware of normal and abnormal features post-transplant and the variations which can be seen in Doppler traces. This ensures that any acute features which may impact on the success of the transplant are quickly highlighted to the referring team.

Causes of free intraperitoneal fluid	
Organ failure	Chronic liver disease with portal hypertension Acute liver failure Renal failure Cardiac failure
Malignancy	
Inflammatory	Acute pancreatitis Acute cholecystitis Peritonitis, tuberculosis Crohn's disease
Budd-Chiari Syndrome	
Postoperative	Blood, urine, bile, or lymphatic fluid
Organ damage	Biliary perforation Urinary tract perforation Bowel perforation (e.g., in diverticulitis) Trauma to liver, spleen or pancreas
CAPD Fluid	Patients on peritoneal dialysis
Ruptured ectopic pregnancy	Hemoperitoneum
Gynecological	Ruptured ovarian cyst, ovarian carcinoma, ovarian fibroma (Meigs syndrome), ovarian torsion, pelvic inflammatory disease

It is recommended that post-transplant scans are performed on day 1 , 5 and 14 plus, as clinically indicated and at an annual follow-up.[48]

Basic Doppler Principles

TIP BOX

Settings for Optimization
Scale: scale should roughly be set between:
- 10–20 cm/s for venous
- 20–30 cm/s for arterial
- 15–25 cm/s for portal venous

Note that it is normal to have velocities of around 40–50 cm/s in a recently transplanted liver's portal vein.

Obtain a good position to assess the vessel and switch on the color Doppler. Adjust your Doppler gain just after you lose "twinkling artifact." Use power Doppler if you struggle to get a Doppler signal.

If you use the Doppler angle button, make sure it is between 60–45 degrees running parallel within the vessel. Heel-toe the probe to achieve this. While angling, the machine will tell you how many degrees you are at, and the angle line will change color to red if the angle is suboptimal.

When scanning low-velocity or small vessels, drop your scale (sometimes <10 cm/s) and adjust your gain. Be aware of your waveform, and if you are struggling to get end-diastolic flow, drop the "filter," which is normally situated next to the scale button. Sometimes the filter or wall thump filter is pre-set to high, and it is actually filtering out the useful Doppler signal. However, be aware that you will also increase the amount of artifact the probe will receive by doing this.

To clarify for optimization for low-velocity flow
- Decrease color velocity scale
- Increase color and/or power Doppler gain
- Decrease wall filter
- Focal zone at the level of the area of interest
- Doppler angle between 60–45 degrees
- Adjust sample volume gate

Waveform Interpretation

The waveform itself represents the distance of blood (cm) and the speed of blood (seconds); hence cm/s in the scale.

It is also representing how the blood is flowing with relationships to the heart contracting and relaxing and organ perfusion (Fig. 2.58A).

Acceleration Times (ms)

When analyzing an arterial waveform, the acceleration time is important in helping rule out arterial stenosis. You are measuring the speed of the systolic upstroke in milliseconds (ms). Normal acceleration times are <80 ms. Between 80 and 100 ms is raised, and anything above 100 ms is clinically significant.[49]

In order to obtain an accurate acceleration time, good image optimization of the Doppler waveform is required.

You can get a good idea of an increased acceleration time just by "eyeballing" the waveform. You will observe a slow rise in the systolic phase causing a "Tardus Parvus" waveform (Fig. 2.58B).

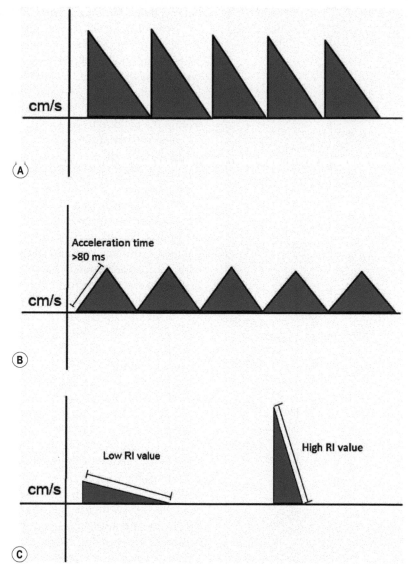

Fig. 2.58 (A) An example of a normal HA waveform. (B) An example of an increased acceleration time or "Tardus Parvus" waveform. Tardus means slow/late, and parvus means small/little. (C) An example of a low and high RI value.

Resistive Index (RI) Values

The RI value is obtained by placing the caliper on the peak systolic velocity and the lowest diastolic velocity. Normal ranging RI values in a transplanted kidney should be between 0.55 and 0.75 within the HA (Fig. 2.58C).[50,51]

A RI value is a way to give the referrer more information about the HA other than if it is patent or not. Reduced RI values can indicate issues with arterial inflow, whereas raised RI values can indicate issues with graft outflow (Fig. 2.58C).

Liver transplantation has now become an accepted treatment for patients with end-stage liver disease, and it is also used in the treatment of fulminant hepatic failure. Improvements in both surgical techniques and immunosuppression have led to an increasing range of indications for transplantation (Table 2.9). The majority of hepatic transplants (80%) are still performed in patients

TABLE 2.9   Indications for Liver Transplantation

Hepatitis C, hepatitis B Alcohol-related disease NASH Cryptogenic cirrhosis Chronic cholestatic disease (PBC, PSC, secondary biliary cirrhosis)	Transplantation is considered once irreversible end-stage liver failure is present, usually with complications such as portal hypertension and encephalopathy
HCC	Usually, on a background of cirrhosis
Metabolic Diseases	
Pediatric	Biliary atresia, cholestatic diseases, metabolic disorders, some malignancies
Budd-Chiari syndrome	Non-malignant occlusion of the hepatic veins, especially total venous occlusion and/or patients with cirrhosis resulting from Budd-Chiari syndrome
Fulminant hepatic failure	Due to drug (usually paracetamol) overdose, acute hepatitis, Budd-Chiari syndrome, Wilson's disease or massive hepatic trauma
Others	Rarely, transplant is undertaken for benign lesions such as polycystic disease, adenoma, or large hemangiomas

with cirrhosis, most commonly from hepatitis C and primary cholestatic disease.[52]

Lack of organ availability has, to some extent, driven the progress of alternative surgical procedures. The use of live related donor organ transplantation, in which part of the liver of a healthy (usually) related donor is transplanted into the recipient, and the use of split liver transplantation, in which the cadaveric organ is split to be transplanted into two recipients (one of which is usually pediatric – see pediatric chapter) has effectively enlarged the organ pool and allowed continuing

improvements in overall survival.[53] Contraindications for liver transplantation continue to dwindle. These include active extrahepatic malignancy, diffuse invasive intrahepatic malignancy, and some comorbidities which prevent major surgery.

The prognosis following transplantation is highly dependent upon both the primary disease and the clinical state of the patient. Patient selection is an important issue, as organs are limited. Priority for organ allocation is managed by the use of the model of end-stage liver disease (MELD) score, which prioritizes patients with the highest short-term mortality.[54]

The presence of malignant liver disease is not a contraindication to transplantation, provided the bulk of the tumor remains relatively modest and is confined to the liver.[55] Patients with larger HCCs (3 cm) and those with cholangiocarcinoma have a higher rate of recurrence post-transplantation and are generally not considered for transplantation.

Preoperative Assessment

The ultrasound scan is one of many investigations leading up to transplantation. The diagnosis of liver pathologic conditions usually involves ultrasound scanning as a first-line, augmented by histology and additional cross-sectional imaging. The role of ultrasound includes contributing to, or confirming, the initial diagnosis, assessing the degree of severity and associated complications of the disease, and providing guidance for biopsy. An important objective is to exclude patients for whom liver transplantation is not feasible or of little benefit, for example, those with extrahepatic malignant disease.

The preoperative assessment focuses on the complications of liver disease, such as features of portal hypertension, the presence of suspicious liver nodules, and any other unsuspected extrahepatic conditions that may delay or compromise potential surgery.

In particular, the sonographer should look for:
- Portal vein thrombosis as this may be a contraindication to transplantation if it is extensive or unable to be effectively bypassed by the surgeon.
- Other features of portal hypertension associated with chronic liver disease (see above) including spleen size and varices.
- Focal liver lesions that may represent malignancy. These may require the administration of ultrasound contrast agents or further imaging such as MRI for characterization.

- Extrahepatic malignancy, in cases with an initial diagnosis of carcinoma.
- Degree and scope of vascular thrombosis in cases of Budd-Chiari syndrome.
- Any incidental pathologic conditions which may alter the management plan.
- Doppler is, of course, essential in assessing the patency and direction of blood flow of the portal venous system, the hepatic veins, IVC, and main HA. It may occasionally be possible to demonstrate arterial anomalies.

Although many patients are considered for transplantation and undergo ultrasound assessment, most of these will never actually receive a transplant. This factor has numerous implications for resources when setting up a pre-transplant ultrasound service. The introduction of live donor transplantation also has considerable service implications, including increased use of intraoperative sonography and other radiological services for donor and recipient, which must be factored in.

Operative Procedure – Intraoperative Ultrasound

Most transplants are orthotopic; i.e., the diseased liver is removed and replaced by the donor organ, instead of heterotopic, in which the donor organ is grafted in addition to the native organ (like most kidney transplants). The transplant requires five surgical anastomoses:
- Suprahepatic vena cava
- Infrahepatic vena cava
- HA (either end-to-end or end-to-side to the aorta)
- Portal vein
- CBD (the gallbladder is removed)

IOUS is useful for assessing the size and spread of intrahepatic neoplastic growths and for assessing vascular invasion in the recipient. Mapping of the hepatic vascular anatomy in living-related donors is also feasible using IOUS.

IOUS with Doppler is also useful for assessing the vascular anastomoses and establishing if portal venous and hepatic arterial flow are adequate.

Postoperative Assessment

Ultrasound plays a key role in the postoperative monitoring of liver transplant patients. Numerous complications are possible (Table 2.10), and many of these can be diagnosed with ultrasound. Ciclosporin immunosuppression is administered, and blood levels of ciclosporin

TABLE 2.10 Postoperative Liver Transplantation Complications

Infection	Abdominal infection-sepsis/ intrahepatic abscess
Vascular	Anastomotic leaks – hematoma Thrombosis or stenosis-ischemia/infarction
Biliary	Bile duct stricture or stenosis leading to dilatation Bile leak – biloma
Rejection	Acute episodes are common in the first two weeks and are of variable severity
Other medical	Neurological Renal dysfunction
Recurrence of the original disease	Hepatitis Cholangiocarcinoma or CC Budd-Chiari syndrome PSC
Post-transplantation lymphoproliferative disorder (PTLD)	More common in children, PTLD is associated with immunosuppression, occurring within the first year of transplantation

are a closely monitored balancing act; too low and the graft may reject, too high, and the toxic effects of the drug may affect the kidneys.

Liver function is biochemically monitored for early signs of complications. Elevated serum bilirubin, alkaline phosphatase, and/or aminotransferase levels are present with most types of graft dysfunction or complication and are investigated first with ultrasound.

Renal dysfunction is a further recognized complication following transplantation. This can be because of various causes, including ciclosporin nephrotoxicity, intraoperative hypotension, or preoperative renal failure.

The hemodynamic changes identified on ultrasound associated with transplantation, from the normal hepatic arterial waveform described earlier, is often not present in the immediate postoperative Doppler ultrasound. The hepatic arterial abnormalities seen in the day one postoperative scans are often normal postoperative appearances and resolve on follow-up scans. Baseline ultrasound and clinical correlation are important to manage patients efficiently.

Complication	Time of Presentation after Transplant
Hepatic artery thrombosis	First 2 weeks
Hepatic artery stenosis	Few weeks to several months
Portal venous thrombosis	Majority within one month
Portal venous stenosis	Usually late (>6 months)
Hepatic venous stenosis	Usually late (>6 months)

Fig. 2.59 The table is showing the complication and time of presentation after a liver transplant.

The RI usually normalizes within seven to 15 days and is not associated with poor graft function (Fig. 2.59).[56]

Postoperative Ultrasound Appearances and Complications

Post-transplant complications may be mechanical (problems with vessels or ducts) or non-mechanical (nonfunction, rejection, infection, or disease recurrence).

Hepatic Artery

The HA is vital to graft success as it is the sole vascular supply to the biliary system. Most HA occlusions occur relatively soon after the operation before a good collateral supply can be established. HA thrombosis or stenosis can lead to bile duct necrosis, causing bile leaks and abscesses or areas of infarction within the liver tissue. Therefore, it is treated as an emergency requiring surgical intervention and, sometimes, retransplantation.

Hepatic Artery Thrombosis (HAT)

HA thrombosis is the most common complication post liver transplant. Early HAT occurs within the first few weeks. Early HAT requires retransplantation in most cases. Ultrasound is used to assess for the presence or absence of flow, with absent flow indicating HAT. It can be challenging to view the HA on ultrasound in early transplant assessment because of allograft edema postoperatively. Good use of Doppler settings and pre-sets are essential, along with reading the operation notes prior so you can understand the transplant's anatomy.

Failure to adequately display the HA with a good spectral trace on ultrasound is often because of inadequate technique. Ensure the artery is scanned intercostally to maintain a low vessel-to-beam angle and that the Doppler sensitivity and filter controls are set for low velocities if arterial flow is not found.

HA stenosis/thrombosis is still a relatively common post-transplant complication in up to 12% of adult patients and up to 40% of pediatric patients. Color Doppler ultrasound has a sensitivity/specificity of 92%/97% for detecting hepatic artery complications,[57] and X-ray angiography is rarely required. Stenosis of the artery at the site of anastomosis is detected by examining the Doppler spectrum (Fig. 2.60).

Hepatic Artery Stenosis (HAS)

HAS can present with similar complications to HAT, but with symptoms developing over days to weeks after transplantation. Patients normally present with increased bilirubin and abnormal-looking bile ducts. Timely detection of HAS is essential as an early intervention to treat the stenosis and prevent any ill effects on the patient. It can be treated by angioplasty and/or stenting. HAS itself causes ischemia to the liver transplant by affecting the quality of arterial blood the graft. HAS usually happens around the HA anastomosis. To be clinically significant, directly after suspected stenosis, there would be a significant increase in the peak systolic velocity (more than double). You would then see a reduction in the RI value <0.55 along with a potential "Tardus Parvus" waveform (acceleration time >80 ms). It is difficult to visualize the velocity increase using ultrasound, but you should see a reduced RI value and increased acceleration time at the porta hepatis, where you would sample the HA normally. The systolic upstroke tends to be delayed (tardus parvus pattern) downstream of the stenosis[58]; the acceleration time is increased (over 0.08 s). The appearance of the HA waveform immediately postoperatively is often one of a small spike with no end-diastolic flow (EDF). This is not a significant finding and will usually develop into the more familiar waveform with forward EDF by 48 h after transplantation.[59]

HA Pseudoaneurysm

However, HA pseudoaneurysms are a rare complication that can be secondary to things like biopsy, angioplasty,

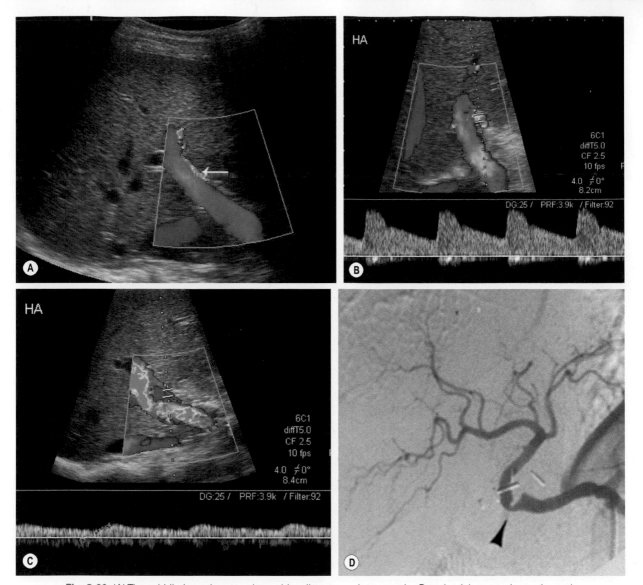

Fig. 2.60 (A) The middle hepatic artery (arrow) in a liver transplant on color Doppler, lying anterior to the main portal vein. (B) Normal HA waveform post-transplantation, demonstrating a steep systolic rise with forward flow throughout the cycle. (C) Slow systolic rise (tardus parvus) and low-velocity flow in hepatic artery stenosis. (D) Angiography confirms and locates the stenosis.

stenting, or infection. They are a cystic structure adjacent or connected to an artery that fills with color on Doppler ultrasound, most giving a "ying and yang" appearance.

The administration of ultrasound contrast media is useful for the detection of flow in difficult examinations (Fig. 2.61).

Portal Vein

Portal Venous Complications

Post liver transplant, it is normal for the portal vein to be sampled at higher than normal velocities ranging between 40 and 60 cm/s. The flow should be hepato-petal (toward the liver). The velocities will reduce over time to about 20 cm/s over a few weeks. Portal vein thrombosis is

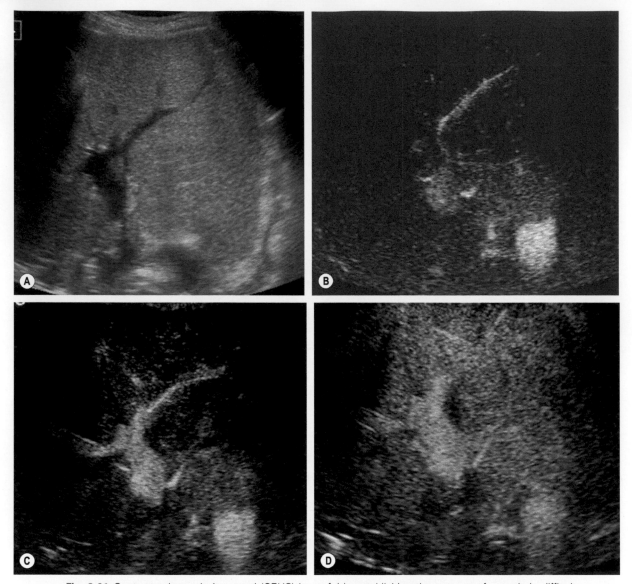

Fig. 2.61 Contrast-enhanced ultrasound (CEUS) is useful in establishing the patency of vessels in difficult cases: (A) Color Doppler was unable to demonstrate flow in the left hepatic artery (HA) in a patient with clinical suspicion of thrombosis. (B) CEUS demonstrates good flow in the HA. (C) The portal vein phase demonstrates the left portal vein posterior to the artery, and (D) the sinusoidal phase demonstrates good contrast take up throughout, confidently excluding the possibility of infarction.

the most common portal vein complication after surgery. It is identified on ultrasound as the absence of flow on color Doppler with anechoic or echogenic material noted within the lumen of the portal vein. Always check with power Doppler and adjust your settings appropriately.

Portal vein stenosis is another complication post liver transplant; however, it can be tricky to diagnose with ultrasound alone as there are high velocities in the portal vein already after transplant. If the velocities do not settle or increase, this could demonstrate portal vein stenosis. Portal vein complications (stenosis or thrombosis) occur in up to 13% of patients. The portal vein anastomosis is readily demonstrated in most patients and shows turbulence associated with

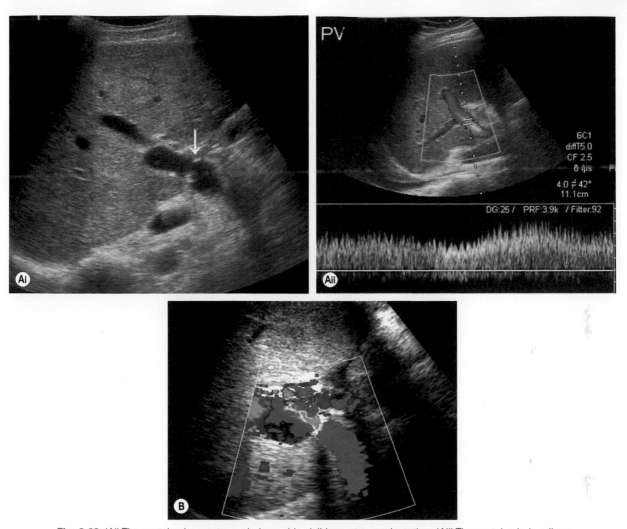

Fig. 2.62 (Ai) The portal vein anastomosis (arrow) is visible post-transplantation. (Aii) The portal vein in a liver transplant demonstrates a turbulent waveform because of the surgical anastomosis. This is not a significant finding. (B) Main portal vein stenosis. A high-velocity jet is seen through the stenosis at the site of the anastomosis, with post-stenotic turbulence.

the anastomotic site (Fig. 2.62), as the diameters of the donor and recipient veins invariably differ. This is not significant in itself but can indicate clinically significant stenosis when accompanied by high velocities of greater than 100 cm/s (Fig. 2.62B). Portal vein stenosis is associated with a steadily increasing spleen size, which is why it is important to have a baseline measurement of the spleen.

Portal vein thrombosis may be occlusive or non-occlusive and may affect intra- and extrahepatic portal

vessels. It is possible to have a blocked MPV with patent intrahepatic portal veins because of collateral formation.

IVC and Hepatic Veins
Hepatic Venous and IVC Complication
End-to-end anastomosis – Conventional method of liver transplantation where the IVC is clamped entirely, surgically removing the diseased liver and IVC. The donor's liver and IVC are then surgically put into the recipient.

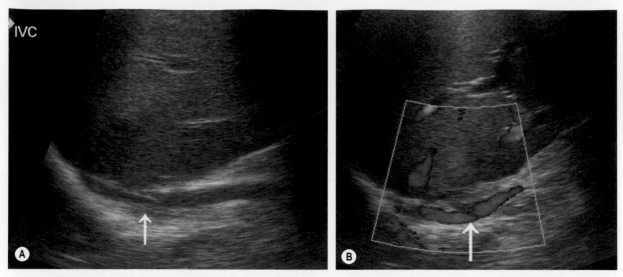

Fig. 2.63 (A) The inferior anastomosis in the inferior vena cava post liver transplantation (arrow). (B) Power Doppler of the same case (arrow).

Piggyback anastomosis – method of liver transplantation which preserves the recipient's IVC at the level of the liver. The donor IVC is then joined to the recipient's vein.

IVC stenosis or thrombosis is uncommon, accounting for less than 3% of patients. The infrahepatic IVC anastomosis is readily seen on ultrasound (Fig. 2.63), but the near-perpendicular angle of the IVC to the beam makes it difficult to assess blood flow velocity and power Doppler, which is less angle-dependent, if often helpful in demonstrating flow in the IVC (Fig. 2.63B). If the transplantation has been performed for Budd-Chiari syndrome, pay particular attention to the hepatic veins, which tend to re-thrombose in some patients.

CBD

Biliary complications account for up to 19% of post-transplantation complications, most occurring in the first three months following the transplantation. A baseline measurement is important to detect small degrees of subsequent dilatation, which may imply stenosis or obstruction. Even relatively minor dilatation can be significant in the transplant recipient; cholestasis can precipitate ascending biliary infection, which may subsequently form liver abscesses, a process which may be aggravated by immunosuppression.

Strictures commonly occur at the anastomosis because of scar tissue, but other non-anastomotic strictures can result from HA insufficiency, causing ischemia. Leakage is a comparatively rare event.

Focal Lesions

The most likely cause of focal lesions in the short-term following transplantation is abscess following infection. Hepatic abscesses may be multiple and are often acoustically subtle in the early stages. Other causes of focal lesions in the early postoperative period may be because of infarction and are associated with interruption of the arterial supply or poor harvesting technique. These can be hyper- or hypoechoic, have well-defined borders, and do not exert a mass effect (Fig. 2.64). In patients with malignancy who have had a transplant, tumor recurrence may also be a serious complication.

Post-Transplantation Malignancy

Patients who are immunosuppressed are at greater risk than normal for developing malignancy. Post-transplantation lymphoproliferative disorder (PTLD) (similar in appearance to non-Hodgkin's lymphoma) is a complication associated with immunocompromise, which affects up to 2% of transplant recipients (Fig. 2.64C). Ultrasound may demonstrate hypoechoic, ill-defined intrahepatic masses, lymphadenopathy, and occasional involvement of the spleen and kidneys.[48]

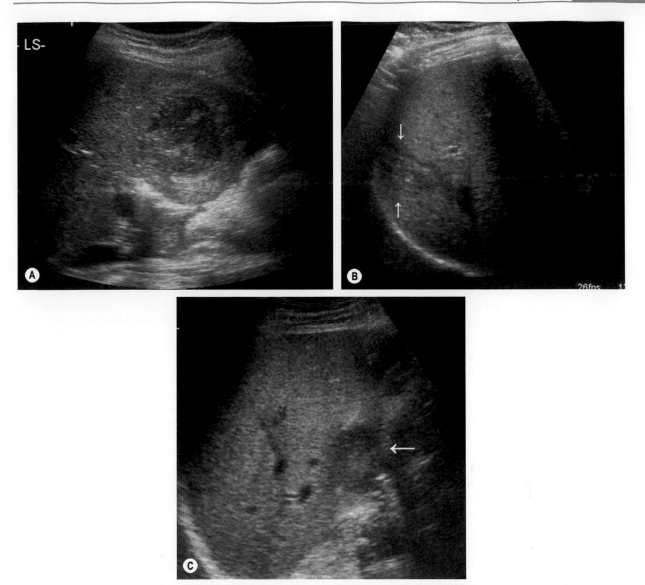

Fig. 2.64 (A) An abscess in a liver transplant. (B) Infarct in a liver transplant (arrows) resulting from hepatic artery thrombosis. (C) Post-transplantation lymphoproliferative disorder, demonstrating a hypoechoic lesion near the porta hepatis in a transplant recipient.

Patients with malignant lesions pre-transplantation, such as HCC or cholangiocarcinoma, have a significant risk of recurrence after transplantation.

Fluid Collections

Following liver transplantation, fluid collections are frequently demonstrated and may be monitored with ultrasound and/or drained under ultrasound guidance. These may represent hematoma (Fig. 2.65), seroma, loculated ascites, or biloma. It is not possible to differentiate different types of collection with ultrasound alone. The appearances are taken in conjunction with the clinical features, and the role of ultrasound is primarily to monitor the gradual resolution of the collection or to establish if an infection is present in a clinically ill patient (by aspiration) and drain the collection if appropriate.

Hematomas usually resolve if left untreated. However, a large hematoma could result from an anastomotic leak

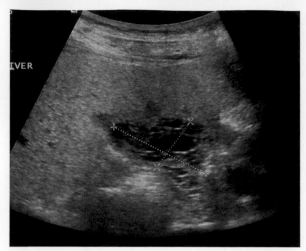

Fig. 2.65 Subphrenic hematoma post liver transplantation. Most resolve spontaneously.

requiring surgical intervention. A leaking bile duct anastomosis is potentially a serious complication that could cause peritonitis. Drainage under ultrasound guidance is a temporary option, but surgical repair is invariably necessary.

Recent recipients of liver transplants often have free intraperitoneal fluid and a right pleural effusion, which resolve spontaneously.

Rejection

Episodes of graft rejection are common in the first two weeks after transplantation. Graft rejection may be acute, in which case the immunosuppression is increased or chronic following several acute episodes. Chronic rejection can only be treated by retransplantation. Rejection does not have any specific ultrasound features on conventional imaging or Doppler, and the diagnosis is made from a liver biopsy following clinical suspicion.

REFERENCES

1. Moorthy K, Mihssin N, Houghton PW. The management of simple hepatic cysts: sclerotherapy or laparoscopic fenestration. *Ann R Coll Surg Engl.* 2001;83:409–414.
2. Adam YG, Nonas CJ. Hepatobiliary cystadenoma. *Southern Med J.* 1995;88:1140–1143.
3. Turgut AT, Akhan O, Bhatt S, Dogra VS. Sonographic spectrum of hydatid disease. *Ultrasound Q.* 2008;24:17–29.
4. Voros D, Katsarelias D, Polymeneas G, et al. Treatment of hydatid liver disease. *Surg Infect (Larchmt).* 2007;8:621–627.
5. Doyle DJ, Hanbidge AE, O'Malley ME. Imaging of hepatic infections. *Clin Radiol.* 2006;61:737–748.
6. Kim TK, Jang HJ, Wilson SR. Benign liver masses: imaging with microbubble contrast agents. *Ultrasound Q.* 2006;22:31–39.
7. Kim TK, Jang HJ, Burns PN, et al. Focal nodular hyperplasia and hepatic adenoma: differentiation with low-mechanical-index contrast-enhanced sonography. *AJR Am J Roentgenol.* 2008;190:58–66.
8. Mortel ÇKJ, Segatto E, Ros PR. The infected liver: radiologic-pathologic correlation. *Radiographics.* 2004;24:937–955.
9. Hicks RJ, Ware RE, Lau EW. PET/CT: will it change the way that we use CT in cancer imaging? *Cancer Imaging.* 2006;6:S52–S62.
10. Adam A. Interventional radiology in the treatment of hepatic metastases. *Canc Treat Rev.* 2002;28:93–99.
11. Zweibel WJ. Sonographic diagnosis of diffuse liver disease. *Semin Ultrasound CT MRI.* 1995;16:8–15.
12. Shapiro RS, Katz R, Mendelson DS, et al. Detection of hepatocellular carcinoma in cirrhotic patients: sensitivity of CT and ultrasound. *J Ultrasound Med.* 1996;15:497–502.
13. Llovet JM, Bruix J. Novel advancements in the management of hepatocellular carcinoma in 2008. *J Hepatol.* 2008;48:S20–S37.
14. Maruyama H, Yoshikawa M, Yokosuka O. Current role of ultrasound for the management of hepatocellular carcinoma. *World J Gastroenterol.* 2008;14:1710–1719.
15. Wu F, Wang ZB, Chen WZ, et al. Advanced hepatocellular carcinoma: treatment with high-intensity focused ultrasound ablation combined with transcatheter arterial embolization. *Radiology.* 2005;235:659–667.
16. Preiss D, Sattar N. Non-alcoholic fatty liver disease: an overview of prevalence, diagnosis, pathogenesis and treatment considerations. *Clin Sci (Lond).* 2008;115:141–150.
17. Chuah SK, Changchien CS, Chiu KW, et al. Changes of hepatic vein waveform in chronic liver diseases. *J Med Ultrasound.* 1995;3:75–80.
18. Thompson Coon J, Rogers G, Hewson P, et al. Surveillance of cirrhosis for hepatocellular carcinoma: a cost-utility analysis. *Br J Cancer.* 2008;98:1166–1175.
19. Thompson Coon J, Rogers G, Hewson P, et al. Surveillance of cirrhosis for hepatocellular carcinoma: systematic review and economic analysis. *Health Tech Assess.* 2007;11:1–206.
20. EFSUMB study group. *Guidelines for the use of contrast agents in ultrasound*; 2004. Available at: www.efsumb.org/guidelines.
21. Ward J, Robinson PJ. How to detect hepatocellular carcinoma in cirrhosis. *Eur Radiol.* 2002;12:2258–2272.
22. Kim SH, Choi BI, Lee JY, et al. Diagnostic accuracy of multi-/single-detector row CT and contrast-enhanced MRI in the detection of hepatocellular carcinomas

meeting the Milan criteria before liver transplantation. *Intervirol.* 2008;51:52–60.

23. World Health Organization. Global surveillance and control of hepatitis C. Report of a WHO consultation organized in collaboration with the viral hepatitis prevention board, Antwerp, Belgium. *J Viral Hepat.* 1999;6:35–47.

24. Blonski W, Reddy KR. Hepatitis C virus infection and hepatocellular carcinoma. *Clin Liver Dis.* 2008;12:661–674.

25. Kumagi T, Heathcote EJ. Primary biliary cirrhosis. *Orphanet J Rare Dis.* 2008;3:1.

26. Dietrich C, Leuschner M, Zeuzem S, et al. Perihepatic lymphadenopathy in primary biliary cirrhosis reflects progression of the disease. *Eur J Gastroenterol Hepatol.* 1999;11:747–753.

27. Talwalkar JA, Kurtz DM, Schoenleber SJ, et al. Ultrasound-based transient elastography for the detection of hepatic fibrosis: systematic review and meta-analysis. *Clin Gastroenterol Hepatol.* 2007;5:1214–1220.

28. Lovet J, Fuster J, Bruix J. The Barcelona approach: diagnosis, staging and treatment of hepatocellular carcinoma. *Liver Transpl.* 2004;10:S115–S120.

29. Kok T, van der Jagt EJ, Haagsma EB, et al. The value of Doppler ultrasound in cirrhosis and portal hypertension. *Scand J Gastroenterol Suppl.* 1999;230:82–88.

30. Gorg C, Riera-Knorrenschild J, Dietrich J. Pictorial review: colour Doppler ultrasound flow patterns in the portal venous system. *Br J Radiol.* 2002;75:919–929.

31. Zweibel WJ. Sonographic diagnosis of hepatic vascular disorders. *Semin Ultrasound CT MRI.* 1995;16:34–48.

32. Wu CC, Yeh YH, Hwang MH. Observation of portal venous flow in liver cirrhosis by Doppler ultrasound: the significance of PVH index. *J Med Ultrasound.* 1994;2:180–184.

33. Konno K, Ishida H, Uno A, et al. Cavernous transformation of the portal vein (CTPV): role of color Doppler sonography in the diagnosis. *Eur J Ultrasound.* 1996;3:231–240.

34. Bach AM, Hann LE, Brown KT, et al. Portal vein evaluation with US: comparison to angiography and CT arterial portography. *Radiol.* 1996;201:149–154.

35. Lafortune M, Patriquin H, Pomier G, et al. Haemodynamic changes in portal circulation after portosystemic shunts; use of duplex sonography in 43 patients. *AJR Am J Roentgenol.* 1987;149:701–706.

36. Colombato L. The role of transjugular intrahepatic portosystemic shunt (TIPS) in the management of portal hypertension. *J Clin Gastroenterol.* 2007;41:S344–S351.

37. Chong WK, Malisch TW, Mazer MJ. Sonography of transjugular intrahepatic portosystemic shunts. *Semin Ultrasound CT MRI.* 1995;16:69–80.

38. Middleton WD, Teefey SA, Darcy MD. Doppler evaluation of transjugular intrahepatic portosystemic shunts. *Ultrasound Q.* 2003;19:56–70.

39. Kravetz D. Prevention of recurrent esophageal variceal hemorrhage: review and current recommendations. *J Clin Gastroenterol.* 2007;41:S318–S322.

40. Baldo V, Baldovin T, Trivello R, Floreani A. Epidemiology of HCV infection. *Curr Pharm Des.* 2008;14:1646–1654.

41. Gomaa A, Khan S, Toledano M, et al. Hepatocellular carcinoma: epidemiology, risk factors and pathogenesis. *World J Gastroenterol.* 2008;14:4300–4308.

42. Aydinli M, Bayraktar Y. Budd-Chiari syndrome: etiology, pathogenesis and diagnosis. *World J Gastroenterol.* 2007;13:2693–2696.

43. Vogel J, Gorich J, Kramme E, et al. Alveolar echinococcosis of the liver: percutaneous stent therapy of Budd-Chiari syndrome. *Gut.* 1996;39:762–764.

44. Mahadeva R, Webb K, Westerbeek R, et al. Clinical outcome in relation to care in centres specialising in cystic fibrosis: cross sectional study. *BMJ.* 1998;316:1771–1779.

45. Nash KL, Allison ME, McKeon D, et al. A single centre experience of liver disease in adults with cystic fibrosis 1995–2006. *J Cyst Fibros.* 2008;7:252–257.

46. Kawooya M, Muyinda Z, Byanyima R, Malwadde E. Abdominal ultrasound findings in HIV: a pictorial review. *Ultrasound.* 2008;16:62–72.

47. Geary M. The HELLP syndrome. *Br J Obst Gynaecol.* 1997;104:887–891.

48. Shaw AS, Ryan SM, Beese RC, Sidhu PS. Ultrasound of non-vascular complications in the post liver transplant patient. *Clin Radiol.* 2003;58:672–680.

49. Crossin JD, Muradali D, Wilson SR. US of liver transplants: normal and abnormal. *Radiographics.* 2003;23(5):1093–1114. https://doi.org/10.1148/rg.235035031. PMID: 12975502.

50. Sanyal R, Lall CG, Lamba R, et al. Orthotopic liver transplantation: reversible Doppler US findings in the immediate postoperative period. *Radiographics.* 2012;32(1):199–211. https://doi.org/10.1148/rg.321115006. PMID: 22236901.

51. Platt JF, Yutzy GG, Bude RO, Ellis JH, Rubin JM. Use of Doppler sonography for revealing hepatic artery stenosis in liver transplant recipients. *AJR Am J Roentgenol.* 1997;168(2):473–476. https://doi.org/10.2214/ajr.168.2.9016229. PMID: 9016229.

52. O'Leary J, Lepe R, Dais G. Indications for liver transplantation. *Gastroenterol.* 2008;34:1764–1776.

53. Måller S, Mehrabi A, Schmied B, et al. Partial liver transplantation? Living donor liver transplantation and split liver transplantation. *Nephrol Dial Transplant.* 2007;22:viii13–viii22.

54. Weisner R, Edwards E, Freeman R. Model for end-stage liver disease (MELD) and allocation of donor livers. *Gastroenterol.* 2003;124:91–96.

55. Bruix J, Sherman M, Llovet JM, et al. Clinical management of hepatocellular carcinoma. Conclusions of the Barcelona-2000 EASL conference. *J Hepatol.* 2001;35:421–430.

56. Sanyal R, Zarzour JG, Ganeshan DM, et al. Postoperative Doppler evaluation of liver transplants. *Indian J Radiol Imaging.* 2014;24(4):360–366. https://doi.org/10.4103/0971-3026.143898.

57. Tamsel S, Demirpolat G, Killi R, et al. Vascular complications after liver transplantation: evaluation with Doppler US. *Abdom Imaging.* 2007;32:339–347.

58. Dodd 3rd GD, Memel DS, Zajko AB, et al. Hepatic artery stenosis and thrombosis in transplant recipients: Doppler diagnosis with resistive index and systolic acceleration time. *Radiol.* 1994;192:657–661.

59. Holbert BL, Campbell WL, Skolnick ML. Evaluation of the transplanted liver and postoperative complications. *Radiol Clin North Am.* 1995;33:521–540.

EXTRANEOUS REFERENCES

1. United Kingdom Association of Sonographers. *Guidelines for professional working standards – ultrasound practice.* London: United Kingdom; 2001.

2. Couinaud C. Lobes et segments hepatiques, note sur l'architecture anatomique et chirugicale du foie. *Presse Med.* 1954;62:709.

3. Conlon RM, Bates JA. Segmental localisation of focal hepatic lesions – a comparison of ultrasound and MRI. In: *Conference proceedings of BMUS, Edinburgh*; 1996.

4. Cheng Y, Huang T, Chen C, et al. Variations of the middle and inferior right hepatic vein: application in hepatectomy. *J Clin Ultrasound.* 1997;25:175–182.

5. Goyal AK, Pokharna DS, Sharma SK. Ultrasonic measurements of portal vasculature in diagnosis of portal hypertension. *J Ultrasound Med.* 1990;9:45.

6. Gaiani S, Bolondi L, Li Bassi S, et al. Effect of meal on portal hemodynamics in healthy humans and in patients. *Hepatol.* 1989;9:815–819.

7. Kabiri H, Domingo OH, Tzarnas CD. Agenesis of the gallbladder. *Curr Surg.* 2006;63:104–106.

8. Davies RP, Downey PR, Moore WR, et al. Contrast cholangiography versus ultrasonographic measurement of the 'extrahepatic' bile duct: a two-fold discrepancy revisited. *J Ultrasound Med.* 1991;10:653–657.

APPENDIX 2.1: LS THROUGH THE RIGHT LOBE OF THE LIVER

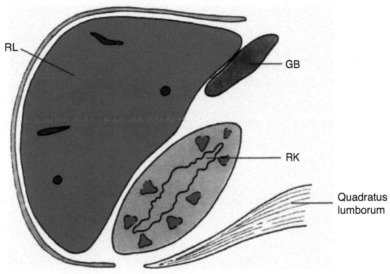

LS through the right lobe of the liver.

APPENDIX 2.2: LS THROUGH THE INFERIOR VENA CAVA

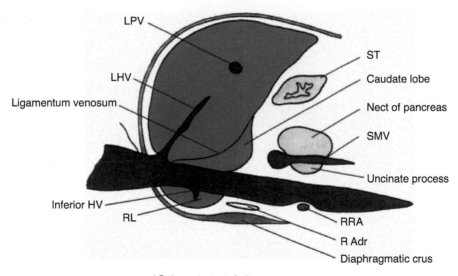

LS through the inferior vena cava.

APPENDIX 2.3: LS THROUGH THE MIDLINE, LEVEL OF THE AORTA

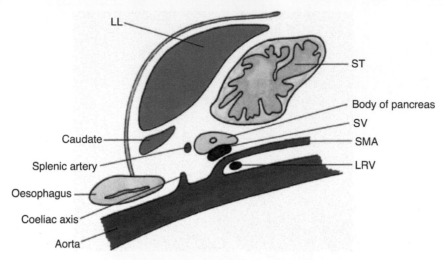

LS through the midline, level of the aorta.

APPENDIX 2.4: LONGITUDINAL, OBLIQUE SECTION ALONG THE CBD

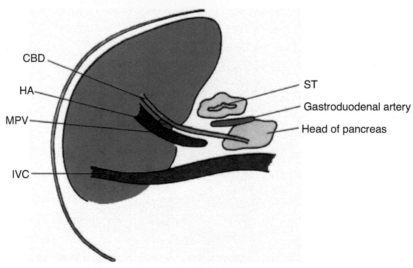

Longitudinal, oblique section along the CBD.

APPENDIX 2.5: TRANSVERSE OBLIQUE SECTION THROUGH THE HEPATIC VENOUS CONFLUENCE

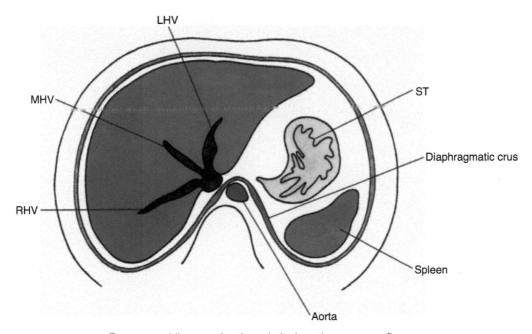

Transverse oblique section through the hepatic venous confluence.

APPENDIX 2.6: TS THROUGH THE LEVEL OF THE PORTA HEPATIS

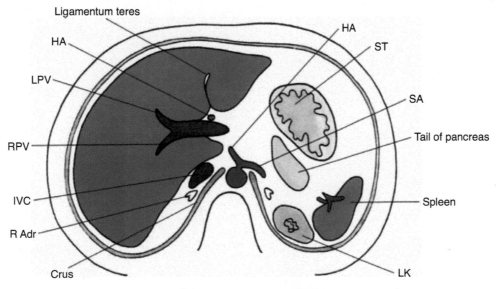

TS through the level of the porta hepatis.

APPENDIX 2.7: TS AT THE LEVEL OF THE PANCREAS

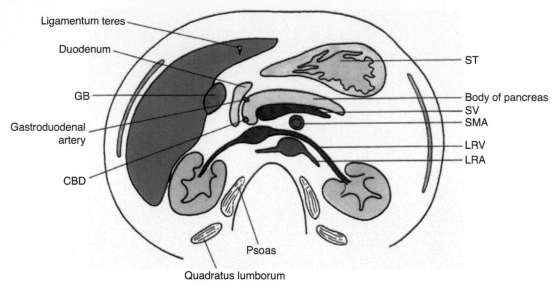

TS at the level of the pancreas.

3

Ultrasound of the Gallbladder and Biliary Tree

James R. Michael

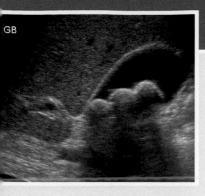

CHAPTER OUTLINE

The Gallbladder and Biliary Tree, 94
  Normal Variants of the Gallbladder, 95
    Pitfalls in Scanning the Gallbladder, 95
    Pathology or Artifact?, 97
  The Bile Ducts, 97
    Bile Duct Measurements, 98
  Techniques, 99
  Common Referral Patterns for Hepatobiliary
    Ultrasound, 99
    Jaundice, 99
    Abnormal Liver Function Tests, 101
Gallbladder Pathologic Conditions, 101
  Cholelithiasis, 101
    Ultrasound Appearances, 101
  Choledocholithiasis, 105
    Biliary Reflux and Gallstone Pancreatitis, 107
    Further Management of Gallstones, 108
  Enlargement of the Gallbladder, 108
    Mucocele of the Gallbladder, 110
    Mirizzi's Syndrome, 110
  The Contracted or Small Gallbladder, 111
    Post-Prandial, 111
    Pathological Causes of a Small Gallbladder, 111
    Porcelain Gallbladder, 112
Hyperplastic Conditions of the Gallbladder Wall, 112
  Adenomyomatosis, 112
    Polyps, 113
    Cholesterolosis, 115
Inflammatory Gallbladder Disease, 116
  Acute Cholecystitis, 116
    Further Management of Acute Cholecystitis, 116

  Chronic Cholecystitis, 117
  Acalculous Cholecystitis, 118
  Complications of Cholecystitis, 119
    Acute on Chronic Cholecystitis, 119
    Gangrenous Cholecystitis, 119
    Emphysematous Cholecystitis, 120
    Gallbladder Empyema, 120
Biliary Tree Dilatation, 123
  Obstructive Jaundice and Biliary Duct Dilation, 123
    Assessment of the Level of Obstruction, 123
    Early Ductal Obstruction, 123
    Diagnosis and Assessment of the Cause of
      Obstruction, 124
    Management of Biliary Obstruction, 126
    Intrahepatic Tumors Causing Biliary
      Obstruction, 127
    Choledochal Cysts, 128
    Cholangitis, 128
  Biliary Dilatation Without Jaundice, 128
    Post-Surgical CBD Dilatation, 128
  Obstruction Without Biliary Dilatation, 129
    Early Obstruction, 129
    Fibrosis of the Duct Walls, 129
Other Biliary Diseases, 129
    Primary Sclerosing Cholangitis (PSC), 129
    Primary Biliary Cirrhosis (PBC), 132
    Caroli's Disease (Congenital Intrahepatic Biliary
      Dilatation), 132
    Parasites, 133
  Echogenic Bile, 134
    Biliary Stasis and Bile Crystals, 134

Obstructive Causes of Biliary Stasis, 135
Haemobilia, 135
Pneumobilia, 135
Malignant Biliary Disease, 136
  Primary Gallbladder Carcinoma, 136

Cholangiocarcinoma, 137
  Management of the Patient with
    Cholangiocarcinoma, 137
Gallbladder Metastases, 138
References, 139

THE GALLBLADDER AND BILIARY TREE

Ultrasound is an essential first-line investigation in suspected gallbladder and biliary duct disease. It is highly sensitive, accurate, and comparatively cheap, and is the imaging modality of choice.[1] Gallbladder pathologic conditions are common and asymptomatic in over 13% of the population.[2]

The normal gallbladder is best visualized after fasting to distend it. It should have a hyperechoic, thin wall (<2 mm) and contain anechoic bile (Fig. 3.1). Measure

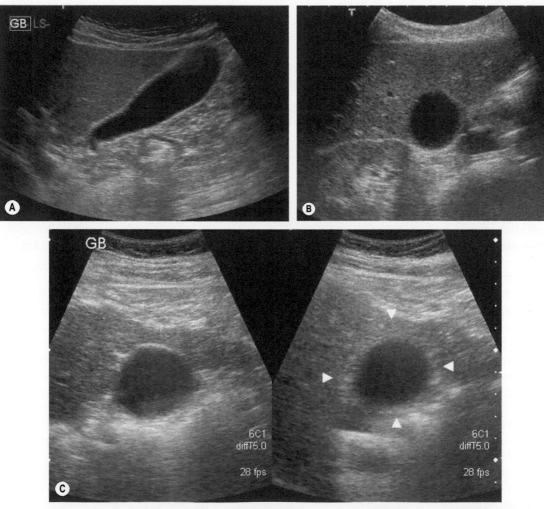

Fig. 3.1 The gallbladder: (A) long section (LS), (B) Transverse section (TS). (C) False appearance of wall thickening is apparent on the right hand image (arrowheads) when the angle of intonation is not perpendicular to the gallbladder wall. The left hand image shows that the wall is normal.

the wall thickness in a longitudinal section of the gallbladder, with the calipers perpendicular to the wall itself. (A transverse section may not be perpendicular to the wall and can overestimate the thickness.)

After fasting for around 6 h, the gallbladder should be distended with bile into an elongated pear-shaped sac. The size is too variable to allow direct measurements to be of any use, but a tense, rounded shape can indicate pathological, rather than physiological dilatation.

Because the size, shape, and position of the gallbladder are infinitely variable, so are the techniques required to scan it. There are, however, several useful pointers to maximize visualization of the gallbladder:

Use the highest frequency possible – 5.0 MHz or higher is especially useful for anterior gallbladders; in this instance, a high-frequency linear probe may be useful.

Use a high line density to pick up tiny stones or polyps. (Reduce the sector angle and the frame rate if possible.) Make sure the focal zone is set over the back wall of the gallbladder to maximize your chances of identifying small stones.

Alter the time gain compensation (TGC) to eliminate or minimize anterior artifacts and reverberation echoes inside the gallbladder, particularly in the near field.

Use tissue harmonic imaging to reduce artifact within the gallbladder and sharpen the image of the wall (particularly in a large abdomen).

Ensure any compounding software is switched off if you are unsure if the small lesion is a stone; removing the compounding software will allow posterior shadowing to be seen more clearly.

Always scan the gallbladder in at least two planes (find the gallbladder's long axis, incorporating the neck and fundus; sweep from side to side, then transversely from neck to fundus) and two patient positions. You will almost certainly miss pathologic conditions if you do not.

The gallbladder may be "folded" (the so-called Phrygian cap). To be able to view this in it is entirety, it may be necessary to turn the patient into various positions (Fig. 3.2).

Bowel gas over the fundus can also be moved by various patient positions; consider scanning with the patient erect to try and move the bowel away from the gallbladder.

Normal Variants of the Gallbladder

The mesenteric attachment of the gallbladder to the inferior surface of the liver is variable in length. This gives rise to large variations in position; at one end of the spectrum, the gallbladder, attached only at the neck, may be fairly remote from the liver, even lying in the pelvis; at the other, the gallbladder fossa deeply invaginates the liver, and the gallbladder appears to lie "intrahepatically" enclosed on all sides by liver tissue.

The presence of a true septum in the gallbladder is rare. A folded gallbladder frequently gives the impression of a septum, but this can be distinguished by positioning the patient to unfold the gallbladder. Occasionally a gallbladder septum completely divides the lumen into two parts. True gallbladder duplication is a rare entity (Fig. 3.3), and it is important not to mistake this for a gallbladder with a pericholecystic collection in a symptomatic patient. Occasionally the gallbladder is absent altogether.

Pitfalls in Scanning the Gallbladder

If the gallbladder cannot be found:

Check for previous surgery – evidence of laparoscopic surgery may be difficult to see in the darkened scanning room.

Check that the patient has fasted.

Look for an ectopic gallbladder – positioned low in the pelvis, for example.

Check that near field artifact has not obscured an anterior gallbladder – a particular problem in very thin patients.

If you still cannot find it, ensure the scanner frequency and settings are optimized, find the porta hepatis, and scan just below it in the transverse section. This is the area of the gallbladder fossa, and you should see at least the anterior gallbladder wall if the gallbladder is present (Fig. 3.4).

A contracted, stone-filled gallbladder, producing heavy shadowing, can be difficult to identify because of the lack of any contrasting fluid in the lumen.

True agenesis of the gallbladder is rare.

Duodenum mimicking gallbladder pathologic conditions:

The close proximity of the duodenum to the posterior gallbladder wall often causes it to invaginate the gallbladder. Maximize your machine settings to visualize the posterior gallbladder wall separate from the duodenum and turn the patient to cause the duodenal contents to move.

Other segments of the fluid-containing gastrointestinal tract can also cause confusion (Fig. 3.5).

Stones that do not shadow:

This is likely to be because of poor settings, rather than any lack of stone reflectivity.

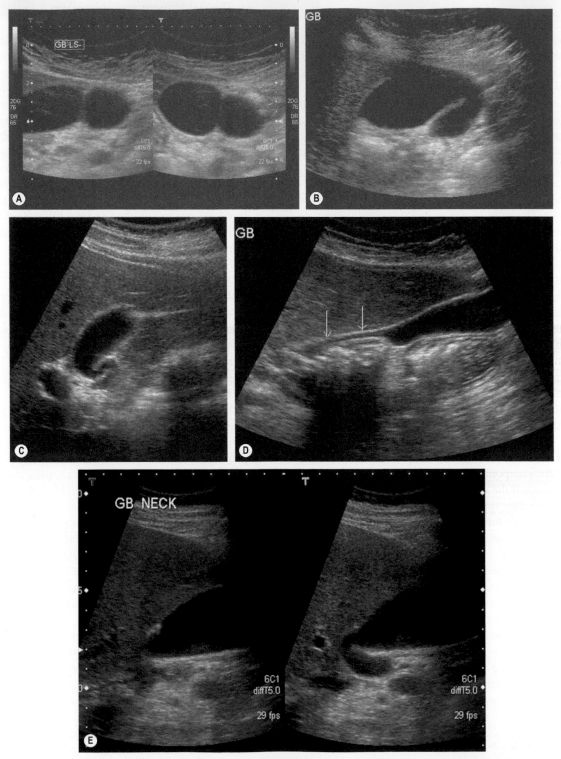

Fig. 3.2 (A) A folded gallbladder is difficult to examine with the patient supine, and the fold may mimic septation. (B) Scanning from a different angle (coronally) demonstrates the true nature of the folded gallbladder. (C) Many gallbladder necks can be tortuous, potentially hiding pathology. (D) Turning the patient decubitus, the right side is raised, unfolds the gallbladder, enabling the neck to be fully examined (arrows). (E) shows how hidden a gallbladder neck can be.

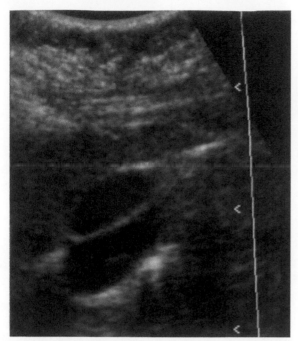

Fig. 3.3 Double gallbladder: an incidental finding in a young woman.

Ensure they are stones and not polyps by positioning the patient erect and watching them move with gravity (beware – polyps on long stalks also move around).
The stones may be smaller than the beamwidth, making the shadow difficult to display.

Ensure the focal zone is set at the back of the gallbladder.
Increase the line density, if possible, by reducing the field of view.
Scan with the highest possible frequency to ensure the narrowest beamwidth.
Reduce the TGC and/or power to ensure you have not saturated the echoes distal to the gallbladder.

Beware of the folded gallbladder! If the gallbladder is folded and the fundus lies underneath the bowel, you may miss pathologic conditions. Always try to unfold it by positioning the patient. A fold in the gallbladder may mimic a septum. Septations are comparatively rare and have been overreported in the past because of the presence of folding.

Pathology or Artifact?

Sometimes the gallbladder may contain some echoes of doubtful significance or be insufficiently distended to evaluate accurately. A rescan, after a meal followed by further fasting, can be useful. This can flush out sludge, redistending the gallbladder with clear bile. It may also help to clarify any confusing appearances of adjacent bowel loops.

The Bile Ducts

The common duct can be easily demonstrated in its intrahepatic portion just anterior and slightly to the right of the portal vein. A cross-section of the main hepatic artery can usually be seen passing between the vein and

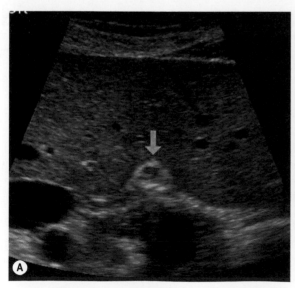
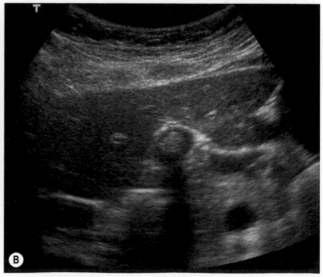

Fig. 3.4 (A) A postprandial, contracted gallbladder located in the gallbladder fossa on TS. (B) A contracted stone-filled gallbladder in TS.

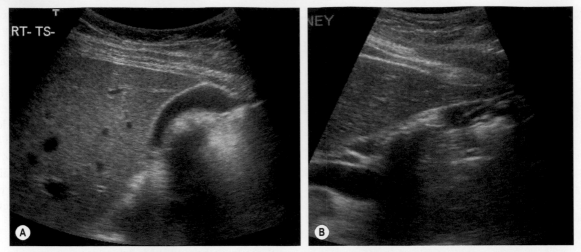

Fig. 3.5 (A & B) The duodenum frequently invaginates the posterior wall of the gallbladder and may mimic stones if the machine settings are not correctly manipulated.

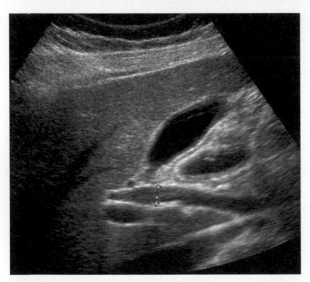

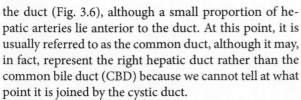

Fig. 3.6 Normal CBD at the porta hepatis. The lower end is frequently obscured by shadowing from the duodenum. The duct should be measured at its widest portion.

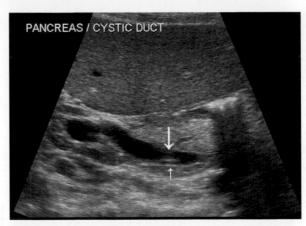

Fig. 3.7 Visualisation of the lower end of the duct often requires the operator to persevere with technique and patient positioning. The normal duct (large arrow) is seen in the head of the pancreas. The cystic duct (small arrow) is just visible posterior to the CBD, in an example of an abnormally low insertion, often associated with pancreatitis.

the duct (Fig. 3.6), although a small proportion of hepatic arteries lie anterior to the duct. At this point, it is usually referred to as the common duct, although it may, in fact, represent the right hepatic duct rather than the common bile duct (CBD) because we cannot tell at what point it is joined by the cystic duct.

The extrahepatic portion of the duct is less easy to see as it is often obscured by overlying duodenal gas. Good visualization of the duct usually requires perseverance

on the part of the operator. It is insufficient just to visualize the intrahepatic portion of the duct, as early obstruction may be present with a normal caliber intrahepatic duct and dilatation of the distal end (Fig. 3.7).

Bile Duct Measurements

The internal diameter of the common duct is usually taken as 6 mm or less. However, it is age-dependent and can be 8-9 mm in an older adult because of degeneration of the elastic fiber in the duct wall. Ensure this is not early obstruction by thoroughly examining the distal CBD or rescanning after a short time interval.

The diameter can vary quite considerably, not only between subjects but along an individual duct. The greatest measurement should be recorded in the longitudinal section. Never measure the duct in a transverse section (for example, at the head of the pancreas); it is invariably an oblique plane through the duct, which will overestimate the diameter. Intrahepatically, the duct diameter decreases. The right and left hepatic ducts are just visible, but more peripheral branches are usually too small to see.

TIP BOX

Patients post cholecystectomy who have had previous duct dilatation frequently also have a persistently dilated but non-obstructed duct (Fig. 3.8). Be suspicious of a diameter of 10 mm or more as this is associated with obstruction because of the formation of stones in the duct.

Techniques

The main, right, and left hepatic ducts tend to lie anterior to the portal vein branches. However, as the biliary tree spreads out, the position of the duct relative to the portal branches is highly variable. Do not assume that a channel anterior to the portal vein branch is always a biliary duct. The walls of the ducts are hyperechoic and can help

distinguish the ducts from vessels however, if in doubt, use color Doppler to distinguish the bile duct from the portal vein or hepatic artery. The proximal bile duct is best seen either with the patient supine, using an intercostal approach from the right, or turning the patient oblique, right side raised. This projects the duct over the portal vein, which is used as an anatomic marker.

Scanning the distal duct usually requires more effort. Right oblique or decubitus positions are useful. Gentle pressure to ease the duodenal gas away from the duct can also be successful. Sometimes, filling the stomach with water (which also helps to display the pancreas) and allowing it to trickle through the duodenum does the trick. Try also identifying the duct in the pancreatic head (Fig. 3.9) and then tracing it retrogradely toward the liver. Asking the patient to take deep breaths is occasionally successful but may make matters worse by filling the stomach with air. It is definitely worth persevering with your technique, particularly in jaundiced patients.

Common Referral Patterns for Hepatobiliary Ultrasound
Jaundice

Jaundice is a frequent cause of referral for an abdominal ultrasound. Therefore, it is essential for the sonographer to have a basic understanding of the various mechanisms to maximize the diagnostic information from the ultrasound scan.

Jaundice or hyperbilirubinemia, is an elevated level of bilirubin in the blood. It is recognized by a characteristic

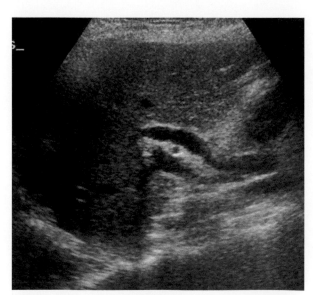

Fig. 3.8 A persistently, mildly dilated duct post-cholecystectomy (8.5 mm). The duct is baggy, rather than under any pressure, and there is no intrahepatic duct dilatation.

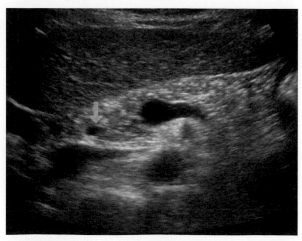

Fig. 3.9 The common bile duct (arrow) is seen in the head of the pancreas on TS.

yellow coloration of the skin and sclera of the eye, often accompanied by itching if prolonged. Bilirubin is derived from the hem portion of hemoglobin. Red blood cells are broken down in the liver into hem and globin, releasing their bilirubin which is non-soluble. This is termed unconjugated bilirubin. This is then taken up by the liver cells and converted to a water-soluble form – conjugated bilirubin, which is excreted via the biliary ducts into the duodenum to aid fat digestion.

By knowing which of these two types of bilirubin is present in the jaundiced patient, the clinician can narrow the diagnostic possibilities. The ultrasound then further refines the diagnosis (Fig. 3.10).

Jaundice can fall into one of two categories:

Obstructive (sometimes called posthepatic) – in which the bile is prevented from draining out of the liver because of obstruction to the biliary duct(s).

Non-obstructive (prehepatic or hepatic) – in which the elevated bilirubin level is because of hemolysis (the breakdown of the red blood cells) or a disturbance in the mechanism of the liver for uptake and storage of bilirubin, such as in inflammatory or metabolic liver diseases.

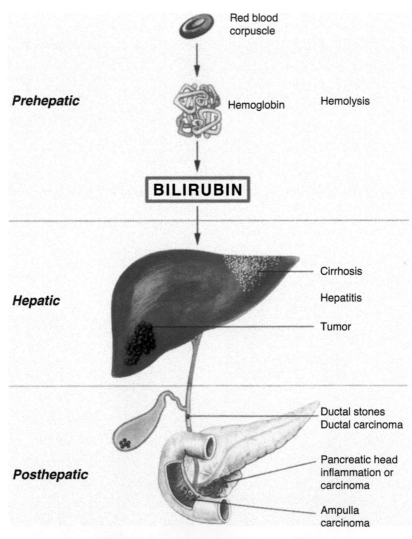

Fig. 3.10 Some common causes of jaundice.

Abnormal Liver Function Tests

Altered or deranged liver function tests (LFTs) are another frequent cause of referral for an abdominal ultrasound. Biochemistry from a simple blood test is often a primary pointer to pathologic conditions and is invariably one of the first tests performed as it is quick and easily accessible. Raised bilirubin in combination with elevated alkaline phosphatase (Alk Phos) is suggestive of obstruction, where an isolated raised bilirubin is more likely to represent a metabolic condition. Ultrasound can be used in cases of obstructive jaundice, which demonstrates some degree of biliary duct dilatation.

Most of the other markers are highly unspecific, being associated with many types of diffuse and focal liver pathologic conditions and may not be relevant in gallbladder disease.

GALLBLADDER PATHOLOGIC CONDITIONS

Cholelithiasis

The most commonly and reliably identified gallbladder pathologic condition is gallstones. More than 10% of the population of the United Kingdom have gallstones. Many of these are asymptomatic (Box 3.1), which is important to remember. When scanning a patient with abdominal pain, it should not automatically be assumed that when gallstones are present, they are responsible for the pain. It is not uncommon to find further pathologic conditions in the presence of gallstones, and a comprehensive upper abdominal survey should always be carried out. However, up to 35% of patients who have gallstones require surgery to relieve symptoms (Table 3.1).[3]

Gallstones are associated with a number of conditions. They occur when the normal ratio of components making up the bile is altered, most commonly when

TABLE 3.1 Causes of a Thickened Gallbladder Wall	
Physiological	**Post-Prandial**
Inflammatory	Acute or chronic cholecystitis
	Sclerosing cholangitis
	Crohn's disease
	AIDS
Adjacent inflammatory causes	Pancreatitis
	Hepatitis
	Pericholecystic abscesses
Non-inflammatory	Adenomyomatosis
	Gallbladder carcinoma
	Focal areas of thickening because of metastases or polyps
	Leukemia
Edema	Ascites from a variety of causes, including organ failure, lymphatic obstruction, and portal hypertension
Varices	Varices of the gallbladder wall in portal hypertension

there is increased secretion of cholesterol in the bile. Conditions that are associated with increased cholesterol secretion and therefore the formation of cholesterol stones include obesity, diabetes, pregnancy, and estrogen therapy. The incidence of stones also rises with age, probably because the bile flow slows down.

An increased secretion of bilirubin in the bile, as in patients with cirrhosis, is associated with pigment (black or brown) stones.

Ultrasound Appearances

There are three classic acoustic properties associated with stones in the gallbladder; they are *highly reflective, mobile,* and cast a *distal acoustic shadow.* In most cases, all these properties are demonstrated (Figs. 3.11–3.13).

Shadowing. The ability to display a shadow posterior to a stone depends on several factors:

1. The reflection and absorption of sound by the stone. This is fairly consistent, regardless of the composition of the stone.

BOX 3.1 Gallstones – Clinical Features

- Often asymptomatic
- Biliary colic – RUQ pain, fatty intolerance
- Positive ultrasound Murphy's sign (if inflammation is present)
- Recurring RUQ pain in chronic cholecystitis
- Jaundice (depending on the degree of obstruction)
- Fluctuating fever (if an infection is present)

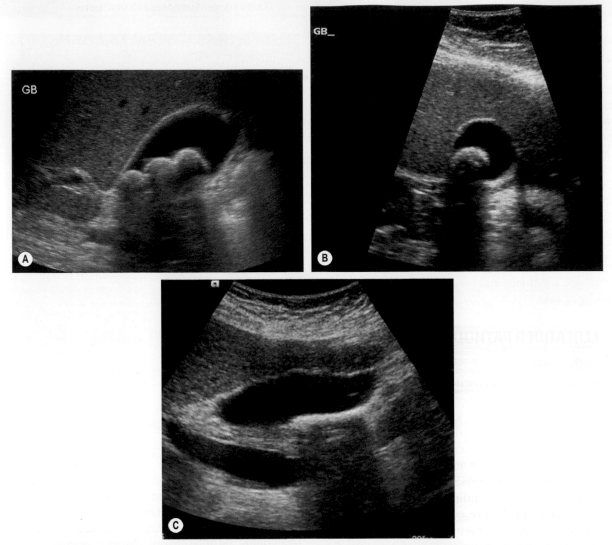

Fig. 3.11 (A) LS and (B) TS through a gallbladder demonstrating stones with posterior acoustic shadowing. (C) Tiny stones lie together to form a block of acoustic shadow behind the gallbladder.

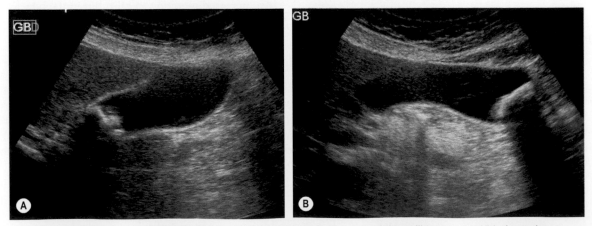

Fig. 3.12 Gallstone mobility: (A) Shadowing from a stone in the neck of the gallbladder. (B) With the patient erect, the stone drops to the fundus of the gallbladder.

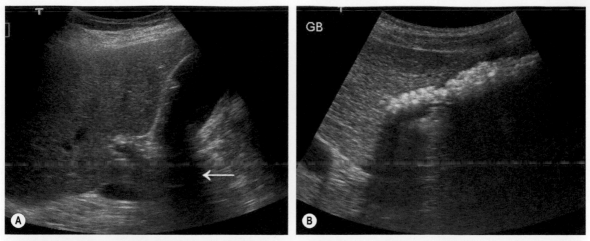

Fig. 3.13 (A) Floating gallstones cast a shadow from the anterior gallbladder (arrow). (B) Floating stones in the gallbladder lumen mimicking gas-filled bowel.

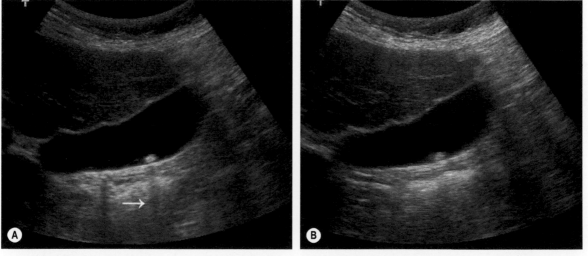

Fig. 3.14 (A) This small stone is wider than the beamwidth and casts an acoustic shadow (arrow). (B) The shadow is no longer evident when the beam focusing is moved anterior to the gallbladder as the beam is now wider than the stone.

2. The size of the stone in relation to the beamwidth. A shadow occurs when the stone fills the width of the beam (Fig. 3.14). This will happen easily with large stones, but a small stone may occupy less space than the beam, allowing sound to continue behind it, so a shadow is not seen. Small stones must therefore be within the focal zone (narrowest point) of the beam and in the center of the beam to shadow (Fig. 3.15). Higher frequency transducers have better resolution and are therefore more likely to display fine shadows than lower frequencies.

3. The machine settings must be compatible with demonstrating narrow bands of shadowing. The fluid-filled gallbladder often displays posterior enhancement or increased through transmission. If the echoes posterior to the gallbladder are "saturated," this will mask fine shadows. Turn the overall gain down to display this better (Fig. 3.16). Some image processing options may reduce the contrast between the shadow and the surrounding tissue, so make sure a suitable dynamic range and image program are used.

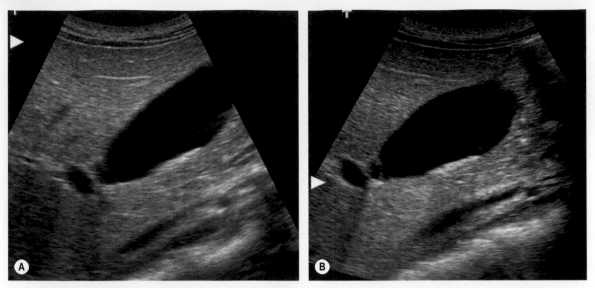

Fig. 3.15 (A) A layer of tiny stones does not shadow when the focal zone is placed incorrectly (arrow), but the shadow is easily demonstrated (B) when the focal zone is placed at the posterior wall of the gallbladder, narrowing the beam at this point.

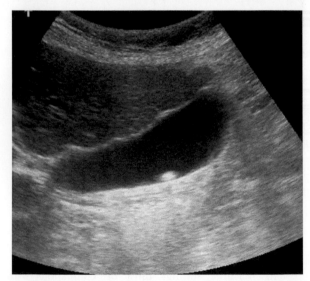

Fig. 3.16 The shadow from the stone in Fig. 3.14 is obscured by the overamplification of the echoes behind the gallbladder.

4. Bowel posterior to the gallbladder may cast its own shadows from gas and other contents, making the gallstone shadow difficult to demonstrate (Fig. 3.17). This is a particular problem with stones in the CBD. Try turning the patient to move the gallbladder away from the bowel. The shadow cast by gas in the duodenum, which contains reverberation, should usually

be distinguishable from that cast by a gallstone, which is sharp and clean.

Reflectivity. The reflective nature of the stone is enhanced by its being surrounded by echo-free bile. In a contracted gallbladder, the reflectivity of the stone is often not appreciated because the hyperechoic gallbladder wall is collapsed over it.

Some stones are only poorly reflective but should still cause a distal acoustic shadow.

Mobility. Most stones are gravity-dependent, and this may be demonstrated by scanning the patient in an erect position (Fig. 3.12) when a mobile calculus will drop from the neck or body of the gallbladder to lie in the fundus. However, some stones will float, forming a reflective layer just beneath the anterior gallbladder wall with shadowing that obscures the rest of the lumen (Fig. 3.13B). When the gallbladder lumen is contracted, either because of physiological or pathological reasons, any stones present are unable to move, and this is also the case in a gallbladder packed with stones (Fig. 3.17D).

Occasionally a stone may become impacted in the neck, and movement of the patient is unable to dislodge it. Stones lodged in the gallbladder neck or cystic duct may result in a permanently contracted gallbladder, a gallbladder full of fine echoes because of inspissated (thickened) bile (Fig. 3.18), or a distended gallbladder because of a mucocele (see below).

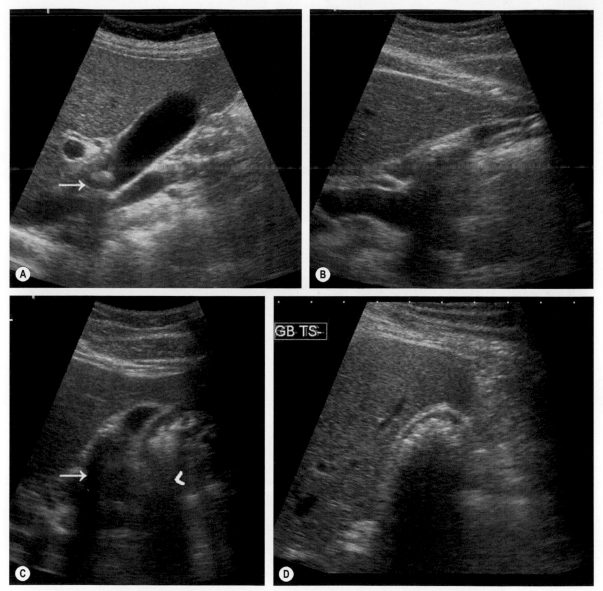

Fig. 3.17 (A) Shadowing from the stone in the neck of the gallbladder (arrow) is less obvious because of the structures lying behind the gallbladder. (B) Shadowing from the duodenum posterior to the gallbladder can obscure the shadowing from tiny stones within the gallbladder lumen. Changing patient position and angle of scanning moves the gas away from the gallbladder. (C) Shadowing from stones in the contracted gallbladder lumen (arrow) is stronger and better defined than the "dirty" shadowing from the adjacent bowel (arrowhead). (D) A contracted gallbladder full of stones casts a strong acoustic shadow from the gallbladder fossa. Note that the echoes from the anterior gallbladder wall are distinct from the echoes from the stones.

Choledocholithiasis

Choledocholithiasis develops in up to 20% of patients with gallstones.[4] Stones may pass from the gallbladder into the common duct or may develop *de novo* within the duct. Stones in the CBD may obstruct the drainage of bile from the liver causing obstructive jaundice. Due to shadowing from the adjacent duodenum, ductal stones are often difficult to demonstrate, and care must be taken to visualize the lower end of the duct if possible (Fig. 3.19).

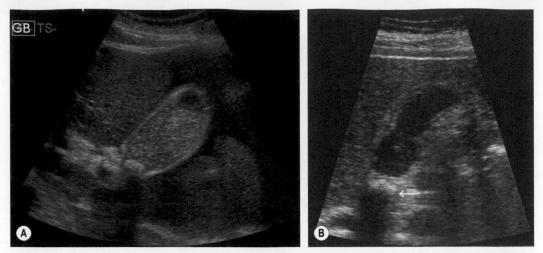

Fig. 3.18 (A) A stone lodged in the gallbladder neck with thickened, inspissated bile filling the gallbladder lumen. (B) The gallbladder neck is curled round, and a stone is lodged within it (arrow).

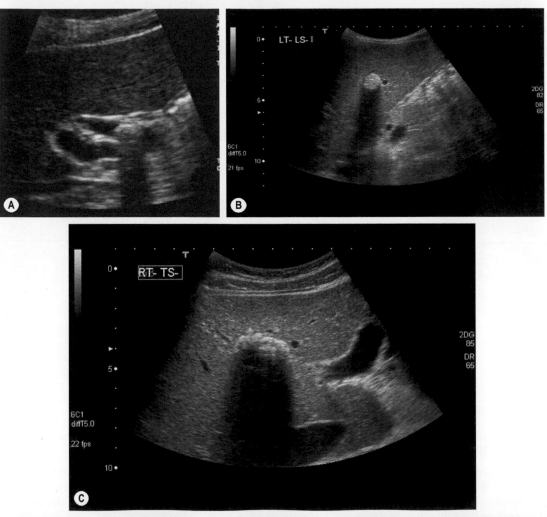

Fig. 3.19 (A) A stone in a dilated CBD with posterior shadowing. The gallbladder was dilated but did not contain stones. (B & C) Stone formation in the intrahepatic ducts.

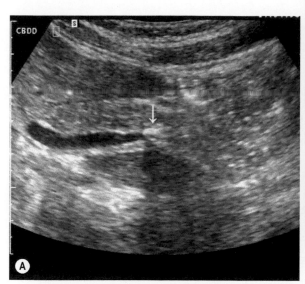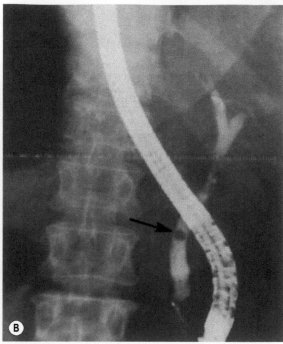

Fig. 3.20 (A) Small stone in the CBD causing intermittent obstruction. At the time of scanning, the CBD was normal in caliber. (B) ERCP of a stone in a normal caliber (5 mm) duct.

Usually, CBD stones are accompanied by stones in the gallbladder and a degree of dilatation of the CBD. In these cases, the operator can usually persevere and demonstrate the offending article at the lower end of the duct. However, the duct may be dilated but empty, the stone having recently passed. Stones may be seen to move up and down a dilated duct. This can create a ball-valve effect so that obstruction may be intermittent. It is not unusual to demonstrate a stone in the CBD without stones in the gallbladder, a phenomenon that is also well documented following cholecystectomy. This may be because of a single calculus in the gallbladder having moved into the duct, or stone formation, de novo, within the duct.

It is also important to remember that stones in the CBD may be present *without* duct dilatation, and attempts to image the entire common duct with ultrasound should *always* be made, even if it is of normal caliber at the porta (Fig. 3.20).

Other ultrasound signs to look for are shown in Box 3.2.

Possible complications of gallstones are outlined in Fig. 3.21. In rare cases, stones may perforate the inflamed gallbladder wall to form a fistula into the small

---

BOX 3.2 Gallstones – Other Ultrasound Signs to Look for

- Acute or chronic cholecystitis
- Complications of cholecystitis, e.g., pericholecystic collection
- Stone impacted in the neck of the gallbladder – mucocele, hydrops
- CBD stones
- Biliary obstruction – dilatation of the CBD and/or intrahepatic ducts
- Pancreatitis
- Other causes of RUQ pain unrelated to stones

---

intestine or colon. A large stone passing into the small intestine may impact the ileum, causing an intestinal obstruction.

Biliary Reflux and Gallstone Pancreatitis

A stone may become lodged in the distal CBD near the ampulla. If the main pancreatic duct joins the CBD proximal to this, bile and pancreatic fluid may reflux up the pancreatic duct, causing inflammation and severe pain. Reflux up the CBD may also result in ascending

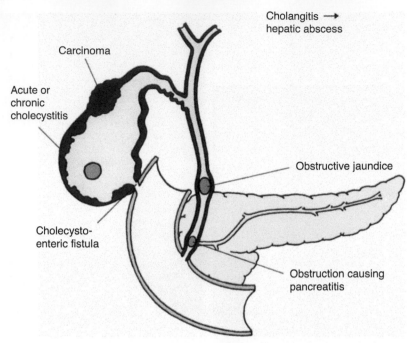

Fig. 3.21 The possible complications of gallstones.

cholangitis, particularly if the obstruction is prolonged or repetitive. Cholangitis may result in dilated bile ducts with mural irregularity on ultrasound, but magnetic resonance cholangiopancreatography (MRCP) is usually superior in demonstrating intrahepatic ductal changes of this nature.

Bile reflux is also associated with anomalous cystic duct insertion (Fig. 3.22A, B), which is more readily recognized on MRCP than ultrasound.

Further Management of Gallstones

MRCP and endoscopic retrograde cholangiopancreatography (ERCP) demonstrate stones in the duct with greater accuracy than ultrasound, particularly at the lower end of the CBD, which may be obscured by duodenal gas on ultrasound (Fig. 3.22C, D).[5] ERCP is invasive, carrying a small risk of morbidity or rarely mortality because of perforation, infection, or pancreatitis but has the advantage of providing the therapeutic option of sphincterotomy and stone removal. This is the modality of choice when stones are known to exist in the duct (for example, following MRCP) and has supplanted surgical removal in many cases.[6]

Laparoscopic cholecystectomy is the preferred method of treatment for symptomatic gallbladder disease in an elective setting. Acute cholecystitis is also increasingly managed by early laparoscopic surgery, with a slightly higher rate of conversion to open surgery than elective cases.[7] Laparoscopic ultrasound may be used as a suitable alternative to operative cholangiography to examine the common duct for residual stones during surgery.[8] It compares well to cholangiography, with a sensitivity and specificity of 96% and 100%, and avoids any radiation dose, but has been slow to be adopted in the United Kingdom, as it requires specialized equipment and training.[9] Both ultrasound and cholescintigraphy are used in monitoring postoperative biliary leaks or hematoma (Fig. 3.23).

Other less common options include dissolution therapy and extracorporeal shock wave lithotripsy. However, these treatments are often only partially successful, require careful patient selection, and also run a significant risk of stone recurrence.[10]

Enlargement of the Gallbladder

Due to the enormous variation in size and shape of the normal gallbladder, it is impossible to diagnose pathological enlargement by simply using measurements. Three-dimensional techniques may prove useful in

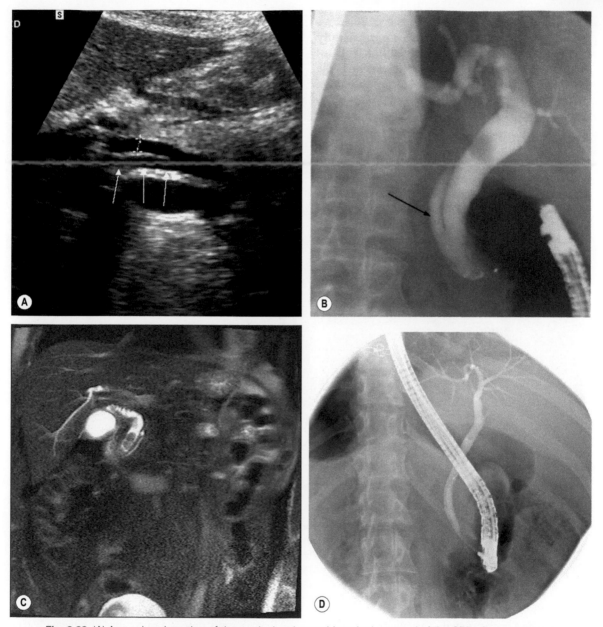

Fig. 3.22 (A) Anomalous insertion of the cystic duct (arrows) into the lower end of the CBD. (B) Appearances of the case in (A) are confirmed on ERCP. A stone is also present in the duct. (C) MRCP showing stones in the CBD. (D) ERCP can be used for therapeutic purposes, such as stone removal or stent insertion.

assessing gallbladder volume,[11] but this is a technique that is only likely to be clinically useful in a minority of patients with impaired gallbladder emptying.

An enlarged gallbladder is frequently referred to as *hydropic*. It may be because of obstruction of the cystic duct (see below) or associated with numerous disease processes such as diabetes, primary sclerosing cholangitis (PSC), leptospirosis, or in response to some types of drugs. A pathologically dilated gallbladder, as opposed to one which is physiologically dilated, usually assumes a more rounded, tense appearance (Fig. 3.24).

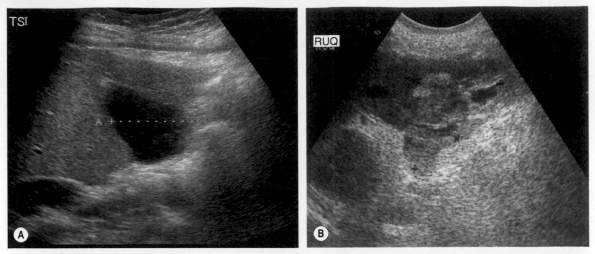

Fig. 3.23 (A) Postoperative bile collection in the gallbladder bed. (B) Hyperechoic, irregular "mass" in the gallbladder bed, which represents a resolving hematoma after laparoscopic cholecystectomy.

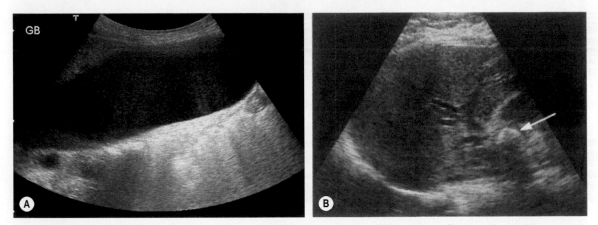

Fig. 3.24 (A) A dilated gallbladder in a patient with obstruction of the CBD because of pancreatic carcinoma. The gallbladder is large, tense, and contains low-level echoes from thickened bile. (B) Mirizzi's syndrome: a large stone in the gallbladder neck compresses the adjacent bile duct, causing an obstruction.

Mucocele of the Gallbladder

If the cystic duct is obstructed – usually by a stone that has failed to pass through to the CBD – the normal flow of bile from the gallbladder is interrupted. Chronic cystic duct obstruction causes the bile to be replaced by mucous secreted by the lining of the gallbladder, resulting in a mucocele. The biliary ducts remain normal in caliber.

If the gallbladder is dilated in the absence of duct dilatation, do a careful search for an obstructing lesion at the neck; a stone in the cystic duct is more difficult to identify on ultrasound as it is not surrounded by echo-free bile (Fig. 3.18).

Mirizzi's Syndrome

Mirizzi's syndrome is a rare cause of biliary obstruction in which compression of the biliary tree is caused by a stone in the adjacent cystic duct. This usually happens in combination with a surrounding inflammatory process which compresses and obstructs the adjacent common hepatic duct, causing distal biliary duct dilatation. This is associated with a low insertion of the cystic duct into the common hepatic duct. Occasionally a fistula forms between the hepatic duct and the gallbladder because of erosion of the duct wall by the stone. Ultimately this may lead to gallstone ileus – small bowel obstruction resulting from migration of a large stone through the cholecystoenteric fistula. If the condition is not promptly diagnosed, recurring cholangitis leading to secondary biliary cirrhosis may result.

On ultrasound, the gallbladder is typically contracted and contains debris. A stone impacted at the neck may be demonstrated together with dilatation of the intrahepatic ducts with a normal caliber lower common duct (Fig. 3.24). The diagnosis is difficult, as it is frequently impossible to rule out carcinoma. Computed tomography (CT) or magnetic resonance imaging (MRI) may assist in this distinction, and ERCP is still considered the "gold standard" especially as it can offer therapeutic stone removal and/or stent placement.[12] Endoscopic or intraductal ultrasounds, if available, have improved the diagnostic accuracy of suspected cases.[13] Although rare, it is an important diagnosis as cholecystectomy in these cases has a higher rate of operative and postoperative complications.[14]

The Contracted or Small Gallbladder
Post-Prandial
The most likely cause of a contracted gallbladder is physiological, following a meal. (This may still occur despite instructions to fast, and it is always worth enquiring when and what the patient has last eaten or drunk.) The normal gallbladder wall is thickened when contracted, and this must not be confused with a pathological process (Fig. 3.25).

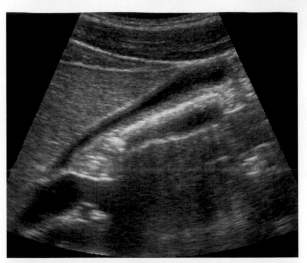

Fig. 3.25 Normal, post-prandial gallbladder with a consequently thickened wall.

Pathological Causes of a Small Gallbladder
Most pathologically contracted gallbladders contain stones. When the gallbladder cannot be identified, try scanning transversely through the gallbladder fossa, just caudal to the porta hepatis. Strong shadowing alerts the sonographer to the possibility of a contracted gallbladder full of stones.

The reflective surface of the stones and distal shadowing are apparent, and the anterior gallbladder wall can be demonstrated with correct focusing and good technique (Figs. 3.17D, 3.26). Do not confuse the

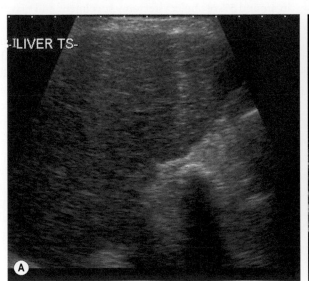

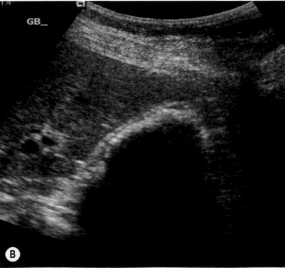

Fig. 3.26 (A) Shadowing from the gallbladder fossa indicates a contracted gallbladder packed with stones. (B) A small layer of bile is visible between the stones and the anterior gallbladder wall.

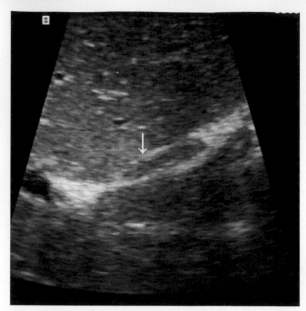

Fig. 3.27 Microgallbladder in cystic fibrosis.

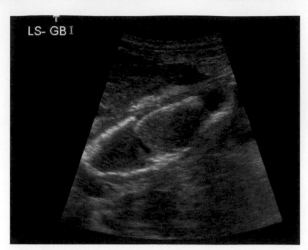

Fig. 3.28 Porcelain gallbladder demonstrating a calcified inner layer of the wall.

appearances of a previous cholecystectomy when bowel in the gallbladder fossa casts a shadow for a contracted stone-filled gallbladder.

A less common cause of a small gallbladder is the *microgallbladder* associated with cystic fibrosis (Fig. 3.27). The gallbladder itself is abnormally small, rather than just contracted. Cystic fibrosis also carries an increased incidence of gallstones because of the altered composition of the bile and bile stasis, and the wall might be thickened and fibrosed from cholecystitis.

Porcelain Gallbladder

When the gallbladder wall becomes calcified, the resulting appearance is of a solid reflective structure, causing a distal shadow in the gallbladder fossa (Fig. 3.28). (This can be distinguished from a gallbladder full of stones where the wall can usually be seen anterior to the shadowing [Fig. 3.17D].)

A porcelain gallbladder probably results from a gallbladder mucocele – a long-standing obstruction of the cystic duct, usually from a stone. The bile inside the non-functioning gallbladder is gradually replaced by watery fluid. The wall becomes fibrotic and thickened, and ultimately calcifies.

There is an association between porcelain gallbladder and gallbladder carcinoma; therefore, a prophylactic cholecystectomy is usually performed to preempt malignant development.[15]

Shadowing from the calcified anterior gallbladder wall can obscure the gallbladder contents and can mimic bowel in the gallbladder fossa. A plain X-ray also clearly demonstrates the porcelain gallbladder.

HYPERPLASTIC CONDITIONS OF THE GALLBLADDER WALL

Adenomyomatosis

This is a common, non-inflammatory, hyperplastic condition that causes gallbladder wall thickening. It occurs in around 5% of cholecystectomy specimens and may be mistaken for chronic cholecystitis on ultrasound.

The epithelium that lines the gallbladder wall undergoes hyperplastic change – extending diverticula into the adjacent muscular layer of the wall. These diverticula or sinuses (known as Rokitansky-Aschoff sinuses) are visible within the wall as fluid-filled spaces (Fig. 3.29), which can bulge eccentrically into the lumen and may contain echogenic material or even (normally pigment) stones.

The wall thickening may be focal or diffuse, and the sinuses may be little more than hypoechoic "spots" in the thickened wall or may become quite large cavities in some cases.[16] Deposits of crystals in the gallbladder wall frequently result in distinctive "comet-tail" artifacts because of rapid small reverberations of the sound.[17]

Focal adenomyomatosis most often occurs at the fundus (Fig. 3.29C) and may be difficult to distinguish from carcinoma. [^{18}F]2-fluoro-2-deoxy-D-glucose positron emission tomography (FDG-PET) may be useful in

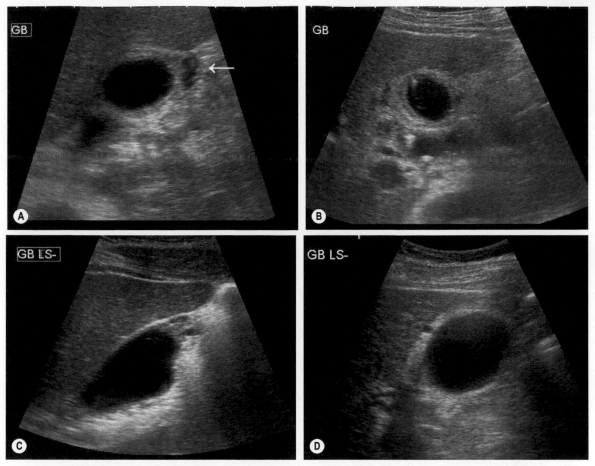

Fig. 3.29 Adenomyomatosis: (A) TS of the gallbladder demonstrating a thickened gallbladder wall with a Rokitansky-Aschoff sinus (arrow). (B) TS of another gallbladder demonstrating a thickened hyperplastic wall with a comet-tail artifact because of crystal deposits. (C) A focal region of adenomyomatosis at the gallbladder fundus. This can sometimes be difficult to distinguish from early gallbladder carcinoma. (D) TS through the gallbladder showing a hyperplastic thickened wall with a small Rokitansky-Aschoff sinus.

the diagnosis of problem cases.[18] Often asymptomatic, it may present with biliary colic, although it is unclear whether this is caused by co-existent stones. Its distinctive appearance allows the diagnosis to be made easily, whether or not stones are present.

Cholecystectomy is performed in symptomatic patients – usually those who also have stones. Although essentially a benign condition, a few cases of associated malignant transformation have been reported, usually in patients with associated anomalous insertion of the pancreatic duct.[19]

Polyps

Gallbladder polyps are common, usually asymptomatic lesions which are incidental findings in up to 5% of the population. Occasionally they are the

cause of biliary colic. They are reflective structures projecting into the gallbladder lumen, which do not cast an acoustic shadow. Unless on a long stalk, they will remain fixed on varying the patient position and are therefore usually distinguishable from stones (Fig. 3.30).

Several types of polyps exist, the most common being cholesterol polyps, which account for around 60% of gallbladder polyps. Others are adenomyomatosis and inflammatory polyps, both of which are also usually benign. True adenomas are less common. There is an association between larger adenomatous gallbladder polyps (>10 mm) and subsequent carcinoma, especially in patients over 50 years of age. Therefore, the finding of a solitary polyp poses

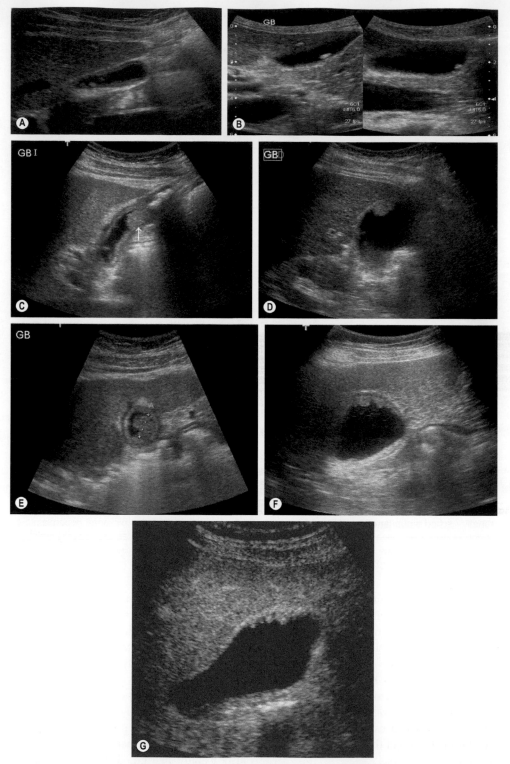

Fig. 3.30 (A) Small polyps in the gallbladder lumen – no posterior shadowing is evident. (B) A gallbladder polyp remains in a fixed position on the gallbladder wall, despite moving the patient erect. (C) Large, sessile gallbladder polyp (arrow) in a thick-walled gallbladder. Stones are present in the gallbladder fundus. (D) Large, broad-based, solitary gallbladder polyp. (E) Such polyps are generally considered at greater risk of malignant transformation, and patients generally undergo cholecystectomy. (F) Multiple gallbladder polyps pre-contrast and (G) post-contrast scan demonstrating take up of contrast in the polyps.

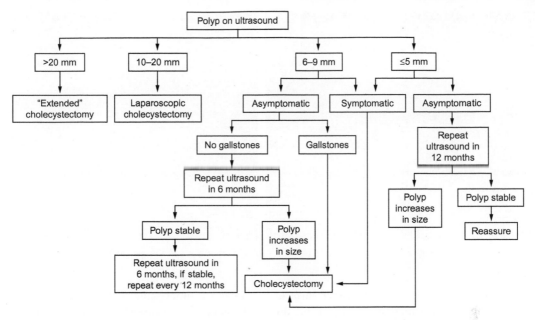

Diagram 3.1 Gallbladder Polyp Pathway. Source: ©West Midlands Cancer Alliance 2019. https://wmcanceralliance. nhs.uk/images/Documents/Hepatobiliary_HPB/HPB_Gallbladder_polyps_guidelines_04_2020.pdf.

a diagnostic dilemma, and cholecystectomy is often advised (Fig. 3.30D, E). Endoscopic ultrasound (EUS) may provide further information in such cases,[20] as it provides high-resolution images of tiny polyps and the layers of the gallbladder wall, and there is some evidence that there is a correlation between EUS appearances and gallbladder polyp histology. Generally, gallbladders in asymptomatic patients with polyps of >1 cm should undergo rescanning to identify subsequent polyp growth and increased risk of carcinoma, and many clinicians advocate cholecystectomy to preempt malignant transformation.[21] In particular, gallbladder polyps in patients with primary sclerosing cholangitis (PSC) have a much greater likelihood of malignancy (40%–60%).[22] Smaller polyps of less than 1 cm in diameter may also be safely monitored with ultrasound.[23]

There is some evidence to suggest that ultrasound contrast agents are useful in demonstrating tumor vascularity in potentially malignant polyps, such as adenomatous polyps.[24] However, so far, this technique has proved non-specific, as some benign cholesterol polyps also demonstrate increased vascularity (Fig. 3.30F, G).

Algorithms are being developed for guidance on the management of gallbladder polyps, with collaboration with primary care, hepatobiliary surgeons, and radiology departments. You should make yourself aware of your local departmental policies and guidelines on the management of gallbladder polyps.

Other guidelines also consider the risk factors that the patient may have included being >50 years old, if they have other conditions such as PSC, and if the patient is of Indian ethnicity. Factors such as sessile (broad-based) polyps are also considered a risk factor (Diagram 3.1). These factors, polyp size and whether the patient is symptomatic then develop a pathway of surgery or surveillance, with small stable polyps only followed up for a maximum of five years. Due to the variations in guidance, it is important that departments develop local protocols to ensure continuity.

Cholesterolosis

Also known as the "strawberry gallbladder," this gets its name because of the multiple tiny nodules on the surface of the gallbladder mucosal lining. These nodules result from a buildup of lipids in the gallbladder wall and are often not visible on ultrasound. However, in some

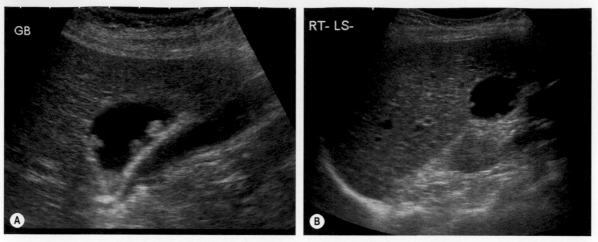

Fig. 3.31 Cholesterolosis (A & B): multiple tiny polyps in the gallbladder.

cases, multiple polyps also form on the inner surface, projecting into the lumen, which are clearly visible on ultrasound (Fig. 3.31). Cholesterolosis may be asymptomatic or may be accompanied by stones and consequently require surgery to alleviate symptoms of biliary colic. The finding of multiple gallbladder polyps should trigger ultrasound follow-up in the asymptomatic patient (see above).

INFLAMMATORY GALLBLADDER DISEASE

Cholecystitis is usually associated with gallstones; the frictional action of stones on the gallbladder wall causes some degree of inflammation in almost all cases. The inner mucosa of the wall is injured, allowing the access of enteric bacteria. The inflammatory process may be long-standing and chronic, acute, or a combination of acute inflammation on a chronic background.

Acute Cholecystitis

Acute inflammation of the gallbladder presents with severe right upper quadrant (RUQ) pain localized to the gallbladder area. The pain can be elicited by (gently!) pressing the gallbladder with the ultrasound transducer – a positive ultrasound Murphy's sign. (This sign, although a useful pointer to acute inflammation, is not specific and can be frequently elicited in other conditions, such as chronic inflammatory cases.)

On ultrasound, the gallbladder wall is thickened – greater than 2 mm. This is not in itself a specific sign

(Table 3.1), but characteristically the thickening in acute cholecystitis is symmetrical, affecting the entire wall, and there is an echo-poor "halo" around the gallbladder as a result of edematous changes (Fig. 3.32). However, this is not invariable, and focal thickening may be present, or the wall may be uniformly hyperechoic in some cases.

Pericholecystic fluid may also be present, and the inflammatory process may spread to the adjacent liver. Complications may occur if the acute inflammation progresses (see below) because of infection, the formation of pericholecystic abscesses, and peritonitis.

Further Management of Acute Cholecystitis

In uncomplicated acute cholecystitis, analgesia to settle the patient in the short term is followed by laparoscopic removal of the gallbladder. Open surgery is reserved for more complex cases.[25,26]

If unsuitable for immediate surgery, for example, in cases complicated by peritonitis, the patient is managed with antibiotics and/or percutaneous drainage of pericholecystic fluid or infected bile from the gallbladder usually under ultrasound guidance. This allows the patient's symptoms to settle and reduces morbidity from the subsequent elective operation. Ultrasound is also useful in guiding bedside cholecystostomy or abscess drainage prior to elective surgical treatment.[27]

The gallbladder may appear thick-walled in the presence of adjacent inflammatory processes, such

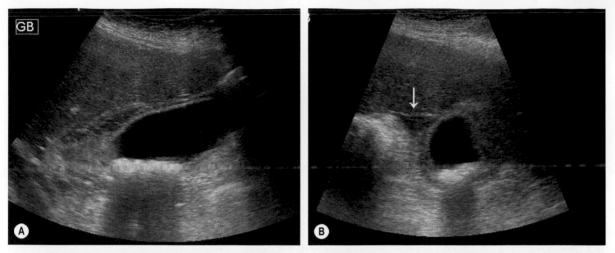

Fig. 3.32 Acute cholecystitis: (A) The gallbladder contains stones, has an edematous, thickened wall, and is tender on scanning. (B) TS of an acutely inflamed gallbladder, with a thickened wall and stones. Pericholecystic fluid is present (arrow).

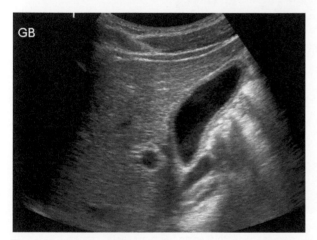

Fig. 3.33 A normal gallbladder in a patient with hepatitis C demonstrates a thickened wall, which should not be confused with acute cholecystitis.

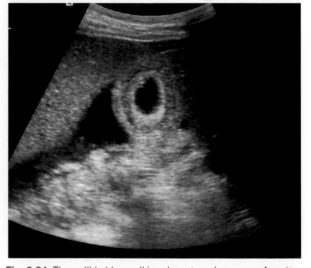

Fig. 3.34 The gallbladder wall is edematous because of ascites resulting from liver failure.

as hepatitis (Fig. 3.33). Ascites will often cause a normal gallbladder wall to look edematous and thickened (Fig. 3.34).

Chronic Cholecystitis

Usually associated with gallstones, chronic cholecystitis presents with lower grade, recurring RUQ pain. The action of stones on the wall causes it to become fibrosed and irregularly thickened, frequently appearing hyperechoic (Fig. 3.35). The gallbladder may be shrunken and contracted, having little or no recognizable lumen around the stones.

Chronic cholecystitis may be complicated by episodes of acute inflammation on a background of the chronic condition.

Most gallbladders that contain stones show at least some histological degree of chronic cholecystitis, even if wall thickening is not apparent on ultrasound.

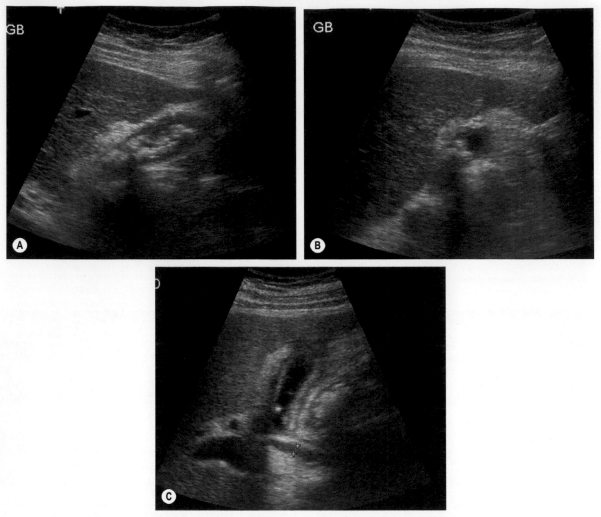

Fig. 3.35 Chronic cholecystitis; (A) A hyperechoic, irregular, thickened wall. The gallbladder is contracted and contains numerous stones. (B) TS demonstrating irregular wall thickening with multiple stones. (C) Considerable wall thickening in chronic cholecystitis. Mildly tender on scanning.

Acalculous Cholecystitis

Inflammation of the gallbladder without stones is relatively uncommon, accounting for around 10% of cases of acute cholecystitis.[28] A thickened, tender gallbladder wall in the absence of any other obvious cause of thickening may be because of acalculous cholecystitis. Traditionally this condition is associated with patients who are already hospitalized and have been fasting, including post-trauma patients, those recovering from surgical procedures, and patients with diabetes. It is brought about by bile stasis leading to a distended gallbladder and subsequently decreased blood flow to the

gallbladder. This, especially in the weakened postoperative state, can lead to infection. However, it also occurs in otherwise healthy patients with no history of acute illness or trauma.[28]

Because no stones are present, the diagnosis is more difficult and may be delayed. Patients with acalculous cholecystitis are more likely to have severe pain and fever by the time the diagnosis is made, increasing the incidence of complications such as perforation.

The wall may appear normal on ultrasound in the early stages but progressively thickens (Fig. 3.36). Biliary sludge is usually present, and a pericholecystic abscess

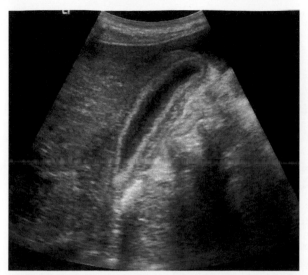

Fig. 3.36 Acalculous cholecystitis. The gallbladder wall is markedly thickened and tender on scanning.

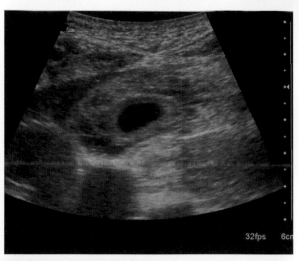

Fig. 3.37 Acute on chronic cholecystitis. A patient with known gallstones and chronic cholecystitis presents with an episode of acute gallbladder pain. The wall is considerably more thickened and hyperechoic than on previous scans and is now tender on scanning.

may develop in the later stages. A positive Murphy's sign may help to focus on the diagnosis, but in unconscious patients, the diagnosis is a particularly difficult one.

In patients already critically ill with their presenting disease or following surgery, ultrasound plays a role in guiding percutaneous cholecystostomy at the bedside to relieve the symptoms.[29]

Chronic acalculous cholecystitis implies a recurrent presentation with typical symptoms of biliary colic but no evident stones on ultrasound. Patients may also demonstrate a low ejection fraction during a cholecystokinin-stimulated hepatic iminodiacetic acid scan. The symptoms are relieved by elective laparoscopic cholecystectomy in most patients, with similar results to those for gallstone disease (although some are found to have a biliary pathologic condition at surgery which might explain the symptoms – such as polyps, cholesterolosis, or biliary crystals/tiny stones, in addition to chronic inflammation).[30]

Complications of Cholecystitis

Acute on Chronic Cholecystitis

Patients with a long-standing history of chronic cholecystitis may experience (sometimes repeated) attacks of acute inflammation. The gallbladder wall is thickened, as for chronic inflammation, and may become focally thickened with both hypo- and hyperechoic regions. Stones are usually present (Fig. 3.37).

Gangrenous Cholecystitis

In a small percentage of patients, acute gallbladder inflammation progresses to gangrenous cholecystitis. Areas of necrosis develop within the gallbladder wall. The wall itself may bleed, and small abscesses form (Fig. 3.38). This severe complication of the inflammatory process requires immediate cholecystectomy.

The gallbladder wall is friable and may rupture, causing a pericholecystic collection and possibly peritonitis. Inflammatory spread may be seen in the adjacent liver tissue as a hypoechoic, ill-defined area. Loops of the adjacent bowel may become adherent to the necrotic wall, forming a cholecystoenteric fistula. This condition is rare but tends to be associated with older patients, often with a background of diabetes or cardiovascular disease, and carries increased morbidity and mortality.[31]

The wall is asymmetrically thickened, and areas of abscess formation may be demonstrated. The damaged inner mucosa sloughs off, forming the appearance of membranes in the gallbladder lumen. The gallbladder frequently contains infected debris. The presence of a bile leak may also be demonstrated with hepatobiliary scintigraphy, using technetium[99M], which is useful in identifying a bile collection that may otherwise be obscured by bowel on ultrasound.

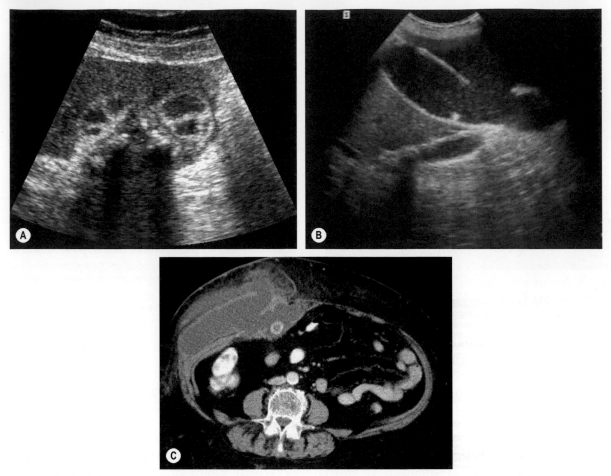

Fig. 3.38 Gangrenous cholecystitis: (A) The gallbladder wall is irregularly thickened, and an intramural abscess has formed on the anterior aspect. (B) The gallbladder has perforated, and a large pericholecystic bile collection has formed. (C) CT of the case in (B), showing perforation of the gallbladder.

Emphysematous Cholecystitis

This is a form of acute gangrenous cholecystitis in which the inflamed gallbladder may become infected, particularly in diabetic patients with gas-forming organisms. Both the lumen and the wall of the gallbladder may contain air, which is highly reflective, but which casts a "noisy," less definite shadow than that from stones. Discrete gas bubbles have been reported on ultrasound within the gallbladder wall[32] and may also extend into the intrahepatic biliary ducts.[33] The air rises to the anterior part of the gallbladder, obscuring the features behind it (Fig. 3.39). This effect may mimic air-filled bowel on ultrasound.

Emphysematous cholecystitis has traditionally had a much higher mortality rate than other forms of cholecystitis, requiring immediate cholecystectomy. However, improvements in ultrasound resolution and the early clinical recognition of this condition suggest that it is now being diagnosed earlier and may be managed more conservatively. The gas in the gallbladder may be confirmed on a plain X-ray (Fig. 3.40), but ultrasound is more sensitive in demonstrating the earlier stages.

Gallbladder Empyema

Empyema is a complication of cholecystitis in which the gallbladder becomes infected behind an obstructed cystic duct. Fine echoes caused by pus are present in the bile (Fig. 3.41). These patients may initially present with the usual features of acute cholecystitis but may then progress to become very ill with fever and acute pain. Localized perforation of the gallbladder wall may cause leakage of infected bile to form a pericholecystic gallbladder collection with subsequent peritonitis.

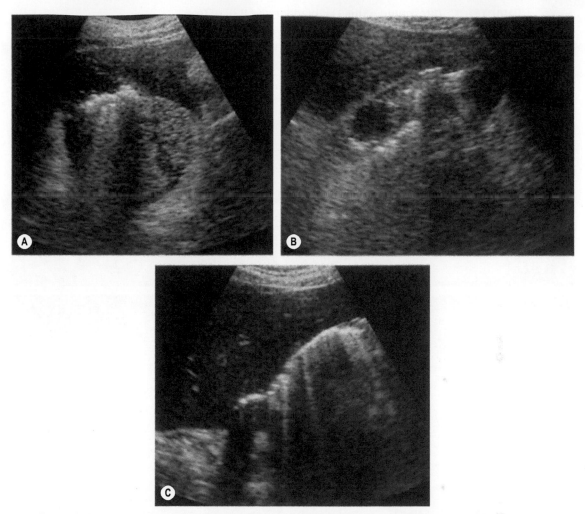

Fig. 3.39 Emphysematous cholecystitis. (A & B) TS and LS with gas and debris in the gallbladder lumen. (C) Gas in the gallbladder lumen completely obscures the contents.

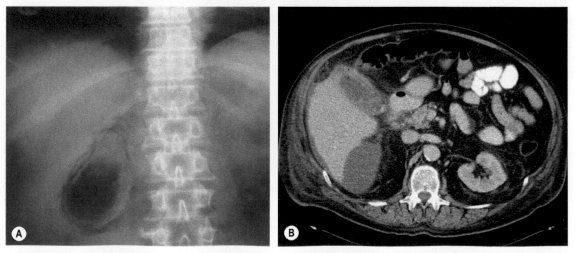

Fig. 3.40 Emphysematous cholecystitis. (A) X-ray demonstrating gas in the gallbladder in emphysematous cholecystitis. (B) CT shows small gas bubbles in the wall of the gallbladder.

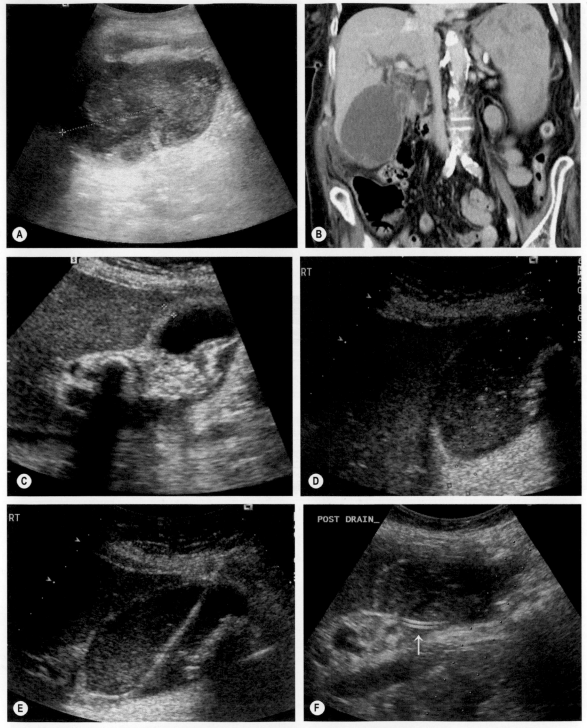

Fig. 3.41 Gallbladder empyema. (A) Dilated tender gallbladder full of pus. (B) CT of the case in (A). (C) Another case of gallbladder empyema with stones blocking the neck of the gallbladder. (D) A gallbladder empyema is about to undergo ultrasound-guided drainage. (E) The guidewire is inserted. (F) A drain (arrow) has been inserted into another case of gallbladder empyema under ultrasound guidance.

Ultrasound may be used to guide bedside drainage (Fig. 3.41D–F) to allow the patient's symptoms to settle before surgery is attempted.[34]

BILIARY TREE DILATATION

Obstructive Jaundice and Biliary Duct Dilation

Obstruction of the biliary tree most commonly occurs around the distal (lower) end of the common duct and almost always results in dilatation of the bile ducts within the liver. In a few cases, it is possible to have an obstruction that fails to dilate the biliary tree, and it is also possible for the biliary tree to be dilated but not obstructed. However, most cases of biliary duct dilatation are caused by obstruction of the common duct, the most common causes being stones or a neoplasm of the bile duct, ampulla, or head of the pancreas. Up to 20% of patients with gallbladder stones will develop choledocholithiasis.[4]

The patient with obstructive jaundice may present with upper abdominal pain, abnormal LFTs (see Chapter 2), and if the obstruction is not intermittent, the sclera of the eye and the skin adopt a yellow tinge.

Assessment of the Level of Obstruction

It is possible for the sonographer to work out where the obstructing lesion is situated by observing which parts of the biliary tree are dilated (Fig. 3.42):

- Dilatation of the CBD (i.e., that portion of the duct below the cystic duct insertion) implies obstruction at its lower end.

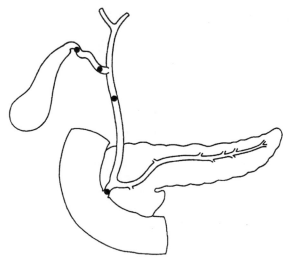

Fig. 3.42 Sites of possible gallstone obstruction.

- Dilatation of both biliary and pancreatic ducts implies obstruction distally at the head of the pancreas or ampulla of Vater. This is more likely to be because of carcinoma of the head of the pancreas, ampulla, or acute pancreatitis than a stone. However, it is possible for a stone to be lodged just distal to the confluence of the biliary and pancreatic ducts.
- Dilatation of the gallbladder alone (i.e., without ductal dilatation) is usually caused by obstruction at the neck or cystic duct (Fig. 3.18).

To assess whether the gallbladder is pathologically dilated may be difficult on ultrasound. The dilated gallbladder will have a rounded, bulging shape because of the increase in pressure inside it.

A gallbladder whose wall has become fibrosed from chronic cholecystitis because of stones will often lose the ability to distend so that the biliary ducts can look grossly dilated despite the gallbladder remaining "normal" in size or contracted.

Early Ductal Obstruction

Beware of very early common duct obstruction before the duct becomes obviously dilated, the duct may be mildly dilated at the lower end, just proximal to a stone, but normal in its intrahepatic portion. Likewise, intermittent obstruction by a small stone at the lower end of the duct may be non-dilated when the scan is performed (Fig. 3.20).

A significant ultrasound feature in the absence of any other identifiable findings is that of thickening of the wall of the bile duct. This not only represents an inflammatory process in the duct wall, which may be found in patients with small stones in a non-dilated duct but is also associated with sclerosing cholangitis.[35]

It is sometimes technically difficult in some patients (particularly those with diffuse liver disease) to determine whether a tubular structure on ultrasound represents a dilated duct or a blood vessel. Color Doppler will differentiate the dilated bile duct from a branch of the hepatic artery or portal vein (Fig. 3.43), provided that the vein is not thrombosed, of course.

It is not useful to use color Doppler routinely to locate the CBD; the angle of insonation is frequently perpendicular to the beam, so the vein may display no color signal, confusing the operator further. In addition, the application of color Doppler reduces the line density and image resolution – exactly the opposite of what you require when searching for a small duct.

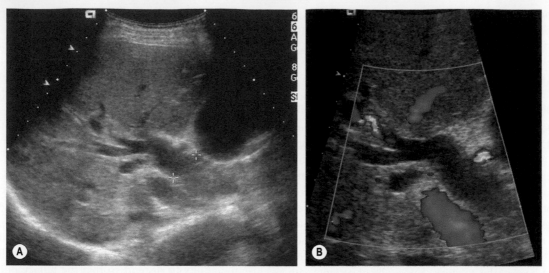

Fig. 3.43 (A & B) Dilated biliary ducts do not demonstrate flow on color or power Doppler, differentiating them from portal vessels.

Diagnosis and Assessment of the Cause of Obstruction

The numerous causes of biliary dilatation are summarized in Table 3.2. Frequently, ultrasound diagnoses the obstruction but does not identify the cause. This is a case for perseverance by the operator, as the lower end of the CBD is visible in most cases once the overlying duodenum has been moved away (Figs. 3.19, 3.20, 3.44). However, ultrasound is not generally regarded as a reliable tool for identifying ductal stones and is frequently unable to diagnose ductal strictures, especially those from benign causes. In the absence of a definite diagnosis of stones, MRCP is an effective, non-invasive technique in the diagnosis of CBD stones and strictures (Fig. 3.44F),[5,36] avoiding the need for the more invasive ERCP.

Although diagnostically highly accurate, the use of ERCP is usually reserved for occasions when therapeutic stone removal or stent insertion may be required, as it is an invasive procedure with attendant risks of pancreatitis, cholangitis, and rarely, perforation of the bile duct or duodenum.[37,38] Complications occur in up to 8% of patients undergoing ERCP, with a mortality rate of up to 0.5%,[39] so the technique should ideally be reserved for those requiring therapeutic intervention.

EUS also has accuracy in detecting CBD stones comparable with ERCP while avoiding the risks associated

TABLE 3.2	Causes of Biliary Duct Dilatation
Intrinsic	Stones
	Carcinoma of the ampulla of Vater
	Cholangiocarcinoma
	Stricture (associated with chronic pancreatitis)
	Biliary atresia/choledochal cyst
	Post liver transplantation bile duct stenosis (usually anastomotic)
	Parasites
	Age-related or post-surgical mild CBD dilatation
Extrinsic	Carcinoma of the head of the pancreas
	Acute pancreatitis
	Lymphadenopathy at the porta hepatis
	Other masses at the porta, e.g., hepatic artery aneurysm, gastrointestinal tract mass
	Intrahepatic tumors (obstructed distal segments)
Diffuse hepatic conditions	Sclerosing cholangitis
	Caroli's disease

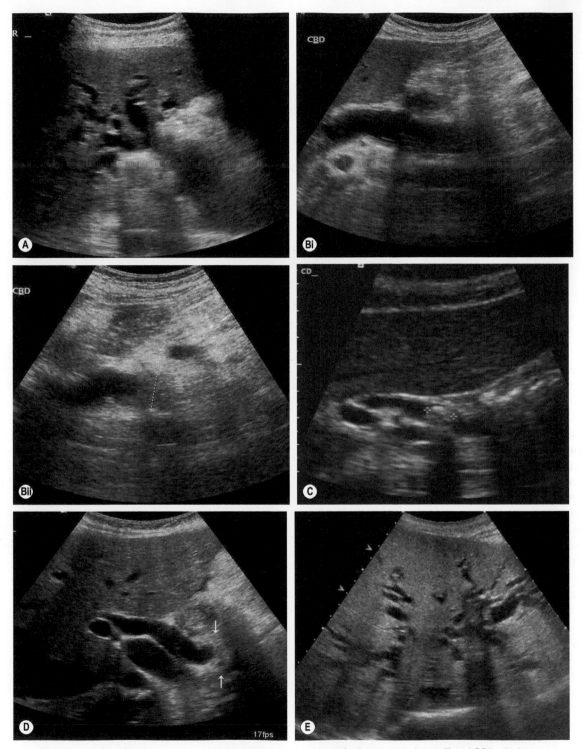

Fig. 3.44 (A) Duodenal gas obscures the cause of obstruction at the lower end of this dilated CBD. (B) Patient positioning can move bowel gas away from the duct (Bi), demonstrating the cause of obstruction (Bii) – a carcinoma of the ampulla confirmed on EUS. (C) A mildly dilated CBD with a stone (calipers). (D) Dilated CBD caused by a lymph node mass at the porta hepatis (arrows). (E) Intrahepatic bile duct dilatation.

Continued

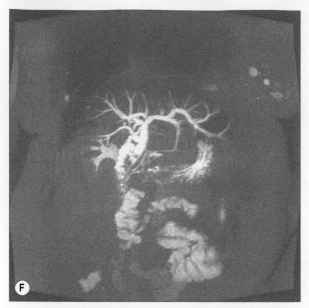

Fig. 3.44, cont'd (F) MRCP demonstrates a stone in the lower end of the duct.

with radiation and biliary instrumentation. It is not yet as readily available as ERCP and requires specialist skills and equipment with a significant learning curve.[40] CT and MRI are useful for staging purposes if the obstructing lesion is malignant. Cholangiocarcinomas spread to the lymph nodes and the liver – and small liver deposits are particularly difficult to recognize on ultrasound if the intrahepatic biliary ducts are dilated.

In hepatobiliary scintigraphy, technetium[99M]-labeled derivatives of iminodiacetic acid are excreted in the bile and may help to demonstrate sites of obstruction, e.g., in the cystic duct – or abnormal accumulations of bile, e.g., choledochal cysts. The technique is also useful in demonstrating postoperative bile leaks.[41]

Courvoisier's law, to which there are numerous exceptions, states that if the gallbladder is dilated in a jaundiced patient, then the cause is *not* because of a stone in the common duct. The reasoning behind this is that gallstones cause a degree of wall fibrosis from chronic cholecystitis, which would prevent it from distending. There are many exceptions to this "law," which include the formation of stones in the duct, without gallbladder stones, and obstruction by a pancreatic stone at the ampulla.

- Do not assume that obstructive jaundice in a patient with gallstones is because of a stone in the CBD. Jaundice may be attributable to other causes.

- Do not assume that obstructive jaundice cannot be because of a stone in the CBD if the gallbladder does not contain stones. A solitary stone can be passed into the duct from the gallbladder, or stones can form within the duct.

Management of Biliary Obstruction

Management of biliary obstruction obviously depends on the cause and the severity of the condition. Radiological imaging may be used for both diagnostic and therapeutic purposes. The first line of investigation tends to be ultrasound. Patients may then be directed either for further imaging, such as MRCP or CT, to clarify the diagnosis or proceed straight to therapeutic intervention. Removal of stones in the CBD may be performed by ERCP with sphincterotomy. Elective, laparoscopic cholecystectomy may occur if gallstones are present in the gallbladder.

Laparoscopic ultrasound is a useful adjunct to the surgical exploration of the biliary tree, and its accuracy in experienced hands equals that of X-ray cholangiography. Its potential has been slow to be realized in many centers, as it requires training and has a steep learning curve. However, the lack of ionizing radiation, together with its accuracy in experienced hands, has allowed it to replace fluoroscopic cholangiography in some centers.[42]

EUS can also be used to examine the CBD, avoiding the need for laparoscopic exploration of the duct. It is highly accurate in diagnosing ductal stones, particularly in experienced hands[43] and may be more sensitive than MRCP in the detection of small ductal stones (depending on the MRCP slice thickness).[44] However, its invasive nature means it is usually reserved for cases when MRCP is negative in patients where the probability of stones or an obstructing lesion remains high.

The treatment of malignant obstruction is determined by the stage of the disease. Accurate staging is best performed using CT and/or MRI. If surgical removal of the obstructing lesion is not a suitable option because of local or distant spread or other comorbidities, palliative stenting may be performed endoscopically to relieve the obstruction and decompress the ducts (Fig. 3.45). The patency of the stent may be subsequently monitored with ultrasound by assessing the degree of duct dilatation.

Clinical suspicion of early obstruction should be raised if the serum alkaline phosphatase is elevated (often more sensitive in the early stages than a raised serum bilirubin). In the presence of ductal dilatation on

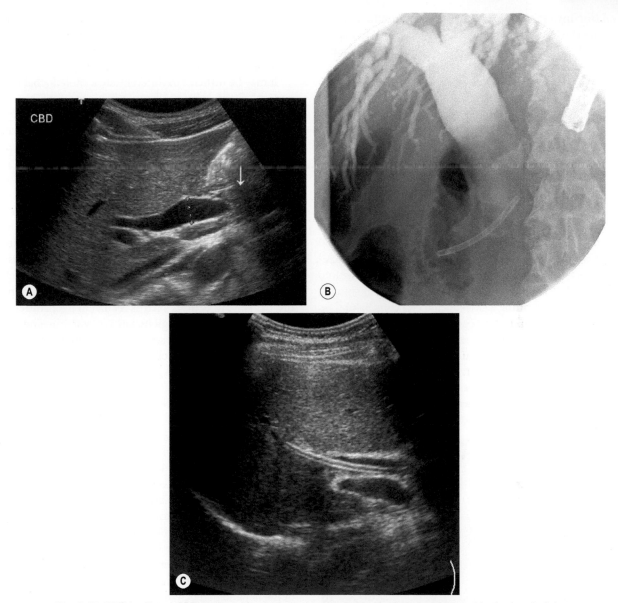

Fig. 3.45 (A) This dilated CBD (calipers) is obstructed by a mass at the lower end (arrow) in the head of the pancreas. (B) ERCP demonstrates a tight, malignant stricture from an ampullary carcinoma. A palliative stent is positioned. (C) Stent in the CBD of a patient with a cholangiocarcinoma. Decompression of the dilated biliary tree has been achieved, and ultrasound can be used to monitor the patency of the stent.

ultrasound, further imaging, such as CT, MRCP, or EUS, may then refine the diagnosis.

Intrahepatic Tumors Causing Biliary Obstruction

Focal masses that cause segmental intrahepatic duct dilatation are usually intrinsic to the duct itself, e.g., cholangiocarcinoma. It is also possible for a focal intrahepatic mass, whether benign or malignant, to compress an adjacent biliary duct, causing subsequent obstruction of that segment. However, this is not a common cause of biliary dilatation and occurs most usually with hepatocellular carcinomas.[45] Most liver metastases deform, rather than compress, adjacent structures, and biliary obstruction only occurs if the metastases are very large and/or invade the biliary tree. A hepatocellular carcinoma (HCC) or metastatic deposit at the porta hepatis may obstruct the common duct by squeezing it against adjacent extrahepatic structures.

Benign intrahepatic lesions rarely cause ductal dilatation, but occasionally their sheer size obstructs the biliary tree.

Choledochal Cysts

Most commonly found in children, this is associated with biliary atresia, in which the distal "blind" end of the duct dilates into a rounded, cystic mass in response to raised intrahepatic pressure. Choledochal cysts in adults are rare and tend to be asymptomatic unless associated with stones or other biliary diseases. They tend to be associated with an anomalous insertion of the CBD into the pancreatic duct, which allows pancreatic enzymes to reflux into the bile duct resulting in inflammation and weakening of the duct wall, forming a choledochal cyst (Fig. 3.46).[46]

The dilatation is less common because of a non-obstructive cause in which the biliary ducts become ectatic and can form diverticula. This may be because of a focal stricture of the duct, which causes reflux and a localized enlargement of the duct proximal to the stricture (see also "Caroli's Disease" below).

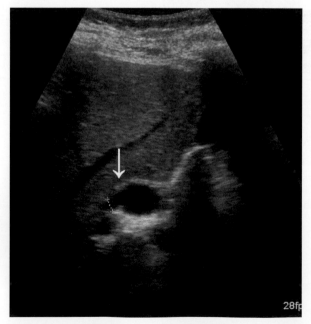

Fig. 3.46 A small choledochal cyst (arrow) at the porta can be seen communicating with the biliary tree (calipers).

Complications of choledochal cysts include cholangitis, formation of stones, and progression of the condition to secondary biliary cirrhosis, which may be associated with portal hypertension.

It may be difficult to differentiate a choledochal cyst, particularly if solitary, from other causes of hepatic cysts. The connection between the choledochal cyst and the adjacent biliary duct may be demonstrated with careful scanning, but further imaging, including MRCP, is frequently required.

Cholangitis

Cholangitis is an inflammation of the biliary ducts. It most commonly occurs secondary to obstruction, where stasis of bile in the biliary tree may lead to infection and acute inflammation of the ducts. Other causes of cholangitis include strictures or stenosis of ducts, post-ERCP, or duct manipulation, AIDS cholangiopathy, parasitic infections such as recurrent pyogenic cholangitis (oriental cholangiohepatitis), which is endemic in Southeast Asia, and sclerosing cholangitis (see also "Primary Sclerosing Cholangitis" below).

Duct dilatation may be present, depending on the cause of the cholangitis. In severe cases, the duct walls appear thickened and irregular, and debris can be seen in the larger ducts (Fig. 3.47). Care should be taken to differentiate ductal wall thickening from tumor invasion, and further imaging may be necessary to exclude malignancy.

Bacterial cholangitis is the most common form because of ascending bacterial infection from the duodenum or portal vein. Bacterial cholangitis is also associated with biliary enteric anastomoses and may be complicated by abscesses if the infection is progressive and untreated. Small abscesses may be difficult to diagnose on ultrasound, as they are frequently isoechoic and ill-defined in the early stages, and biliary dilatation makes evaluation of the hepatic parenchyma notoriously difficult.

Contrast CT may identify small abscesses not visible on ultrasound, and MRCP or ERCP demonstrates mural changes in the ducts.

Biliary Dilatation Without Jaundice
Post-Surgical CBD Dilatation

In patients who have had cholecystectomy associated with previous dilatation of the CBD, it is common to find a persistent (but non-significant) mild dilatation of the duct postoperatively. The serum alkaline phosphatase and bilirubin levels should be normal in the absence

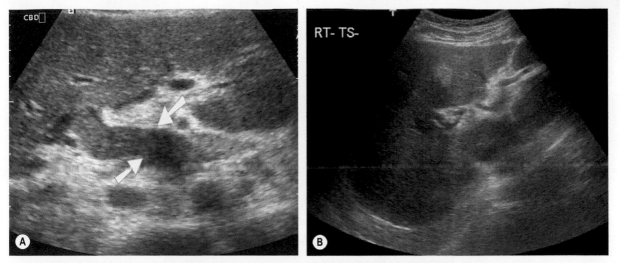

Fig. 3.47 (A) Cholangitis with debris present in the dilated CBD (arrows). (B) Hyperechoic thickened and inflamed portal tracts in a patient with chronic cholangitis.

of a pathologic condition. Because stones may be found in the duct postoperatively, it is important to differentiate non-obstructive from truly obstructive dilatation in a symptomatic patient (Fig. 3.48A). If in doubt, the patient may be rescanned at a suitable interval to assess any increase in ductal diameter.

Focal obstruction. Intrahepatic tumors, such as cholangiocarcinoma, may obstruct a segment of the biliary tree while the remainder of the liver and biliary tree appears normal. Focal duct dilatation should trigger the operator to examine the proximal area of dilatation for a possible mass. Such tumors may be present before jaundice is clinically apparent.

Pitfalls. Patients with cirrhosis and portal hypertension may have dilated hepatic arteries, which can mimic the appearances of dilated ducts (Fig. 3.48B, C). Color or power Doppler will readily differentiate between these, as the bile duct lacks a Doppler signal. However, care must be taken to use an appropriate angle of insonation to display the Doppler signal in the blood vessels, as both duct *and* patent vessels may display no color if perpendicular to the sound beam.

Pneumobilia (air in the ducts) casts a distal acoustic shadow and may obscure ductal dilatation.

Obstruction Without Biliary Dilatation
Early Obstruction
It is possible to scan a patient at the time of recent onset of obstruction from a stone before the ducts have had time to dilate, leading to a false-negative diagnosis. If clinical suspicion persists, a rescan is frequently useful in these cases.

Occasionally, stones have a ball-valve effect in the duct, causing an intermittent obstruction which may not demonstrate ductal dilatation on the ultrasound scan.

Fibrosis of the Duct Walls
Several chronic pathological conditions cause the walls of the ducts to become fibrotic and stiff. These include PSC (see below), hepatitis, and other chronic hepatic diseases leading to cirrhosis. The liver itself becomes rigid, and this prevents biliary dilatation. In such cases, the lack of dilated bile ducts does not necessarily imply an absence of obstruction.

OTHER BILIARY DISEASES

Primary Sclerosing Cholangitis (PSC)
PSC is a rare form of chronic, cholestatic hepatobiliary disease in which the walls of the bile ducts become inflamed, causing narrowing. It predominantly affects young men (with a 2:1 male to female ratio) and is characterized by multiple biliary strictures and bead-like dilatations of the ducts. The cause of PSC remains unclear, but it is associated with inflammatory bowel disorders or may be idiopathic.

Clinical features include jaundice, itching, and fatigue. Twenty-five percent of patients also have

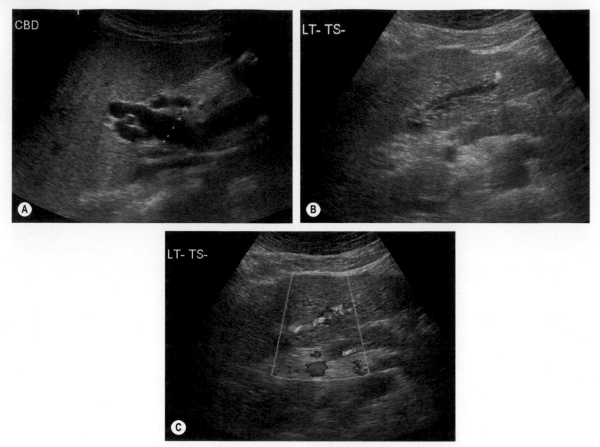

Fig. 3.48 (A) Biliary dilatation following laparoscopic cholecystectomy because of a surgical clip across the CBD. (B) The appearance of dilated ducts is a pitfall in patients with portal hypertension. (C) Color Doppler reveals that the dilated "tube" is actually an enlarged artery, not a duct.

gallstones, complicating the diagnosis; 70% of affected patients also have ulcerative colitis. Progressive, gradual fibrosis causes strictures and eventually obliterates the biliary tree. Untreated, this leads to hepatic failure. PSC has a strong association with cholangiocarcinoma, and it is this, rather than hepatic failure, which may lead to death. In the absence of malignancy, however, hepatic transplantation has a 70%-90% five-year survival rate,[47] although recurrence of the disease is a recognized complication.[48]

Ultrasound appearances. The ultrasound appearances in PSC may be normal, particularly in the early stages, or may demonstrate a coarse, hyperechoic liver texture. Ductal strictures may cause downstream dilatation in some segments (Fig. 3.49), and in some cases, there is marked biliary dilatation. However, in most patients, the biliary ducts are prevented from dilatation by the surrounding fibrosis and so appear unremarkable on

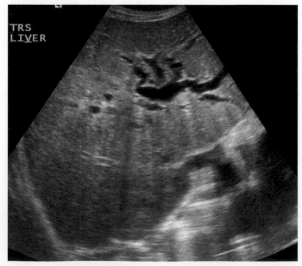

Fig. 3.49 Localized biliary dilatation because of a ductal stricture in a patient with PSC.

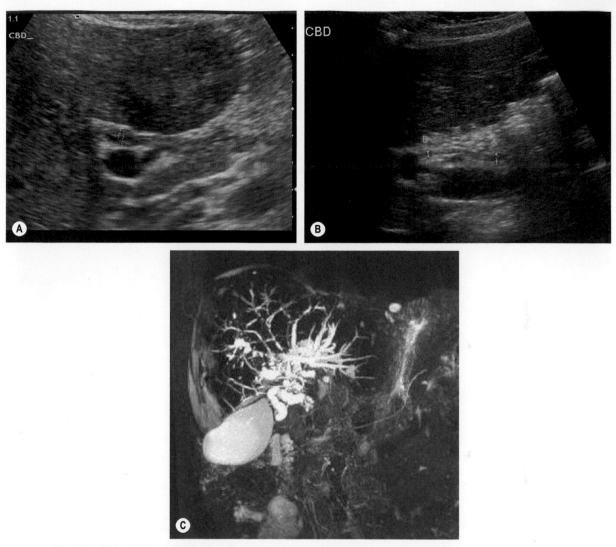

Fig. 3.50 PSC: (A) Mural thickening in this normal caliber CBD is typical of PSC (proven on biopsy). (B) Another case of PSC demonstrating thickening of a very narrow duct (calipers) and strictures in the CBD. (C) MRCP demonstrating numerous bile duct strictures in PSC.

ultrasound. MRCP is superior at demonstrating intrahepatic ductal strictures (Fig. 3.50). Mural thickening, particularly in the CBD, may be demonstrated with careful scanning (Fig. 3.50A),[49] and may be the only ultrasound sign. Ultrasound also demonstrates the effects of portal hypertension in advanced disease. The gallbladder may also have a thickened wall and can be dilated.[50]

Due to the association between PSC and cholangiocarcinoma, which may be multifocal, a careful search must be done for mass lesions. Because the ultrasound appearances may be those of a coarse, nodular liver texture, it is difficult to identify small cholangiocarcinomas.

Ultrasound contrast may help to highlight suspected lesions (Fig. 3.51), but MRI is the next investigation of choice to stage the disease. The diagnosis is an important one because the patient's prognosis and management are affected by the presence of cholangiocarcinoma. If no masses are identified, the prognosis is favorable, and patients may benefit from the endoscopic removal of stones to relieve symptoms, endoscopic stenting of main duct strictures to relieve jaundice, and subsequent liver transplantation to preempt the formation of carcinoma. However, if carcinoma is already present, five-year survival falls to 10%.

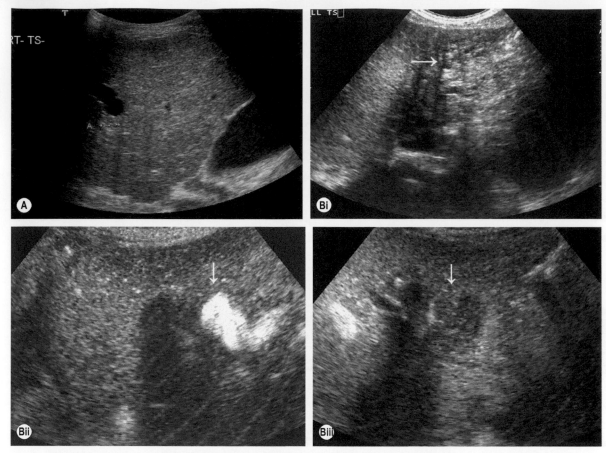

Fig. 3.51 (A) Focally dilated bile ducts are a clue to the tiny cholangiocarcinoma (calipers) in this patient with PSC. (Bi) A cholangiocarcinoma is suspected because of focally dilated intrahepatic ducts (arrow) but not visualized on ultrasound. (Bii) CEUS demonstrates arterial enhancement of the lesions (arrow) with (Biii) sinusoidal phase hypoenhancement.

Primary Biliary Cirrhosis (PBC)

PBC is another example of a cholestatic disease that gradually obliterates the biliary tree and ultimately leads to cirrhosis. It is discussed more fully in Chapter 2.

Caroli's Disease (Congenital Intrahepatic Biliary Dilatation)

This is a rare, congenital condition where the bile ducts are irregularly dilated with diverticula-like projections. These diverticula may become infected and may separate off from the biliary duct, forming choledochal cysts (Fig. 3.52). In most cases, the entire hepatobiliary system is affected to some degree. Sufferers may present in early childhood, with symptoms of portal hypertension,[51] or may remain well until adulthood, presenting with cholangitis. It is generally thought to be an autosomal

recessive, inherited condition, and the prognosis is poor. Medical control of associated portal hypertension with varices can improve the quality of life.

In a few cases, the disease is confined to one or two segments of the liver, in which case a cure can be effected with hepatic resection.[52] The extrahepatic biliary tree is often unaffected.

The ultrasound appearances are usually widespread intrahepatic duct dilatation, with saccular and fusiform biliary ectasia. The diagnosis is often unclear because it is also associated with biliary stone formation. The dilatation is also associated with cholangitis, and signs of infection may be present in the form of debris within the ducts or even abscesses. Sometimes frank choledochal cysts can be located.

Advanced disease is associated with portal hypertension and, in some cases, cholangiocarcinoma.[53]

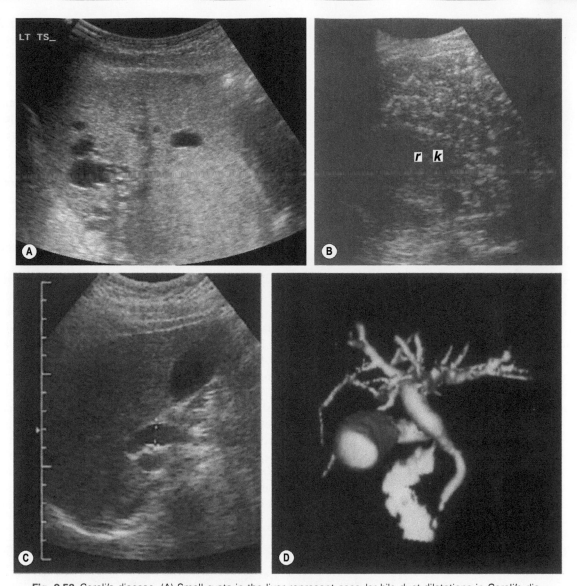

Fig. 3.52 Caroli's disease. (A) Small cysts in the liver represent saccular bile duct dilatations in Caroli's disease. (B) TS of a different patient with end-stage disease. The grossly abnormal liver texture contrasts with the right kidney. (C) A small section of focal CBD dilatation persisted in a symptomatic patient with normal caliber distal CBD. This was confirmed on ERCP and thought to be a dyskinetic segment, causing biliary reflux, but was later diagnosed as a mild form of Caroli's. (D) 3D CT reconstruction of the case in (C), confirming the ultrasound appearances. Note the tiny ectatic "pouchings" of the intrahepatic ducts characteristic of Caroli's.

The presence of multiple cystic spaces on imaging must not be confused with multi- or polycystic disease, and the identification of communication between the cysts and the biliary tree with CT or MRI is an important factor in making the diagnosis.[54]

Parasites

Parasitic organisms, such as the *Ascaris* worm and liver fluke, are extremely rare in the United Kingdom. However, they are a common cause of biliary colic in Africa, the Far East, and South America. Hyperechoic

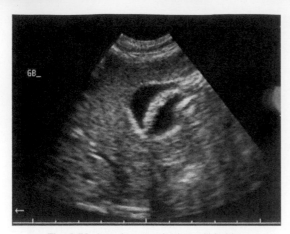

Fig. 3.53 Ascaris worm in the gallbladder.

linear structures in the gallbladder lumen or dilated ducts should raise the sonographer's suspicion in patients native to or those who have visited these countries.[55] Impacted worms in the biliary ducts may also mimic other ductal masses, and they are a rare cause of obstructive biliary dilatation (Fig. 3.53).

Patients may present with acute cholangitis or abdominal pain and vomiting. Endoscopic management is frequently highly effective.[56]

Echogenic Bile
Biliary Stasis and Bile Crystals
Fine echoes in the bile within the gallbladder are not uncommon on an ultrasound scan. This is common because of the inspissation of bile following prolonged starvation – for example, following surgery (Fig. 3.54). These appearances disappear after a normal diet is resumed, and the gallbladder has emptied and refilled. Echogenic bile occurs when the solutes in the bile precipitate, often because of hypomotility of the gallbladder, and can commonly be seen following bone marrow transplantation and in patients who have undergone prolonged periods (4–6 weeks) of total parenteral nutrition.[57]

Prolonged biliary stasis may lead to inflammation and/or infection, particularly in postoperative patients and those in immunosuppression. Its clinical course varies from complete resolution to progression to gallstones. However, following the resumption of oral feeding, the gallbladder may contract and empty the sludge into the biliary tree causing biliary colic, acute pancreatitis, and/or acute cholecystitis.[58] For this reason, cholecystectomy may be considered in symptomatic patients with biliary sludge.

The fine echoes may form a gravity-dependent layer and may clump together, forming "sludge" balls (Fig. 3.54B). To avoid misdiagnosing sludge balls as polyps, turn the patient to disperse the echoes or rescan after the patient has resumed a normal diet.

Biliary stasis is associated with an increased risk of stone formation.[59] Occasionally, echogenic bile persists even with normal gallbladder function (Fig. 3.55). It is likely that there is a spectrum of biliary disease in which gallbladder dysmotility and subsequent saturation of the bile leads to the formation of crystals in the bile and also in the gallbladder wall. Some particles become quite large, forming microlithiasis, which is likely to be an

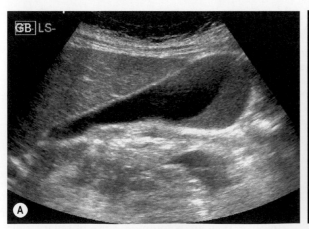

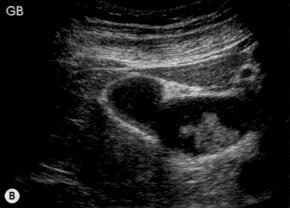

Fig. 3.54 (A) Inspissated bile in the normal gallbladder of a fasting patient. (B) Biliary sludge in a tumefactive "ball" can mimic a polyp. Moving the patient to disperse the sludge avoids this pitfall.

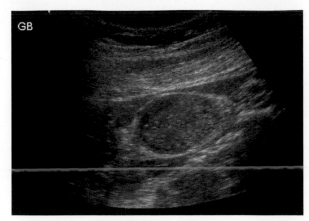

Fig. 3.55 Biliary crystals.

intermediate stage in stone formation.[60] Pain and biliary colic may be present prior to stone formation. Biliary crystals or "microlithiasis" (usually calcium bilirubinate granules) have a strong association with acute pancreatitis,[61] and their presence in patients who do not have gallstones may therefore be highly significant.

Obstructive Causes of Biliary Stasis

Pathological bile stasis in the gallbladder is because of obstruction of the cystic duct (from a stone, for example) and may be demonstrated in a normal-sized or dilated gallbladder. The bile becomes viscous and hyperechoic. The biliary ducts remain normal in caliber. Eventually, the bile turns watery and appears echo-free on ultrasound; this is known as a mucocele (see above).

Bile stasis within the ducts occurs either because of prolonged and/or repetitive obstruction or a cholestatic disease such as PBC (Chapter 2) or PSC. This can lead to cholangitis.

Haemobilia

Blood in the gallbladder can result from gastrointestinal bleeding or other damage to the gallbladder or bile duct wall – for example, iatrogenic trauma from an endoscopic procedure or biopsy – or it may be associated with ruptured hepatic artery aneurysm.

The appearances depend upon the stage of evolution of the bleeding. Fresh blood appears as fine, low-level echoes. Blood clots appear as solid, non-shadowing structures, and there may be hyperechoic, linear strands.[62] A history of trauma may allow the sonographer to differentiate haemobilia from other causes of echogenic bile, particularly those associated with gallbladder inflammation, and there may be other evidence of abdominal trauma on ultrasound – such as a hemoperitoneum.

Pneumobilia

Air in the biliary tree is usually iatrogenic and frequently seen following procedures such as ERCP, sphincterotomy, or biliary surgery. Although it does not usually persist, the air can remain in the biliary tree post-procedure for months, even years, and is not significant.

It is characterized by highly reflective linear echoes (Fig. 3.56), which follow the course of the biliary ducts.

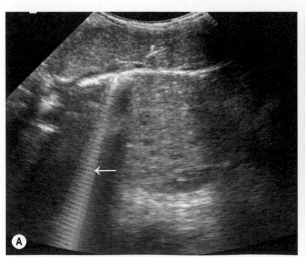

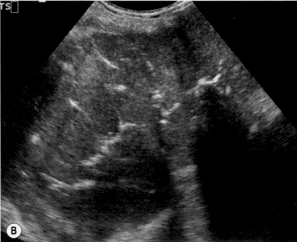

Fig. 3.56 (A & B) Air in the biliary tree following surgery. Note the "reverberative" shadow (arrow).

The air usually casts a shadow that is different from that of stones – often having reverberative artifacts and being much less well-defined or clear. This shadowing obscures the lumen of the duct and can make an evaluation of the hepatic parenchyma difficult.

Pneumobilia may also be present in emphysematous cholecystitis, an uncommon complication of cholecystitis, in which gas-forming bacteria are present in the gallbladder (see above) or in cases where a necrotic gallbladder has formed a cholecystoenteric fistula. Rarely, multiple biliary stones form within the ducts throughout the liver, which can be confused with the appearance of air in the ducts.

MALIGNANT BILIARY DISEASE

Primary Gallbladder Carcinoma

Cancer of the gallbladder is usually associated with gallstones and a history of cholecystitis. Most often, the gallbladder lumen is occupied by a solid mass that may have the appearance of a large polyp. The wall appears thickened and irregular, and shadowing from the stones may obscure it posteriorly. A bile-filled lumen may be absent, further complicating the ultrasound diagnosis (Fig. 3.57). In a porcelain gallbladder (calcification of the gallbladder wall), which is associated with gallblad-

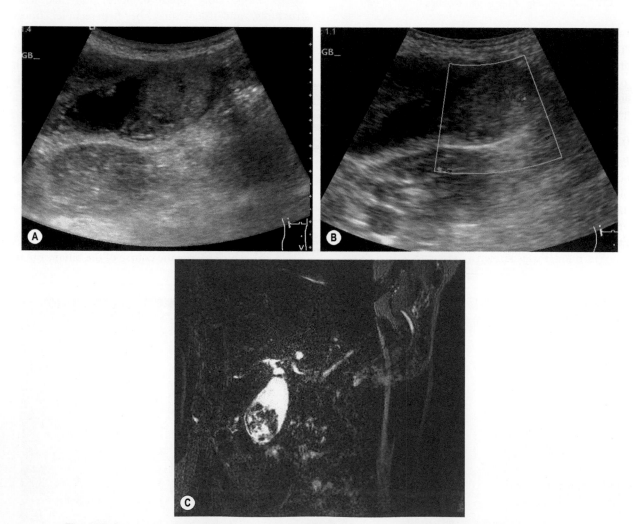

Fig. 3.57 Gallbladder carcinoma: (A) Gallbladder containing solid material, irregular wall thickening. Stones were also present (not shown). (B) Color Doppler shows vascularity in the solid component of the mass. (C) MRCP of gallbladder cancer.

der carcinoma, the shadowing may obscure any lesion in the lumen, making detection almost impossible.

Particular risk factors for gallbladder carcinoma include large stones, polyps of over 1 cm in size, porcelain gallbladder, and occasionally, choledochal cyst because of the anomalous junction of the pancreatobiliary ducts.[15]

The carcinoma itself is frequently asymptomatic in the early stages, and patients tend to present with symptoms relating to the stones. It tends to be an aggressive lesion that quickly metastasizes to the liver and portal nodes and has a very poor prognosis, with a curative surgical resection rate of around 15%–20%. Ultrasound may also demonstrate local spread into the adjacent liver, but further staging with CT is invariably necessary.[63]

Cholangiocarcinoma

This is a malignant lesion arising in the wall of the bile duct. It is readily recognizable from an ultrasound point of view when it occurs in and obstructs the common duct, as the subsequent dilatation outlines the proximal part of the tumor with bile (Fig. 3.58). However, tumors occurring intrahepatically tend to be isoechoic and notoriously difficult to detect. Cholangiocarcinoma may occur at any level along the biliary tree and is frequently multifocal.

A cholangiocarcinoma is referred to as a *Klatskin tumor* when it involves the confluence of the right and left hepatic ducts. These lesions are often difficult to detect on both ultrasound and CT, and the only clue may be the proximal dilatation of the biliary ducts (Fig. 3.59). Contrast-enhanced ultrasound (CEUS) is helpful

in localizing a suspected lesion because of arterial hypervascularity followed by hypoenhancement in the sinusoidal phase (Fig. 3.51).

Although rare, the incidence of cholangiocarcinoma seems to be increasing, and it is strongly associated with PSC (see above).[64]

Multifocal cholangiocarcinoma may spread to the surrounding liver tissue and have a poor prognosis. It may be almost impossible to identify these lesions in a liver with a texture already altered by diffuse disease before they become large. A pattern of dilated ducts distal to the lesion is a good clue (Figs. 3.60, 3.61).

Management of the Patient with Cholangiocarcinoma

These patients have a poor prognosis, as the lesions usually present with jaundice because of invasion and obstruction of the duct. They spread to surrounding tissues, including the portal vein and lymph nodes, metastasize to the liver, and can be multifocal, particularly with PSC.

Staging of the disease is performed with CT or MRI. EUS can outline invasion into the biliary duct, and laparoscopic ultrasound can pick up peritoneal or local spread.

Surgical resection of the tumor is becoming more successful in patients with single lesions,[65] and liver transplantation in patients with PSC has a good prognosis, provided the tumor bulk is low. Palliation is frequently the only feasible option, and the insertion of a stent, either percutaneously or endoscopically, to bypass the obstructing lesion and assist drainage of the liver

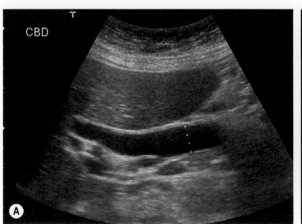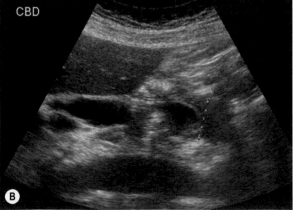

Fig. 3.58 Cholangiocarcinoma: (A) The dilated CBD (calipers) is obstructed by a mass at the lower end, which is largely obscured by the duodenum. (B) Repositioning the patient to move the duodenal gas reveals a cholangiocarcinoma at the lower end of the duct (calipers).

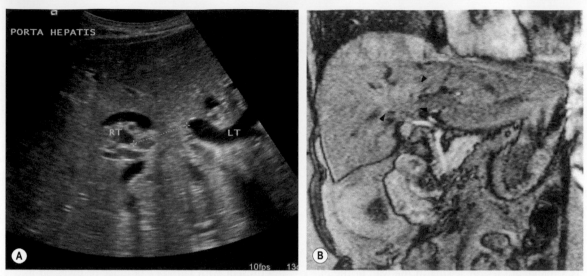

Fig. 3.59 Cholangiocarcinoma. (A) Irregular mass at the porta (calipers) causing right and left biliary duct obstruction – a Klatskin tumor. (B) MRI of the same patient confirming the mass at the porta.

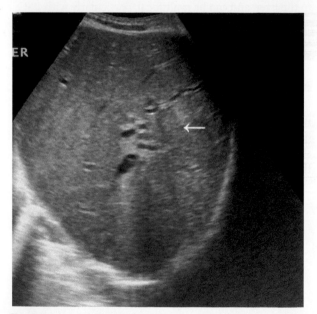

Fig. 3.60 Focally dilated ducts in the peripheral liver are obstructed by a small intrahepatic cholangiocarcinoma (calipers).

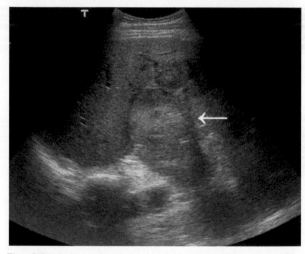

Fig. 3.61 A large intrahepatic cholangiocarcinoma near the porta hepatis (arrow).

will relieve the symptoms and often allows the patient to return home for some months.

Other treatment options, such as chemotherapy, have limited success. Despite improvements in treatment, only a minority of patients survive beyond 12 months after the initial diagnosis.[66]

Gallbladder Metastases

Metastases from other primaries may occasionally be deposited within the gallbladder wall (Fig. 3.62), usually as a late presentation of the disease process. Often, other metastatic deposits, for example, in the liver and lymph nodes, may raise suspicion of gallbladder metastases in an irregularly thickened gallbladder wall.

The ultrasound appearances are of focal thickening and polyp-like lesions in the wall of the gallbladder. This

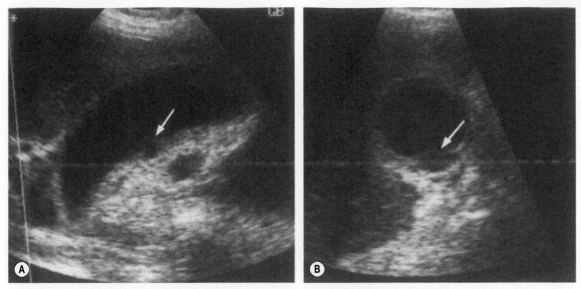

Fig. 3.62 Metastases in the gallbladder wall: (A) LS and (B) TS from advanced ovarian carcinoma.

may mimic primary gallbladder carcinoma, but knowledge of a previously diagnosed primary, for example, melanoma, lung, or breast carcinoma, will point toward the diagnosis.

REFERENCES

1. Shea JA, Berlin JA, Escarce JJ, et al. Revised estimates of diagnostic test sensitivity and specificity in suspected biliary tract disease. *Arch Intern Med.* 1994;154:2573–2581.
2. Pandey M, Khatri AK, Sood BP, et al. Cholecystosonographic evaluation of the prevalence of gallbladder disease: a university hospital experience. *Clin Imaging.* 1996;20:269–272.
3. Schirmer BD, Winters KL, Edlich RF. Cholelithiasis and cholecystitis. *J Long Term Eff Med Implants.* 2005;15:329–338.
4. Freitas M, Bell R, Duffy A. Choledocholithiasis: Evolving standards for diagnosis and management. *World J Gastroenterol.* 2006;12:3162–3167.
5. Hallal AH, Amortegui JD, Jeroukhimov IM, et al. Magnetic resonance cholangiopancreatography accurately detects common bile duct stones in resolving gallstone pancreatitis. *J Am Coll Surg.* 2005;200:869–875.
6. Nathanson LK, O'Rourke NA, Martin IJ, et al. Postoperative ERCP versus laparoscopic choledochotomy for clearance of selected bile duct calculi: a randomized trial. *Ann Surg.* 2005;242:188–192.
7. Liu TH, Consorti ET, Mercer DW. Laparoscopic cholecystectomy for acute cholecystitis: technical considerations and outcome. *Semin Laparosc Surg.* 2002;9:24–31.
8. Tranter SE, Thompson MH. Potential of laparoscopic ultrasonography as an alternative to operative cholangiography in the detection of bile duct stones. *Br J Surg.* 2001;88:65–69.
9. Tranter SE, Thompson MH. A prospective single-blinded controlled study comparing laparoscopic ultrasound of the common bile duct with operative cholangiography. *Surg Endosc.* 2003;17:216–219.
10. Petroni ML, Jazrawi RP, Pazzi P, et al. Risk factors for the development of gallstone recurrence following medical dissolution. The British-Italian Gallstone Study Group. *Eur J Gastroenterol Hepatol.* 2000;12:695–700.
11. Pauletzki J, Sackman M, Holl J, Paumgartner G. Evaluation of gallbladder volume and emptying with a novel three-dimensional ultrasound system: comparison with sum-of-cylinders and the ellipsoid methods. *J Clin Ultrasound.* 1996;24:277–285.
12. Ahlawat SK, Singhania R, Al-Kawas FH. Mirizzi syndrome. *Curr Treat Options Gastroenterol.* 2007;10:102–110.
13. Wehrmann T, Riphaus A, Martchenko K, et al. Intraductal ultrasonography in the diagnosis of Mirizzi syndrome. *Endoscopy.* 2006;38:717–722.
14. Johnson LW, Sehon JK, Lee WC, et al. Mirizzi's syndrome: experience from a multi-institutional review. *Am Surg.* 2001;67:11–14.
15. Sheth S, Bedford A, Chopra S. Primary gallbladder cancer: recognition of risk factors and role of prophylactic cholecystectomy. *Am J Gastroenterol.* 2000;95:1402–1410.
16. Fowler RC, Reid WA. Ultrasound diagnosis of adenomyomatosis of the gallbladder: ultrasonic and pathological correlation. *Clin Radiol.* 1988;39:402–406.

17. Boscak AR, Al-Hawary M, Ramsburgh SR. Adenomyomatosis of the gallbladder. *Radiographics.* 2006;26:941–946.

18. Koh T, Taniguchi H, Kunishima S, Yamagishi H. Possibility of differential diagnosis of small polypoid lesions in the gallbladder using FDG-PET. *Clin Positron Imaging.* 2000;3:213–218.

19. Tanno S, Obara T, Maguchi H, et al. Association between anomalous pancreatobiliary ductal union and adenomyomatosis of the gallbladder. *J Gastroenterol Hepatol.* 1998;13:175–180.

20. Azuma T, Yoshikawa T, Araida T, Takasaki K. Differential diagnosis of polypoid lesions of the gallbladder by endoscopic ultrasonography. *Am J Surg.* 2001;181:65–70.

21. Akyürek N, Salman B, Irkörücü O, et al. Ultrasonography in the diagnosis of true gallbladder polyps: the contradiction in the literature. *HPB (Oxford).* 2005;7:155–158.

22. Buckles DC, Lindor KD, Larusso NF, et al. In primary sclerosing cholangitis, gallbladder polyps are frequently malignant. *Am J Gastroenterol.* 2002;97:1138–1142.

23. Myers RP, Shaffer EA, Beck PL. Gallbladder polyps: epidemiology, natural history and management. *Can J Gastroenterol.* 2002;16:187–194.

24. Numata K, Oka H, Morimoto M, et al. Differential diagnosis of gallbladder diseases with contrast-enhanced harmonic gray scale ultrasonography. *J Ultrasound Med.* 2007;26:763–774.

25. Bhattacharya D, Ammori BJ. Contemporary minimally invasive approaches to the management of acute cholecystitis: a review and appraisal. *Surg Laparosc Endosc Percutan Tech.* 2005;15:1–8.

26. Bellows CF, Berger DH, Crass RA. Management of gallstones. *Am Fam Physician.* 2005;72:637–642.

27. Foley WD, Quiroz FA. The role of sonography in imaging of the biliary tract. *Ultrasound Q.* 2007;23:123–135.

28. Shridhar Ganpathi I, Diddapur RK, Eugene H, Karim M. Acute acalculous cholecystitis: challenging the myths. *HPB (Oxford).* 2007;9:131–134.

29. Babb RR. Acute acalculous cholecystitis: a review. *J Clin Gastroenterol.* 1992;15:238–241.

30. Chen PF, Nimeri A, Pham QH, et al. The clinical diagnosis of chronic acalculous cholecystitis. *Surg.* 2001;130:578–581.

31. Girgin S, Gedik E, Taçyildiz IH, et al. Factors affecting morbidity and mortality in gangrenous cholecystitis. *Acta Chir Belg.* 2006;106:545–549.

32. Coffin CT, Weingardt JP, Drose JA. Sonographic appearances of emphysematous cholecystitis. *JDMS.* 1995;11:204–206.

33. Konno K, Ishida H, Naganuma H, et al. Emphysematous cholecystitis: sonographic findings. *Abdom Imaging.* 2002;27:191–195.

34. Tseng LJ, Tsai CC, Mo LR, et al. Palliative percutaneous transhepatic gallbladder drainage of gallbladder empyema before laparoscopic cholecystectomy. *Hepatogastroenterol.* 2000;47:932–936.

35. Berger J, Lindsell DRM. Case report: Thickening of the walls of non-dilated bile ducts. *Clin Radiol.* 1997;52:474–476.

36. Kim TK, Kim BS, Kim JH, et al. Diagnosis of intrahepatic duct stones: superiority of MR cholangiopancreatography over endoscopic retrograde cholangiopancreatography. *AJR Am J Roentgenol.* 2002;179:429–434.

37. Calvo MM, Bujanda L, Calderon A. Role of magnetic resonance cholangiopancreatography in patients with suspected choledocholithiasis. *Mayo Clin Proc.* 2002;77:407–412.

38. Sakai Y, Tsuyuguchi T, Tsuchiya S, et al. Diagnostic value of MRCP and indications for ERCP. *Hepatogastroenterol.* 2007;54:2212–2215.

39. Ong TZ, Khor JL, Selamat DS, et al. Complications of endoscopic retrograde cholangiography in the post-MRCP era: a tertiary center experience. *World J Gastroenterol.* 2005;11:5209–5212.

40. Norton SA, Alderson D. Prospective comparison of endoscopic ultrasonography and endoscopic retrograde cholangiopancreatography in the detection of bile duct stones. *Br J Surg.* 1997;84:1366–1369.

41. Tripathi M, Chandrashekar N, Kumar R, et al. Hepatobiliary scintigraphy. An effective tool in the management of bile leak following laparoscopic cholecystectomy. *Clin Imaging.* 2004;28:40–43.

42. Perry KA, Myers JA, Deziel DJ. Laparoscopic ultrasound as the primary method for bile duct imaging during cholecystectomy. *Surg Endosc.* 2008;22:208–213.

43. Aljebreen A, Azzam N, Eloubeidi MA. Prospective study of endoscopic ultrasound performance in suspected choledocholithiasis. *J Gastroenterol Hepatol.* 2008;23:741–745.

44. McMahon CJ. The relative roles of magnetic resonance cholangiopancreatography (MRCP) and endoscopic ultrasound in diagnosis of common bile duct calculi: a critically appraised topic. *Abdom Imaging.* 2008;33:6–9.

45. Lau WY, Leung KL, Leung TWT, et al. Obstructive jaundice secondary to hepatocellular carcinoma. *Surg Oncol.* 1995;4:303–308.

46. Sato M, Ishida H, Konno K, et al. Choledochal cyst due to anomalous pancreatobiliary junction in the adult: sonographic findings. *Abdom Imaging.* 2001;26:395–400.

47. Martins E, Chapman RW. Sclerosing cholangitis. *Curr Opin Gastroenterol.* 1996;12:466–470.

48. Alexander J, Lord JD, Yeh MM, et al. Risk factors for recurrence of primary sclerosing cholangitis after liver transplantation. *Liver Transpl.* 2008;14:245–251.

49. Majoie CBLM, Smits NJ, Phoa SSKS, et al. Primary sclerosing cholangitis: sonographic findings. *Abdom Imaging*. 1995;20:109–113.

50. Van de Meeberg PC, Portincasa P, Wolfhagen FHJ, Van Erpecum KJ. Increased gall bladder volume in primary sclerosing cholangitis. *Gut*. 1996;39:594–599.

51. Kawarasaki H, Sato T, Sanjo K, et al. Evaluation of long-term results of Caroli's disease: 21 years' observation of a family with autosomal 'dominant' inheritance, and review of the literature. *Hepato-Gastroenterol*. 1995;42:175–181.

52. Benhidjeb T, Rudolph B, Muller JM. Curative partial hepatectomy in unilobar Caroli's syndrome– report of three cases with long-term follow-up. *Dig Surg*. 1997;14:123–125.

53. Miller WJ, Sechtin AG, Campbell WL, Pieters PC. Imaging findings in Caroli's disease. *AJR Am J Roentgenol*. 1995;165:333–337.

54. Levy AD, Rohrmann Jr CA, Murakata LA, Lonergan GJ. Caroli's disease: radiologic spectrum with pathologic correlation. *AJR Am J Roentgenol*. 2002;179:1053–1057.

55. Al Absi M, Qais AM, Al Katta M, et al. Biliary ascariasis: the value of ultrasound in the diagnosis and management. *Ann Saudi Med*. 2007;27:161–165.

56. Misra SP, Dwivedi M. Clinical features and management of biliary ascariasis in a non-endemic area. *Postgrad Med*. 2000;76:29–32.

57. Chen EY, Nguyen TD. Gallbladder sludge. *N Engl J Med*. 2001;345:2e.

58. Ko CW, Sekijima JH, Lee SP. Biliary sludge. *Ann Intern Med*. 1999;131:630–631.

59. Portincasa P, Di Ciaula A, Vendemiale G, et al. Gallbladder motility and cholesterol crystallization in bile from patients with pigment and cholesterol gallstones. *Eur J Clin Invest*. 2000;30:317–324.

60. Jüngst C, Kullak-Ublick GA, Jüngst D. Gallstone disease: microlithiasis and sludge. *Best Pract Res Clin Gastroenterol*. 2006;20:1053–1062.

61. Kohut M, Nowak A, Nowakowska-Dulawa E. The frequency of bile duct crystals in patients with presumed biliary pancreatitis. *Gastrointest Endosc*. 2001;54:37–41.

62. Lo HW, Yuan CY. Ultrasonic spectrum of hemobilia in the bile duct and gallbladder. *J Med Ultrasound*. 1994;2:77–80.

63. Tsukada K, Takada T, Miyazaki M, et al. Diagnosis of biliary tract and ampullary carcinomas. *J Hepatobiliary Pancreat Surg*. 2008;15:31–40.

64. Fevery J, Verslype C, Lai G, et al. Incidence, diagnosis, and therapy of cholangiocarcinoma in patients with primary sclerosing cholangitis. *Dig Dis Sci*. 2007;52:3123–3135.

65. Figueras J, Llado L, Valla C, et al. Changing strategies in diagnosis and management of hilar cholangiocarcinoma. *Liver Transpl*. 2000;6:786–794.

66. Miller G, Schwartz LH, D'Angelica M. The use of imaging in the diagnosis and staging of hepatobiliary malignancies. *Surg Oncol Clin N Am*. 2007;16:343–368.

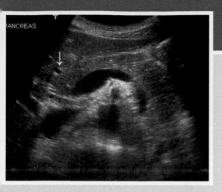

4

Ultrasound of the Pancreas

Sharan Wadhwani

CHAPTER OUTLINE

The Normal Pancreas, 143
 Ultrasound Techniques, 143
 Ultrasound Appearances, 146
 Pitfalls in Scanning the Pancreas, 146
 Biochemical Analysis, 146
 Congenital Anomalies of the Pancreas, 147
 Other Imaging, 148
Endoscopic Ultrasound, 148
Pancreatitis, 150
 Acute Pancreatitis, 150
  Clinical Features, 150
  Ultrasound Appearances, 151
 Management of Acute Pancreatitis, 154
 Recurrent Acute vs Chronic Pancreatitis, 154
  Ultrasound Appearances, 154
Malignant Pancreatic Disease, 156

Pancreatic Carcinoma, 156
  Clinical Features and Management, 156
 Ultrasound Appearances of Pancreatic
  Carcinoma, 159
 Secondary Ultrasound Findings in Pancreatic
  Adenocarcinoma, 160
 Pancreatic Metastases, 160
Benign Focal Pancreatic Lesions, 160
 Focal Fatty Sparing of the Pancreas, 160
 Focal Pancreatitis, 161
 Other Benign Lesions, 161
Trauma of the Pancreas, 162
Pancreatic Transplantation, 162
 Ultrasound Appearances, 163
References, 164

THE NORMAL PANCREAS

Ultrasound Techniques

The pancreas lies posterior to the stomach and duodenum, and therefore a variety of techniques must usually be employed to examine it fully because of the presence of gas which can obscure the organ. Ultrasound may not always be considered the first line of investigation. Computed tomography (CT), magnetic resonance imaging (MRI), endoscopic ultrasound (EUS), and/or endoscopic retrograde cholangiopancreatography (ERCP) may be required to augment and refine, depending on the diagnosis.

To obtain good views, the operator must make the best use of acoustic windows, different patient positions, and various techniques to fully investigate the pancreas. Start by scanning the epigastrium in a transverse plane, using the left lobe of the liver as an acoustic window. Using the splenic vein as an anatomical marker, the body of the pancreas can be identified anterior to this. The tail of the pancreas is slightly cephalic to the head, so the transducer plane should be accordingly oblique to display the whole organ (Fig. 4.1). Different transducer angulations display different sections of the pancreas to best effect.

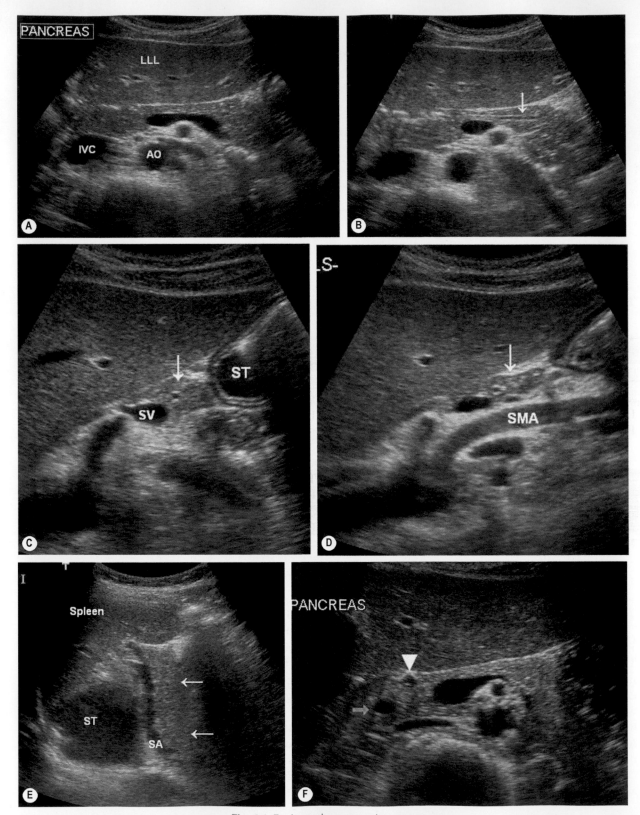

Fig. 4.1 For legend see opposite page.

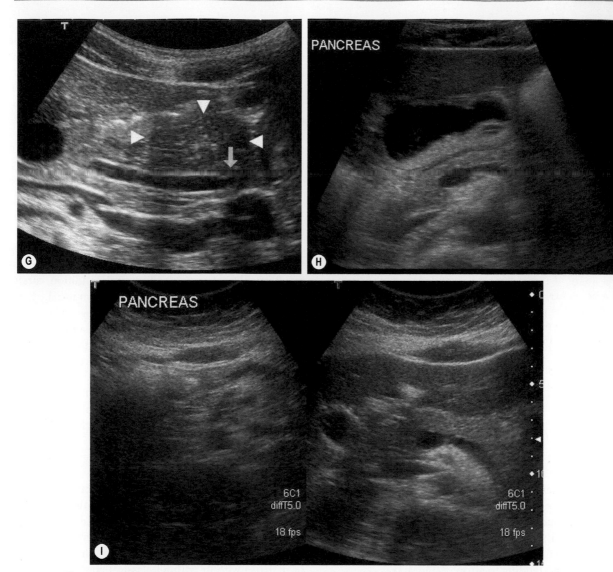

Fig. 4.1, cont'd (A) TS showing through the epigastrium showing the normal pancreas. The left lobe of the liver makes a good acoustic window. (B) The normal pancreatic duct (arrow) is seen in the body of the pancreas. (C) LS in the epigastric midline, demonstrating the body of the pancreas (arrow) with a cross-section through its normal duct. ST, stomach; SV, splenic vein. (D) The body of the pancreas (arrow) lies anterior to the superior mesenteric artery. (E) LS through the left upper quadrant, using the spleen as a window to the tail of the pancreas (arrows). The splenic artery lies against the tail of the pancreas (TOP). (F) The normal common bile duct (CBD) (arrow) can be seen in the head of the pancreas (HOP) in TS. Gastroduodenal artery (arrowhead). (G) The lower end of the CBD (arrow) as it goes through the HOP (arrowheads). (H) A pancreas obscured by overlying bowel gas can be seen through the acoustic window of a water-filled stomach. (I) Abdominal protrusion can be useful for visualizing the pancreas in a gassy abdomen; the right image displays the pancreas when the patient is asked to push the abdomen out.

Identify the echo-free splenic vein and the superior mesenteric artery (SMA) posterior to it. The latter is surrounded by an easily visible, hyperechoic fibrous sheath. The pancreas is "draped" over the splenic vein.

TIP BOX

Where possible, use the left lobe of the liver as an acoustic window to the pancreas, angling slightly caudally.

The tail, which is often quite bulky, may require the transducer to be angled toward the patient's left. The spleen also makes a good window to the tail in the coronal section (Fig. 4.1E). If you cannot see the pancreatic head properly, turn the patient left side raised, which moves the duodenal gas up toward the tail of the pancreas. Right side raised may demonstrate the tail better. If these maneuvers still fail to demonstrate the organ fully, try:

- Asking the patient to perform the Valsalva maneuver with abdominal protrusion (Fig. 4.1I).
- Scanning the patient erect.
- Filling the stomach with a water load to create an acoustic window through which the pancreas can be seen (Fig. 4.1H).

Ultrasound Appearances

The texture of the pancreas is rather coarser than that of the liver.

The echogenicity of the normal pancreas alters according to age. In a child or young person, it may be quite bulky and relatively hypoechoic compared to the liver. In adulthood, the pancreas is hyperechoic compared with a normal liver, becoming increasingly so in the elderly and tending to atrophy (Fig. 4.2).

The pancreas does not have a capsule, and its margins can appear rather ill-defined, becoming infiltrated with fat in later life. These age-related changes are highly significant to the sonographer; what may be considered normal in an elderly person would be abnormally hyperechoic in a younger one and may represent a chronic inflammatory state. Conversely, a hypoechoic pancreas in an older patient may represent acute inflammation, whereas the appearances could be normal in a young person.

The main pancreatic duct is most easily visualized in the body of the pancreas, where its walls are perpendicular to the beam. The normal diameter is up to 5 mm within the head, reducing to up to 2 mm within the tail. Any main duct dilatation over 6 mm should be considered abnormal, likely requiring further investigation with CT, MRI, or EUS depending on clinical circumstance.[1] The common bile duct (CBD) can be seen in the right lateral portion of the head, and the gastroduodenal artery lies anterolaterally (Fig. 4.1F). The size of the uncinate process varies.

Pitfalls in Scanning the Pancreas

The normal stomach or duodenum can mimic pancreatic pathologic conditions, especially if the patient has insufficiently fasted. A fluid-filled stomach can be particularly confusing when looking for pancreatic fluid collections in patients with acute pancreatitis. Giving the patient a drink of water usually differentiates the gastrointestinal tract from a collection. In addition, careful assessment of the wall of a fluid collection usually helps to differentiate. The bowel wall can show a layered appearance with microvascular flow within and peristalses given time. True collections may have a thin/imperceptible wall or a thick, fixed wall that appears homogenous with no internal vascularity.

Epigastric or portal lymphadenopathy may also mimic a pancreatic mass. If careful scanning and appropriate patient positioning are unable to elucidate, CT is usually the next step.

Biochemical Analysis

In many pancreatic diseases, the production of the digestive pancreatic enzymes is compromised either by obstruction of the duct draining the pancreas or by the destruction of the pancreatic cells that produce the enzymes. This can result in malabsorption of food and/or diarrhea with or without classical epigastric pain radiating into the back. Fecal elastase levels can be used to assess for exocrine insufficiency. In positive cases, oral pancreatic enzyme replacement therapy is used to restore intestinal enzyme levels so that absorption improves nutritional status.

The pancreas produces the digestive enzymes amylase, lipase, and peptidase, which occur in trace amounts in the blood. If the pancreas is damaged or inflamed, the resulting release of enzymes into the bloodstream causes an increase in serum amylase and lipase levels. The enzymes also pass from the bloodstream into the urine, and therefore urinalysis can also contribute to the

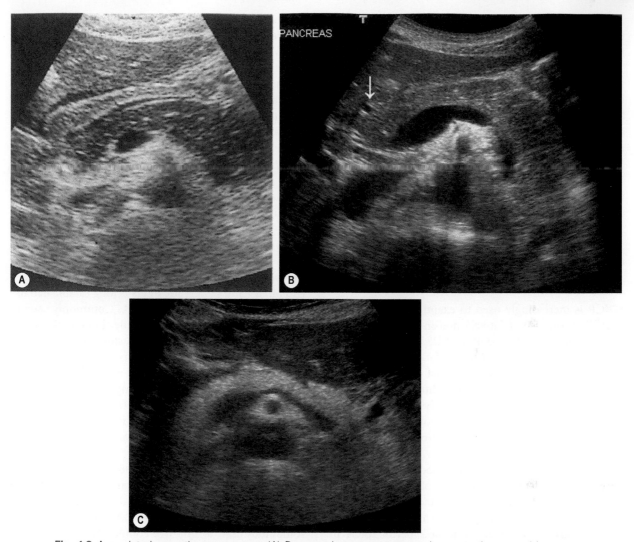

Fig. 4.2 Age-related acoustic appearances: (A) Pancreas in a young person, demonstrating normal hypoechogenicity. (B) The normal adult pancreas is slightly more echogenic than the liver. Note the gastroduodenal artery near the head of the pancreas (arrow). (C) The pancreas becomes hyperechoic and infiltrated with fat in an older patient.

diagnosis. Conversely, where there is atrophy to the pancreas, these enzymes are not produced in sufficient volume, and therefore in cases of acute recurrent or chronic pancreatitis, levels can remain normal or low.

Congenital Anomalies of the Pancreas

The normal pancreas results from the fusion of two embryonic buds – the ventral bud arises from the CBD, forming the uncinate process and part of the head, and the dorsal arises from the posterior wall of the duodenum. This dual can sometimes be clearly seen with ultrasound, whereby there is a clear difference in echogenicity of each component, although underlying architecture remains uniform/undisturbed. Developmental anomalies of the pancreas occur because of a failure of the dorsal and ventral pancreatic ducts to fuse – *pancreas divisum* – which is present in up to 10% of the Western population. In such a configuration, the uncinate duct drains to the major papilla along with the CBD, whereas the main duct within the body drains to the minor papilla, usually slightly cranial to the ampulla. This arrangement may cause inadequate drainage of the pancreatic duct; its causal link with pancreatitis remains uncertain. A rare developmental anomaly of the ventral bud may occur – *pancreas anulare* – in which pancreatic tissue encircles the bowel. In this latter case, patients can present with a proximal small bowel obstruction in infancy, but this may also be an incidental finding at autopsy. These anomalies are rarely diagnosed on ultrasound, better seen on CT and MRI, although divisum is thought to occur in over 10% of the population. Agenesis of the pancreas is very rare, usually associated with other defects, and children with this condition usually die soon after birth.

Other Imaging

MRCP is increasingly used to examine the pancreatic duct[2] because of its relatively non-invasive nature and low risk compared to ERCP[3] or EUS. ERCP is invasive (it requires a wire/catheter to be placed across the ampulla into the bile duct and contrast dye injected) and carries a small risk of post-procedure pancreatitis or, rarely, perforation, and so is generally reserved for therapeutic procedures such as the balloon trawl extraction of stones, placement of a stent, and/or sphincterotomy with diathermy.

EUS is an increasingly useful modality for imaging the pancreas in detail, without the problems of intervening stomach or duodenal gas. This technique is helpful for imaging the ducts and parenchyma in high resolution and has also been shown to be superior to CT in detecting occult neoplasms.[4] The proximity of the endoscope to the pancreas and ducts improves sensitivity and specificity for tiny stones and lesions. It also has the facility to take a biopsy if required (Fig. 4.5D), which can be accurately directed toward the area of interest, improving histological yield.

Current NICE (National Institute for Clinical Excellence, United Kingdom) Guidelines determine CT as the primary modality for pancreatic assessment in the context of potential cancer.[5] Despite this, unexpected malignancies are commonly identified following initial transabdominal ultrasound, especially in the presence of dilated biliary ducts; therefore, a sound knowledge of pancreatic sonography remains an important skill. In addition to identifying pancreatic masses, CT is also used to stage patients with pancreatic carcinoma. CT is generally the imaging of choice in severe acute pancreatitis because of its ability to identify significant complications that require urgent attention, including pseudoaneurysm and portal thrombosis. With specific multiphase techniques, CT can detect pancreatic necrosis, although the use of contrast ultrasound may also have a useful role in assessing vascularity,[6] diagnosing necrosis, and even in identifying tumors, allowing further imaging to be directed more appropriately. The emergence of shear wave elastography also provides the potential for further improvement in sonographic detection rates, especially when applied to EUS.

ENDOSCOPIC ULTRASOUND

Visualization of the ampulla along with the gallbladder and biliary and pancreatic ducts is long established using ERCP, first developed in 1968.[7] Commonly used to explore the bile ducts and provide therapeutic access for common procedures such as stone extraction and cytological brushings of stricturing disease, its usefulness to assess the pancreas is more limited. In the context of pancreatitis with symptomatic main duct obstruction, it can be used to extract calculi that may stimulate recurrent attacks. The risk profile for ERCP is significant, including acute pancreatitis and bowel perforation.

EUS was developed in the 1980s and uses a high-frequency probe placed intraluminally within the esophagus, stomach, or proximal small bowel to assess adjacent structures (Fig. 4.3A). A probe cover is sometimes used to improve contact with the mucosal surface, and fluid distension of the balloon can provide a useful window for transmission of the beam. Initially, a radial array offered a circumferential image perpendicular to the orientation of the probe (Fig. 4.3B). While providing additional information, the beam orientation to the endoscope limited assessment to diagnostic imaging only. Over the next decade, the uptake of EUS increased with the development of a linear crystal array that allows a more versatile and directed assessment of the pancreas and biliary system, with additional access to all adjacent structures within the mediastinum and upper abdomen (Fig. 4.3C, D).[8] Using a linear array also allows passage of instruments via the endoscope that remain visible within the plane of the projected beam – enabling directed access for diagnostic and therapeutic intent (Fig. 4.3). Diagnostic

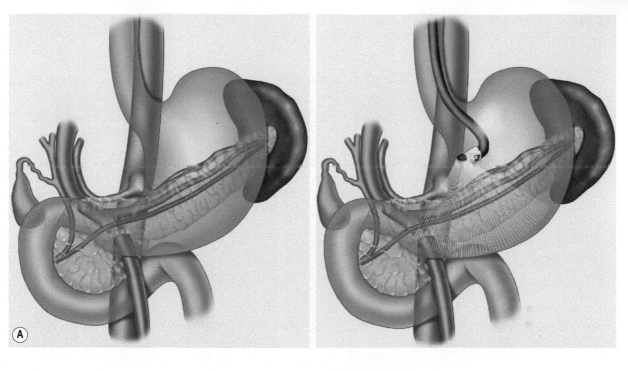

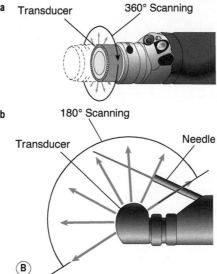

Fig. 4.3 (A) Diagram of EUS pancreas body and tail examination: Linear echoendoscope. (B) a – Distal tip of electronic radial endoscopic ultrasound (EUS) endoscope. b – Distal tip of curvilinear EUS fine-needle aspiration (FNA) endoscope.

Continued

fine-needle aspiration (FNA) and core biopsy (FNB) techniques allow pathological confirmation of suspected malignant and benign disease.

The utility of EUS continues to develop, with the ability to access the pancreas using a minimally invasive technique; procedures currently available include drainage of peripancreatic collections, ablation of solid tumors, biliary diversion, and vascular interventions such as pressure gradient measurements/embolization.

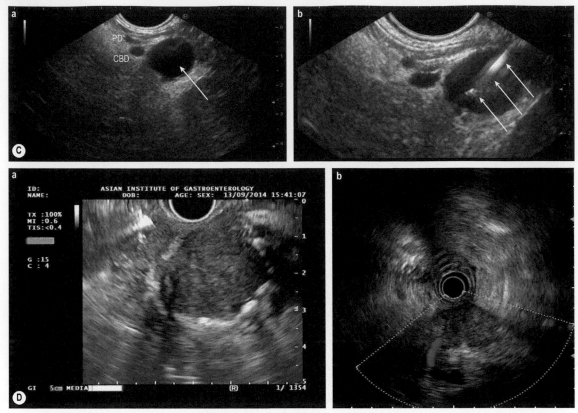

Fig. 4.3, cont'd (C) Linear endoscopic images. a – Cystic lesion (arrowed) in the head of the pancreas; the common bile duct and pancreatic duct are also visible. The lesion is an intraductal papillary mucinous neoplasm. b – Lesion is sampled by FNA. The needle is arrowed. (D) a – Linear EUS of the pancreas – Pancreatic head mass with peripheral calcifications. b – Radial EUS. Pancreatic body mass with celiac artery encasement. (Sources: Endosonography, Fourth Edition, 2019 ; Clinical Gastrointestinal Endoscopy, Second Edition, 2011; Kumar and Clark's Clinical Medicine, Tenth Edition, 2021; Encyclopedia of Gastroenterology, Second Edition.)

PANCREATITIS

Inflammation of the pancreas may be acute or chronic, solitary or recurrent, and is usually a response to the destruction of pancreatic tissue by its own digestive enzymes (*autodigestion*) that have been released from damaged pancreatic cells along with a hyperinflammatory response.

Acute Pancreatitis

Clinical Features

Acute inflammation of the pancreas has several possible causes (Table 4.1) but is most commonly associated with gallstones or excessive alcohol ingestion.

Clinically it presents with severe, rapid-onset epigastric pain, radiating to the back, with or without abdominal distention, nausea, or vomiting. In milder cases, the patient may recover spontaneously. If allowed to progress untreated, a range of complications, including bleeding, sepsis, multi-organ failure, and death, may occur.

Biochemically, amylase and lipase levels (the pancreatic enzymes responsible for the digestion of starch and lipids) in the blood and urine are raised because of cell damage with rupture of the cell membranes and release into the blood capillaries. In cases of chronic or recurrent pancreatitis, the gland may not produce normal levels of such enzymes, and therefore their rise in blood/urine levels during acute episodes may be more limited, sometimes non-detectable. In such instances, CT is recommended to confirm the diagnosis of pancreatitis and exclude another cause for symptoms.

TABLE 4.1	Causes of Acute Pancreatitis
Biliary calculi	Most common cause. Obstructs the main pancreatic duct/papilla of Vater and may cause reflux of bile into the pancreatic duct
Alcoholism	Alcohol overstimulates pancreatic secretions causing overproduction of enzymes, and is toxic to the pancreatic cells
Trauma/ iatrogenic	Damage/disruption of the pancreatic tissue, e.g., in a road traffic accident or by surgery, biopsy, or ESWL[6]
Drug induced	A relatively uncommon cause. Some anti-cancer drugs can cause chemical injury
Infection	E.g., mumps. A rare cause of pancreatitis
Congenital anomaly	Duodenal diverticulum, duodenal duplication, sphincter of Oddi stenosis, or choledochal cyst may obstruct the pancreatic duct, giving rise to pancreatitis
Hereditary	A rare, autosomal dominant condition presenting with recurrent attacks in childhood or early adulthood

ESWL, extracorporeal shock wave lithotripsy.

Ultrasound Appearances

Mild acute pancreatitis may have no demonstrable features on ultrasound, especially if the scan is performed after the acute episode has settled. Although ultrasound is used to assess the pancreas in cases of suspected acute pancreatitis, its main role is in demonstrating the *cause* for pancreatitis, commonly biliary calculi, to plan further management. The ultrasound finding of microlithiasis or sludge in the gallbladder is highly significant in cases of suspected pancreatitis[9] and is often implicated in the cause of recurrent pancreatitis. A finding of biliary dilatation with or without the presence of gallstones in such instances is important and may help determine further diagnostic tests, including MRCP, if the extrahepatic duct is not entirely visualized with ultrasound alone.

Acute idiopathic pancreatitis (AIP) is a term used when the cause of pancreatitis has not been demonstrated, although the majority of these do turn out to have microlithiasis or biliary sludge. Improved ultrasound imaging is more readily able to detect microlithiasis, and EUS is particularly useful in such cases, as it is more sensitive in detecting tiny stones in the CBD. In more severe cases, the pancreas becomes enlarged and hypoechoic because of edema. The main duct may be dilated during the edematous phase of the episode or prominent (Fig. 4.4) in cases of ductal obstruction or chronic pancreatitis.

As the condition progresses, digestive enzymes leak out, forming pockets or collections. Such collections are termed according to the time since onset of symptoms and the pathophysiology of inflammation (interstitial edematous or necrotic) as per the Revised Atlanta classification.[10] Focal uniform/simple fluid in context of edematous pancreatitis without an established, well-circumscribed wall and formed within 4 weeks of onset of symptoms is termed an APFC (acute peripancreatic fluid collection). After 4 weeks, this fluid may develop a capsule—forming a pseudocyst. In the context of necrotizing pancreatitis, initial fluid usually appears complex with solid components/debris and sometimes involving the pancreatic parenchyma. Such fluid formed within the first 4 weeks of onset of symptoms, without a circumscribed capsule/wall, is termed an ANC (acute necrotic collection). After around 4 weeks this fluid may develop a capsule, representing WON (walled off necrosis). These are most frequently found in the lesser sac, near the body/tail of the pancreas, but can extend cranially into the chest through the diaphragmatic hiatus or occur anywhere in the abdomen – within the pancreatic tissue itself, anywhere in the peritoneal or retroperitoneal space or even tracking up the fissures into the liver – so a full abdominal ultrasound survey is essential on each attendance (Fig. 4.4). CT is particularly useful in demonstrating the complications of acute pancreatitis, including retroperitoneal changes, which may be obscured on transabdominal ultrasound.[11]

Pseudocysts are so-called because they do not exhibit a true wall with a viable epithelium like most cysts but are merely collections of fluid surrounded by a tough, fibrous, relatively acellular capsule/wall. Pseudocysts may be echo-free but generally contain echoes from tissue debris and may be loculated. In a small percentage of cases, a collection may become infected, forming an abscess. In such cases, there may be gas components within, which can make differentiation with adjacent bowel loops difficult.

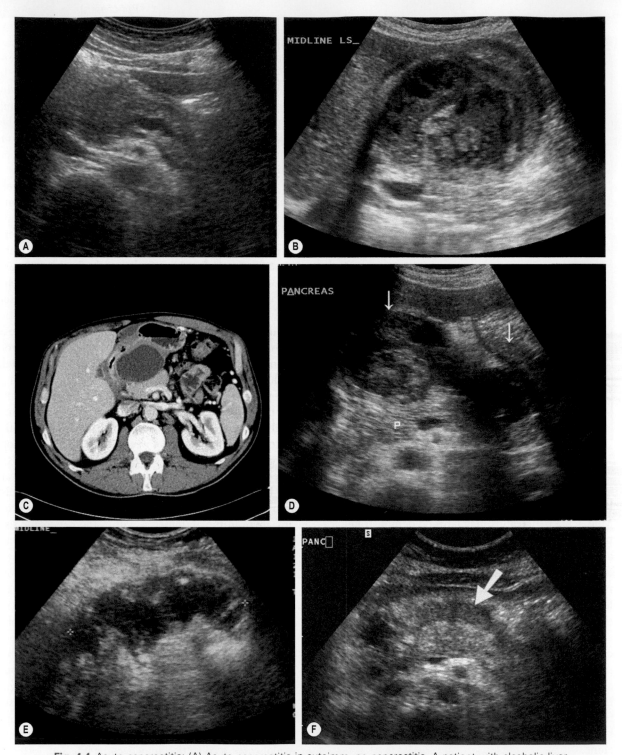

Fig. 4.4 Acute pancreatitis: (A) Acute pancreatitis in autoimmune pancreatitis. A patient with alcoholic liver disease. The pancreas is hypoechoic and bulky with a lobulated outline and dilated main duct. (B) Large pseudocyst near the body of pancreas in acute pancreatitis. (C) Computed tomography of the case in (B), showing pseudocyst anterior to the pancreas. (D) Exudate (arrows) anterior to the body and tail of the pancreas. P, head of the pancreas. (E) The pancreas (calipers) has become necrotic after repeated attacks of pancreatitis. (F) Inflammatory exudate (arrow) is seen around the right kidney in acute pancreatitis.

Continued

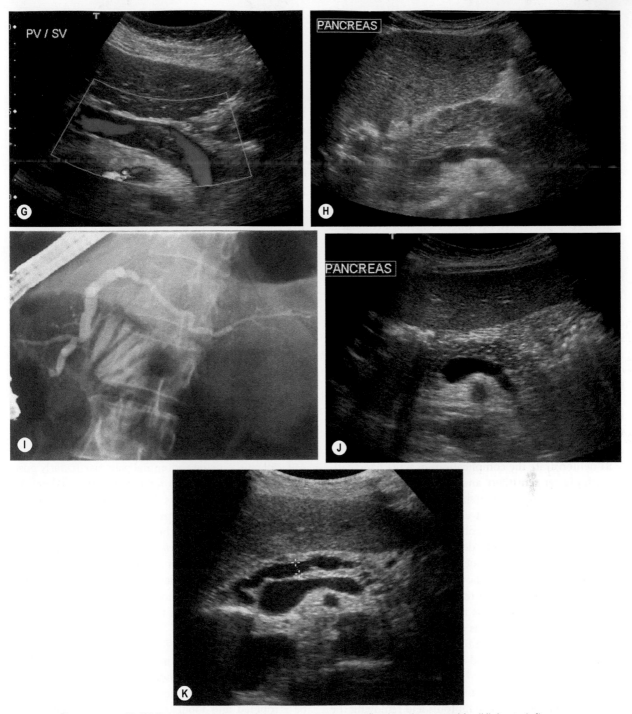

Fig. 4.4, cont'd (G) Splenic and portal vein thrombosis is a complication of pancreatitis. (H) Acute inflammation demonstrating an enlarged, tender edematous pancreas, which is relatively hypoechoic. (I) endoscopic retrograde cholangiopancreatography. A patient with pancreatitis has a dilated proximal pancreatic duct. (J) Human immunodeficiency virus with associated pancreatitis. The pancreas is relatively hypoechoic, and in another case, pancreatic duct dilatation is present (K).

Although acute pancreatitis usually affects the entire organ, it may occur focally. This presents a diagnostic dilemma for ultrasound, as the appearances are indistinguishable from a tumor. The clinical history may help to differentiate; suspicion of focal pancreatitis should be raised in patients with a previous history of chronic pancreatitis or a history of excess alcohol ingestion with normal CA 19-9 (a tumor marker for pancreatic carcinoma) levels.[12] The enlargement of the pancreas in acute pancreatitis may have other consequences; for example, the enlarged pancreatic head may obstruct the CBD, causing biliary dilatation.

Doppler ultrasound is useful in assessing associated vascular complications. Prolonged and repeated attacks of acute pancreatitis may cause the splenic vein to become encased and compressed, causing splenic and/or portal vein thrombosis, with all its attendant sequelae. Furthermore, hepatic or portal venous thrombus in cases of acute pancreatitis is potentially treatable and can prevent further clinical deterioration. Additionally, inflammation of the closely related gastroduodenal or hepatic arteries may cause damage to the wall causing pseudoaneurysms at high risk of catastrophic hemorrhage.

Management of Acute Pancreatitis

While ultrasound is useful in demonstrating associated gallstones, biliary sludge, and fluid collections, CT or MRI demonstrate the complications of acute pancreatitis with greater sensitivity and specificity. Localized areas of necrotic pancreatic tissue can be demonstrated on biphasic contrast-enhanced CT, together with vascular complications, such as thrombosis.

MRCP or CT is used to demonstrate the main pancreatic duct and its point of insertion into the CBD. Anomalous insertions are thought to be associated with pancreatitis because of the reflux of bile into the pancreatic duct. ERCP, which is more invasive and subject to potential complications, is generally reserved for circumstances that require the removal of stones, alleviating the need for surgery, and in the placement of stents in the case of strictures.[13]

Pancreatitis can be difficult to treat and management consists of alleviating the symptoms and removing the cause where possible. Patients with gallstone pancreatitis do well after cholecystectomy, but if the gallbladder is not removed, recurrent attacks of increasingly severe inflammation occur in up to a third of patients.

Walled-off necrosis or pseudocysts that do not resolve spontaneously may be drained percutaneously under ultrasound or CT guidance, or depending on the site of the collection, a drain may be positioned endoscopically from the cyst into the stomach.[14] Pseudocyst formation may cause thrombosis of the splenic vein, spreading to the portal and mesenteric veins in some cases. Other vascular complications include splenic artery aneurysm, which may form because of damage to the artery by the pseudocyst.

Surgery to remove necrotized or hemorrhagic areas of pancreatic tissue may be undertaken in severe cases, although this is decreasingly common with more effective endoscopic drainage/management techniques.

Recurrent Acute vs Chronic Pancreatitis

Patients with acute pancreatitis are at risk of repeated inflammatory episodes that eventually develop through to chronic inflammation. Recurrent acute pancreatitis (RAP) differs from chronic pancreatitis (CP) and is defined as more than two attacks of acute pancreatitis without evidence of chronic pancreatitis. There is no clear consensus regarding the relationship between RAP and CP, although recurrent AIP is frequently associated, likely because of the inherent nature of its unknown cause.[15]

In CP, normal pancreatic tissue is progressively replaced by fibrosis, which may encase the nerves in the celiac plexus, causing abdominal pain, particularly postprandial. The patient has fatty stools (steatorrhea) because of malabsorption, as there is a decreased capacity to produce digestive enzymes.

Diagnosis of CP can be difficult, especially in the early stages.[16] Serum enzyme levels are less elevated than in acute disease (if at all). MRCP is useful but limited in assessing the smaller side ducts. EUS is currently a sensitive and accurate modality in assessing the ductal system and the pancreatic tissue.

Ultrasound Appearances

The pancreas in CP becomes abnormally hyperechoic (Fig. 4.5A). This should not be confused with the normal increase in echogenicity with age. The gland may be atrophied and lobulated, and the main pancreatic duct is frequently dilated and ectatic,[17] with a beaded appearance.

Calcification may be identified in the pancreatic tissue, both on ultrasound and on a plain X-ray, and there

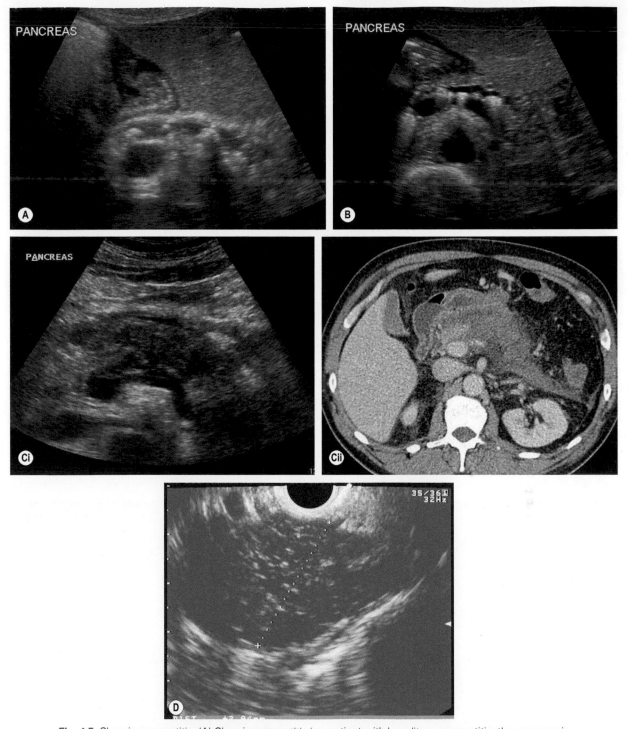

Fig. 4.5 Chronic pancreatitis. (A) Chronic pancreatitis in a patient with hereditary pancreatitis; the pancreas is hyperechoic with stones in the dilated duct. (B) Calcification of the pancreas in alcoholic pancreatitis, with a prominent main duct. (Ci) An acute phase in a patient with a history of repeated acute on chronic pancreatitis. The pancreas is now necrotic, and the SV contains thrombus. (Cii) Computed tomography demonstrates a lack of contrast in the necrotic pancreatic tissue. (D) Endoscopic ultrasound of a patient with autoimmune pancreatitis. The pancreas is swollen and hypoechoic; the operator is lined up to perform an ultrasound-guided biopsy.

may be stones in the duct. Generally speaking, strong shadows are cast from the calcific foci, but small flecks may be too small to shadow (Fig. 4.5B, C). As with acute inflammation, CT is the method of choice for demonstrating the complications of CP.

Obstruction of the duct can cause pseudocyst formation, and other complications include biliary obstruction and portal/splenic vein thrombosis.

MALIGNANT PANCREATIC DISEASE

Pancreatic Carcinoma

Clinical Features and Management

Carcinoma of the pancreas is usually aggressive and is currently the fourth most common cause of cancer-related death. It carries a very poor prognosis – five-year survival is less than 5%.[17,18] Metastatic deposits from primary pancreatic adenocarcinoma occur early in the course of the disease, and 80% of patients already have nodal disease or distant metastases in the lungs, liver, or bone by the time the diagnosis is made, which accounts for the poor prognosis. The emergence and increasing adoption of EUS in the diagnosis of pancreatic cancer and improvements in chemotherapy regimes in recent years is likely to have improved statistics, but outcomes remain poor where curative surgery cannot be performed.

The presenting symptoms depend on the size of the lesion, its position within the pancreas, and the extent of metastatic deposits. Commonly, pancreatic cancers are found incidentally with imaging performed for other reasons or nonspecific symptoms. Most pancreatic carcinomas (60%) are found in the head of the pancreas,[19] and patients can present with the associated symptoms of jaundice because of obstruction of the CBD (Fig. 4.6). Carcinomas located in the body or tail of the pancreas do not cause obstructive jaundice and are therefore more likely to present late when treatment options become more limited.

The majority (80%) of pancreatic cancers are ductal adenocarcinomas, most of which are located in the head of the pancreas. The rest comprise rarer neoplasms and neuroendocrine tumors. Neuroendocrine tumors, which originate in the islet cells of the pancreas, tend to be either insulinomas (generally benign) or gastrinomas (malignant). These can be secreting or non-secreting tumors; when secreting, these generally present with hormonal abnormalities while the tumor is still small and are more amenable to detection by EUS than by conventional sonography.

Cystic neoplasms of the pancreas are frequently asymptomatic and have become increasingly recognized because of better imaging techniques[20] and usually represent serous or mucinous tumors (Fig. 4.6E). Mucinous lesions are more commonly associated

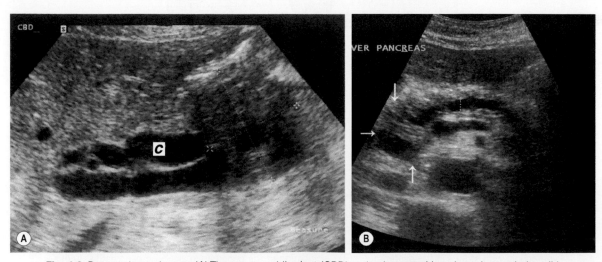

Fig. 4.6 Pancreatic carcinoma: (A) The common bile duct (CBD), c, is obstructed by a large hypoechoic solid mass at its lower end (calipers), which is carcinoma in the head of the pancreas. (B) TS through the pancreas, demonstrating a complex mucinous cystadenocarcinoma in the head (arrows), causing dilatation of the main pancreatic duct (calipers).

Continued

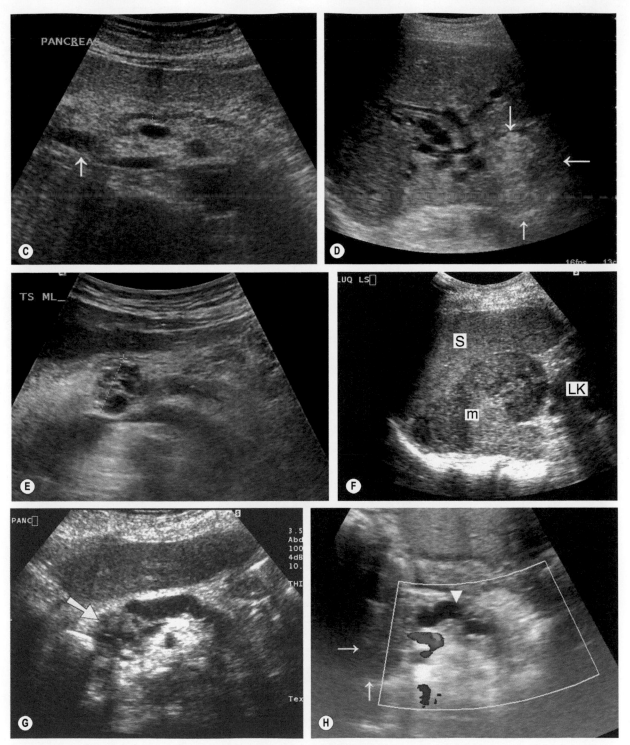

Fig. 4.6, cont'd (C) A small, hypoechoic adenocarcinoma (arrow) in the head of the pancreas (HOP) causing mild pancreatic duct dilatation. (D) Intrahepatic duct dilatation caused by a large tumor in the head of the pancreas (arrows), confirmed by computed tomography. (E) Complex cystic mass in the head of the pancreas, confirmed as a cystadenocarcinoma. (F) A complex mass (m) between the spleen (S) and the left kidney is a large carcinoma of the tail of the pancreas. (G) Dilated pancreatic duct because of carcinoma in the head (arrow). (H) Color Doppler helps differentiate the dilated pancreatic duct (arrowhead), which does not contain flow. The dilatation is caused by carcinoma in the HOP (arrows).

Continued

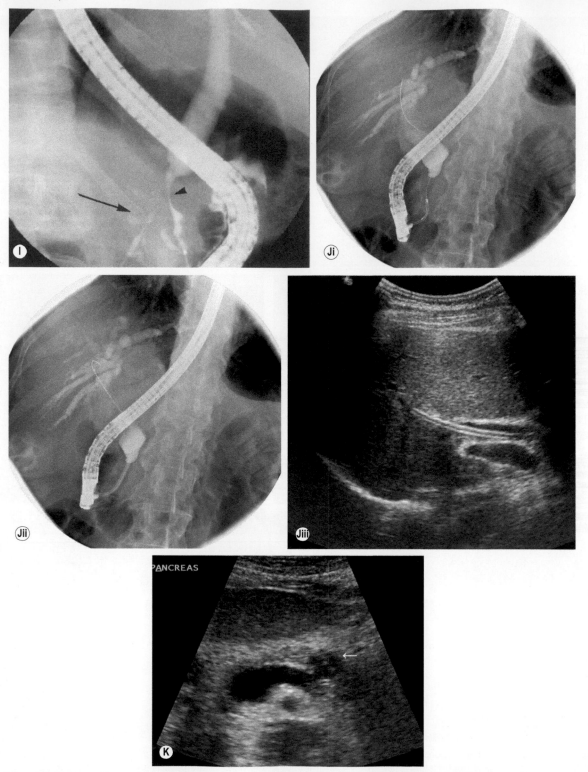

Fig. 4.6, cont'd (I) Endoscopic retrograde cholangiopancreatography (ERCP) demonstrating a long stricture of the pancreatic duct (arrow) involving the side branches in a large pancreatic carcinoma. The CBD is compressed (arrowhead) by nodes, causing biliary dilatation. A palliative stent was inserted. (Ji, ii) ERCP is used to place a stent in the CBD to decompress the ducts, later demonstrated on ultrasound (Jiii). (K) Metastatic deposit (arrow) from primary breast carcinoma in the body of the pancreas.

with the potential for malignancy; prognosis depends upon early detection and effective surveillance. Various strategies exist involving CT/MRI and EUS; the latter allows for aspiration of fluid with biochemical analysis and FNA cytology to assess for cellular features of dysplasia/malignancy. They pose a diagnostic dilemma, appearing predominantly cystic on ultrasound, and can be located anywhere within the pancreas. They follow a much less aggressive course than adenocarcinomas, metastasizing late, and have a much higher curative rate with surgery if performed at the appropriate time.[21] The presence of calcification may be a pointer to malignancy in a cystic lesion but is still difficult to differentiate from an inflammatory mass.

Surgical removal of pancreatic carcinoma within the uncinate, head, neck, or proximal body by partial pancreaticoduodenectomy – the Whipple procedure – may be curative. However, only 20% of patients have a potentially resectable tumor, and the five-year survival rate following resection is less than 5%.[22] Over 70% of patients die from hepatic metastases within three years postoperatively.[23]

Differential diagnoses of pancreatic masses must always be considered (Table 4.2); focal lesions in the pancreas may represent inflammatory, rather than malignant, masses. Ultrasound-guided biopsy of pancreatic masses is limited by low sensitivity[24] because of the inflammatory element surrounding many carcinomas, so a negative biopsy is unhelpful.

Endosonography-guided aspiration or biopsy has high sensitivity and specificity for diagnosing pancreatic cancer and is also useful in patients with a previous negative biopsy in whom malignancy is suspected.[25] ERCP may also be used to insert a palliative stent in the CBD to relieve biliary obstruction.

The detection of pancreatic carcinoma by ultrasound is usefully followed by a CT scan for staging purposes as this will demonstrate invasion of peripancreatic fat, vascular involvement, and lymphadenopathy, and any distant metastasis.

Ultrasound Appearances of Pancreatic Carcinoma

Adenocarcinoma, which comprises 80% of pancreatic neoplasms, is a solid tumor, usually hypoechoic or of mixed echogenicity, with an irregular border (Fig. 4.6). Because the mass is most frequently located in the head

TABLE 4.2 Differential Diagnoses of Focal Pancreatic Masses	
Solid	
Adenocarcinoma	Hypoechoic, usually in the HOP
Focal acute pancreatitis	Hypoechoic. Clinical history of pancreatitis
Focal chronic pancreatitis	Hyperechoic, sometimes with calcification History of pancreatitis
Endocrine tumor	Less common. Small, hypoechoic, well defined
Metastases	Late manifestation, widespread disease
Cystic[17]	
Pseudocyst	History of pancreatitis
Mucinous tumor, serous cystadenoma, intraductal papillary mucinous neoplasm (IPNM)	Less common than adenocarcinoma – tend to form in the body or tail of the pancreas. More favorable prognosis following resection
Necrotic or hemorrhagic tumor	
Simple cyst	Rare. Exclude polycystic disease by scanning the liver and kidneys

of the pancreas, which lies behind the duodenum, it may be difficult to identify at first. A major clue is the dilatation of the CBD, which must be carefully traced to its point of obstruction. Adenocarcinoma is a hypovascular tumor, and Doppler may not demonstrate flow within it in many cases. Contrast-enhanced ultrasound may assist in demonstrating the extent of the tumor,[26] although CT is still widely considered the imaging of choice for staging purposes.[27] The pancreatic duct distal to the mass may be dilated and can be mistaken for the splenic vein. Obstructed ductal appearances are usually more tortuous than the smooth, continuous walls of the splenic vein. Color Doppler is useful in confirming the lack of flow in the duct and in identifying the vein behind it (Fig. 4.6G, H).

Neuroendocrine tumors, which arise from the islet cells in the pancreas, include insulinomas, which are benign, and gastrinomas, which are more often malignant. They are usually hypoechoic, hypervascular, well defined, and exhibit a mass effect, often without a distally dilated main pancreatic duct. They are generally smaller at presentation than adenocarcinomas and tend to arise in the body or tail of the pancreas. Up to 40% of these tumors go undetected by both transabdominal ultrasound and CT, with EUS and laparoscopic ultrasound having the highest detection rates for insulinomas. Gastrinomas tend to be multiple and may also be extrapancreatic.

A small proportion of pancreatic cancers contain an obvious fluid content (see above) and are similar in acoustic appearance to a pseudocyst, but unlike a pseudocyst, a mucinous cystic neoplasm is not usually associated with a history of pancreatitis. However, some low-grade malignancies can cause pancreatitis if the duct is obstructed,[28] and aspiration of fluid by EUS is useful, especially in the presence of elevated carcinoembryonic antigen (CEA), low glucose, and amylase levels.

It is also possible to see areas of hemorrhage or necrosis within a lesion, which look complex or fluid-filled. Calcification is also seen occasionally but is nonspecific.[29]

Secondary Ultrasound Findings in Pancreatic Adenocarcinoma

The most obvious secondary feature of carcinoma of the head of the pancreas is the dilated biliary system. In a series of 62 pancreatic cancers, biliary dilatation occurred in 69%, pancreatic duct dilatation in 37%, and the *double duct sign* (pancreatic and biliary duct dilatation) in 34% of patients.[29]

Although the gallbladder is frequently dilated with no visible stones, this is not always the case; incidental gallstones may be present, causing chronic inflammation, which prevents the gallbladder from dilating. For this reason, it is imperative that the CBD is carefully traced down to the head of the pancreas to identify the cause of obstruction.

A thorough search for lymphadenopathy and liver metastases should always be done. If the mass is large, it is impossible to differentiate whether it arises from the ampulla of Vater or the head of the pancreas. This differentiation, however, is usually academic at this stage. Color Doppler can demonstrate considerable hypo- or hyper-vascularity within the mass and may also identify vascular invasion of the celiac axis; SMA; hepatic, splenic, and/or gastroduodenal arteries; and of the portal and splenic veins – a factor that is particularly important in assessing the suitability of the tumor for curative resection.

The recognition of the involvement of peripancreatic vessels by carcinoma with color Doppler, together with the ultrasound assessment of compression or encasement of these vessels, has been found to be highly sensitive and specific (79% and 89%) for diagnosing unresectability.[30] Palliative care using stent insertion with ERCP (Fig. 4.6J) or with percutaneous trans-hepatic cholangiography using fluoroscopic guidance alleviates the biliary obstruction.

Pancreatic Metastases

The most common source for pancreatic metastases is renal cell carcinoma, although they may also occur from breast, lung, and gastrointestinal tract primary tumors. They are relatively uncommon on ultrasound (Fig. 4.6K) simply because they are a late manifestation in patients who generally already have known malignant disease and in whom investigations are multiple and previous.

Widespread metastatic disease can be demonstrated on ultrasound, particularly in the liver, and there is often considerable epigastric lymphadenopathy, which can be confused with the appearances of pancreatic metastases on the scan.

TIP BOX

Pathology of the pancreas, both benign and malignant, can affect the adjacent vasculature by compression, encasement, or thrombosis.

Doppler of the splenic, portal, and superior mesenteric veins is useful in demonstrating the extent of vascular complication when pancreatic abnormalities are suspected.

BENIGN FOCAL PANCREATIC LESIONS

Focal Fatty Sparing of the Pancreas

The uncinate process and ventral portion of the head of the pancreas may sometimes appear hypoechoic compared to the rest of the gland (Fig. 4.7). This is because of a relative lack of fatty deposition and is often more noticeable in older patients, in whom the pancreas is normally hyperechoic.[31] Similar differences can be seen in cases of pancreas divisum (see above). Its significance

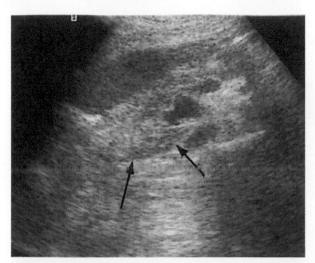

Fig. 4.7 The uncinate process is relatively hypoechoic (arrows) because of fatty sparing.

lies in not confusing it with a focal pancreatic mass. The area of fatty sparing is well defined, with no enlargement or mass effect, and is regarded as a normal variation in the ultrasound appearances. If doubt exists, CT, MRI, or EUS will differentiate fatty sparing from true neoplasm.

Focal Pancreatitis

Inflammation can affect the whole or just part of the gland. Occasionally, hypoechoic, focal acute, or CP areas are present (see pancreatitis above). These are invariably a diagnostic dilemma, as they are indistinguishable on ultrasound from focal malignant lesions (Fig. 4.8). Factors that point toward inflammation include a previous history of symptoms of pancreatitis and a normal CA 19-9 tumor marker level. In such cases, where CT does not offer a resolution, EUS is increasingly used to clarify benign from malignant pathologies.

Other Benign Lesions

Benign cysts in the pancreas are increasingly recognized (Fig. 4.9A). They can rarely be associated with other conditions such as polycystic disease, cystic fibrosis, or von Hippel–Lindau disease (an autosomal dominant disease characterized by pancreatic and renal cysts, renal carcinoma, phaeochromocytoma, and/or hemangioblastomas in the cerebellum and spine). The presence of a solitary cystic lesion in the absence of these conditions should be reported along with any associated high-risk (obstructed CBD with jaundice, main duct dilatation >10 mm, mural nodule) or worrisome (thickened cyst wall, diameter >3 cm, main duct 6-9 mm +/- abrupt

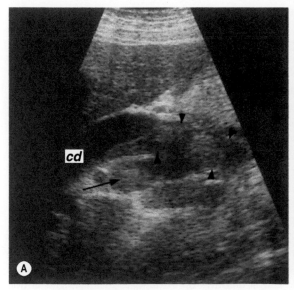

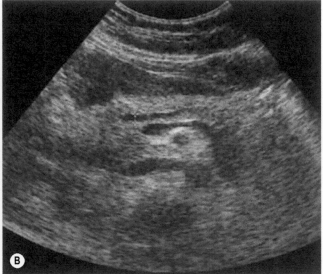

Fig. 4.8 (A) Focal acute pancreatitis in the head of the pancreas. The common bile duct (CBD) is obstructed by a hypoechoic mass in the head, with blood clots and debris within the duct. The differential diagnosis is malignancy. (B) The same patient eight months later. The acute inflammation has resolved, the obstruction is relieved, and the pancreas now appears hyperechoic with a mildly dilated duct, consistent with chronic pancreatitis.

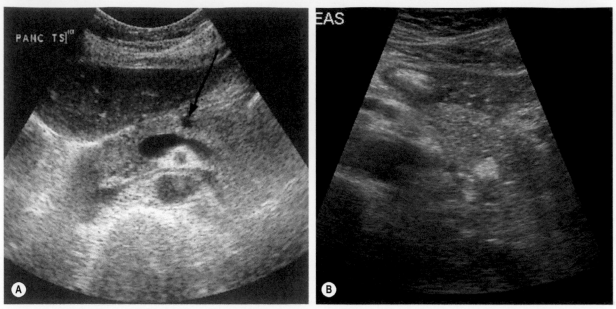

Fig. 4.9 (A) Tiny cyst in the body of the pancreas. This was confirmed on computed tomography and remained stable for two years. (B) Small, well defined, hyperechoic lesion in the tail of the pancreas, which remained stable over a number of years. Assumed to be a rare, benign hemangioma (no histology available), although any solid mass in the pancreas is usually suspected to be malignant until proven otherwise.

caliber change and distal pancreatic atrophy, lymphadenopathy) features to ensure appropriate onward investigations or surveillance are performed with appropriate clinical supervision.

Unlike those in the liver, pancreatic hemangiomas are extremely rare (Fig. 4.9B). Any complex cystic or solid lesion in the pancreas is usually considered suspicious for malignancy until proved otherwise.

TRAUMA OF THE PANCREAS

The pancreas is particularly vulnerable to "blunt" trauma in road traffic accidents, in which the upper abdomen is thrown against the seat belt, resulting in laceration – often at the neck of the pancreas. The duct may be ruptured, with consequent leakage of pancreatic juice into the abdominal cavity, and severe cases result in complete pancreatic transection with pancreatic ascites. The release of pancreatic enzymes triggers pancreatitis and/or peritonitis, with the gland appearing enlarged and hypoechoic.

Ultrasound may be helpful in identifying hemoperitoneum or localizing a collection, but it will not differentiate pancreatic secretions from hematoma.

CT is the method of choice in cases of suspected pancreatic trauma, although even here, the signs of injury can be surprisingly subtle considering the damage.[32]

PANCREATIC TRANSPLANTATION

In patients with insulin-dependent diabetes mellitus with end-stage renal disease, simultaneous pancreatic and kidney transplantation is a recognized successful treatment that improves the quality of life and the survival of the patients.[33] Typically, such patients also have severe complications, such as retinopathy and vascular disease, which may be stabilized, or even reversed, by transplantation. Simultaneous pancreas and kidney transplantation now has a one-year graft survival of almost 90% because of improved organ preservation techniques, surgical techniques, and immunosuppression.[34]

The transplanted kidney is generally placed in the iliac fossa with the pancreas on the contralateral side and can sometimes be difficult to localize. The donor kidney is plumbed in as usual, with anastomoses to the recipient iliac artery and vein. The pancreatic vessels are anastomosed to the contralateral iliac vessels.

The pancreatic secretions are primarily by enteric drainage, as the previous method of bladder drainage was associated with an increased incidence of urological complications such as urinary tract infection, hematuria, and reflux pancreatitis.[35]

Postoperative complications include rejection, sepsis, inflammation, anastomotic leak, or vascular thrombosis. Localized postoperative bleeding usually resolves spontaneously. Ultrasound is useful in locating fluid collections, but CT is most often used to assess pancreatitis or anastomotic leaks.[36]

Ultrasound Appearances

Ultrasound is useful for evaluating renal transplant perfusion; once isolated, the organ is clearly seen and infrequently obscured. Unfortunately, it is less useful for the transplanted pancreas, which is frequently obscured by the overlying bowel. The donor pancreas is usually situated in the iliac fossa but can be placed more centrally, particularly if a renal transplant has also been performed, resulting in difficult localization and limited visualization.

Ultrasound is limited in its ability to assess the transplanted pancreas, even if it can be located among the bowel loops. The lack of an adjacent reference organ, such as the liver, makes the assessment of its echogenicity subjective, and therefore subtle degrees of inflammation are difficult to detect. Fluid collections are frequently concealed beneath the bowel and when identified, their appearance is nonspecific. Contrast CT is more successful in detecting anastomotic leaks and collections and is usually used for guided aspiration.

Color Doppler can display perfusion throughout the pancreas, and the main vessels may be traced to their anastomoses, depending on the overlying bowel (Fig. 4.10).

Neither CT nor ultrasound are particularly helpful in evaluating rejection, and it is difficult to differentiate transplant pancreatitis from true rejection. The Doppler resistance index does not correlate with a rejection process and has not been found useful. MRI can detect vascular occlusion and arterial and venous thrombosis and is particularly useful in patients in whom the pancreas is obscured by overlying bowel.

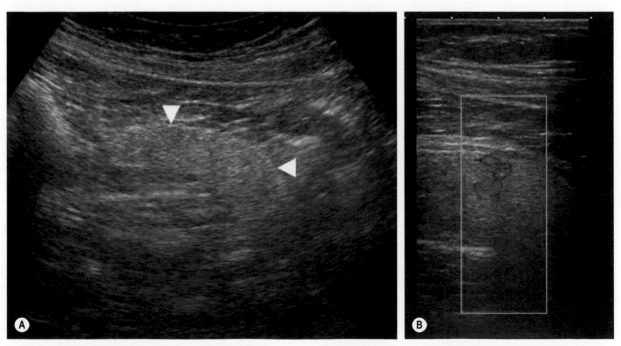

Fig. 4.10 (A) The transplanted pancreas (arrowheads) is difficult to identify in the iliac fossa because of adjacent bowel and lack of the usual anatomical markers. (B) A high frequency helps to identify perfusion in the body of the pancreatic transplant.

REFERENCES

1. Tanaka M, Chari S, Adsay V, et al. International consensus guidelines for management of intraductal papillary mucinous neoplasms and mucinous cystic neoplasms of the pancreas. *Pancreatol.* 2006;6(1-2):17–32.
2. Hallal AH, Amortegui JD, Jeroukhimov IM, et al. Magnetic resonance cholangiopancreatography accurately detects common bile duct stones in resolving gallstone pancreatitis. *J Am Coll Surg.* 2005;200:869–875.
3. Calvo MM, Bujanda L, Calderson A, et al. Comparison between magnetic resonance cholangiopancreatography and ERCP for evaluation of the pancreatic duct. *Am J Gastroenterol.* 2002;97:347–353.
4. Rizk M, Gerke H. Utility of endoscopic ultrasound in pancreatitis: a review. *World J Gastroenterol.* 2007;13:6321–6326.
5. NICE. *Pancreatic cancer in adults: diagnosis and management.* NICE Guideline [NG85]; 2018.
6. Rickes S, Mönkemüller K, Malfertheiner P. Acute severe pancreatitis: contrast-enhanced sonography. *Abdom Imaging.* 2007;32:362–364.
7. ASGE Standards of Practice Committee. Anderson MA, Fisher L et al. Complications of ERCP. *Gastrointest Endosc.* 2012;75(3):467–473.
8. Reddy Yogananda, Willert Robert P. Endoscopic ultrasound; what is it and why should we use it? *Clinical Med.* 2009;9(6):539–543.
9. Pezzilli R, Billi P, Barakat B, et al. Ultrasonic evaluation of the common bile duct in biliary acute pancreatitis patients: comparison with endoscopic retrograde cholangiopancreatography. *J Ultrasound Med.* 1999;18:391–394.
10. Banks PA, Bollen TL, Dervenis C, et al. Classification of acute pancreatitis—2012: revision of the Atlanta classification and definitions by international consensus. *Gut.* 2013;62:102–111.
11. Morgan DE. Imaging of acute pancreatitis and its complications. *Clin Gastroenterol Hepatol.* 2008;6:1077–1085.
12. Yamaguchi K, Chijiiwa K, Saiki S, et al. 'Mass-forming' pancreatitis masquerades as pancreatic carcinoma. *Int J Pancreatol.* 1996;20:27–35.
13. Madhotra R, Lombard M. Endoscopic retrograde cholangiopancreatography should no longer be used as a diagnostic test: the case against. *Dig Liver Dis.* 2002;34:375–380.
14. Gumaste VV, Pitchumoni CS. Pancreatic pseudocyst. *Gastroenterol.* 1996;4:33–43.
15. Machicado JD, Yadav D. Epidemiology of recurrent acute and chronic pancreatitis: similarities and differences. *Dig Dis Sci.* 2017;62(7):1683–1691.
16. Bolondi L, LiBassi S, Gaiani S, Barbara L. Sonography of chronic pancreatitis. *Radiol Clin North Am.* 1989;27:815–833.
17. Garcea G, Dennison AR, Pattenden CJ, et al. Survival following curative resection for pancreatic ductal adenocarcinoma. A systematic review of the literature. *Pancreas.* 2008;9:99–132.
18. Iott MJ, Corsini MM, Miller RC. Evidence-based guidelines for adjuvant therapy for resected adenocarcinoma of the pancreas. *Clin J Oncol Nurs.* 2008;12:599–605.
19. Damjanov I. Pancreatic neoplasms. In: *Pathology for health related professionals.* Philadelphia: Saunders; 1996:324–326.
20. Mulkeen A, Yoo P, Cha C. Less common neoplasms of the pancreas. *World J Gastroenterol.* 2006;12:3180–3185.
21. Lichtenstein DR, Carr-Locke DL. Mucin-secreting tumours of the pancreas. *Gastrointest Endosc Clin N Am.* 1995;5:237–258.
22. Cooperman AM, Kini S, Snady H, et al. Current surgical therapy for carcinoma of the pancreas. *J Clin Gastroenterol.* 2000;31:107–113.
23. Ishikawa O, Ohigashi H, Imaoka S, et al. Is the long-term survival rate improved by preoperative irradiation prior to Whipple's procedure for adenocarcinoma of the pancreatic head? *Arch Surg.* 1994;129:1075–1080.
24. Di Stasi M, Lencioni R, Solmi L, et al. Ultrasound-guided fine needle biopsy of pancreatic masses: results of a multicenter study. *Am J Gastroenterol.* 1998;93:1329–1333.
25. Rafique A, Freeman S, Carroll N. A clinical algorithm for the assessment of pancreatic lesions: utilization of 16- and 64-section multidetector CT and endoscopic ultrasound. *Clin Radiol.* 2007;62:1142–1153.
26. D'Onofrio M, Zamboni G, Faccioli N, et al. Ultrasonography of the pancreas. 4. Contrast-enhanced imaging. *Abdom Imaging.* 2007;32:171–181.
27. Furukawa H, Uesaka K, Boku N. Treatment decision making in pancreatic adenocarcinoma: multidisciplinary team discussion with multidetector-row computed tomography. *Arch Surg.* 2008;143:275–280.
28. Brugge WR. Diagnosis and management of relapsing pancreatitis associated with cystic neoplasms of the pancreas. *World J Gastroenterol.* 2008;14:1038–1043.
29. Yassa N, Yang J, Stein S, et al. Gray-scale and colour flow sonography of pancreatic ductal adenocarcinoma. *J Clin Ultrasound.* 1997;25:473–480.
30. Angeli E, Venturini M, Vanzulli A, et al. Color Doppler imaging in the assessment of vascular involvement by pancreatic carcinoma. *AJR Am J Roentgenol.* 1997;168:193–197.

31. Jacobs JE, Coleman BG, Arger PH, Langer JE. Pancreatic sparing of focal fatty infiltration. *Radiology.* 1994;190:437–439.

32. Craig MH, Talton DS, Hauser CJ, Poole GV. Pancreatic injuries from blunt trauma. *Am Surg.* 1995;61:125–128.

33. Dean PG, Kudva YC, Stegall MD. Long-term benefits of pancreas transplantation. *Curr Opin Organ Transplant.* 2008;13:85–90.

34. Krishnamurthi V, Philosophe B, Bartlett ST. Pancreas transplantation: contemporary surgical techniques. *Urol Clin North Am.* 2001;28:833–838.

35. Sutherland DE, Gruessner RW, Dunn DL, et al. Lessons learned from more than 1000 pancreas transplants at a single institution. *Ann Surg.* 2001;233:463–501.

36. Green SJ, Sidhu PS, Deane CR. Imaging of simultaneous kidney pancreatic transplants. *Imaging.* 2002;14:299–307.

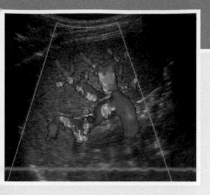

5

Ultrasound of the Spleen and Lymphatic System

Nicola J. Davidson

CHAPTER OUTLINE

The Spleen – Normal Appearances and
  Technique, 167
  Ultrasound Appearances, 168
  Splenic Size, 168
  Splenomegaly, 168
  Splenic Anatomical Variants, 168
  Splenunculi, 168
  Pitfalls in Scanning the Spleen, 171
Malignant Splenic Disease, 171
  Lymphoproliferative
    Disorders, 171
  Clinical Features and Management, 171
  Ultrasound Appearances, 171
  Leukemia, 173
  Metastases, 173

Benign Splenic Conditions, 174
  Cysts, 174
  Abscess, 175
  Calcification, 176
  Hemolytic Anemia, 176
Vascular Abnormalities of the Spleen, 176
  Hemangioma, 176
  Splenic Infarction, 176
    Splenic Vein Thrombosis, 178
    Splenic Artery Aneurysm, 179
    Pseudoaneurysm, 179
  Splenic Trauma, 179
  Lymphatic System, 179
  Lymphangioma, 182
References, 183

THE SPLEEN – NORMAL APPEARANCES AND TECHNIQUE

The spleen is the largest organ within the lymphatic system and has many supporting roles within the body, including being integral in supporting the immune system and with blood filtration, recycling red blood cells, and storage of platelets and white blood cells. The spleen normally lies in the left upper quadrant (LUQ), posterior to the splenic flexure and stomach, which often results in poor views when trying an anterior approach because of the gas from the bowel and stomach. Therefore, it is best approached from the left lateral intercostal aspect with the patient supine. Air within the gas-filled bowel will rise anteriorly to the spleen, providing a clearer view. Gentle respiration is frequently more successful than deep inspiration, as the latter brings the lung bases downwards and may obscure a small spleen altogether.

TIP BOX

If the spleen is still not visualized, positioning the patient decubitus, left side raised, may also be successful but sometimes has the effect of causing the gas-filled bowel loops to rise to the left flank, once again obscuring the spleen. A posterior approach may also be considered in some patients.

Ultrasound Appearances

The normal spleen has a homogeneous texture, with smooth, clearly defined margins and a pointed inferior edge. It is usually of similar echotexture to the liver (but may be slightly hypo- or hyperechoic in some subjects). Sound attenuation through the spleen is less than that through the liver, requiring the operator to "flatten" the time gain compensation controls to maintain an even level of echoes throughout the organ.

The main splenic artery and vein and their branches may be demonstrated at the splenic hilum (Fig. 5.1A–C). The spleen provides an excellent acoustic window to the upper pole of the left kidney, the left adrenal gland, and the tail of the pancreas.

Splenic Size

Ultrasound examination to assess the spleen for size is a common request because of physical examination having low sensitivity and specificity, especially with mild splenomegaly.[1] The size and shape of the spleen can be highly variable between different people because of the variations in each person's height, weight, and physique. When commenting upon size, it is important to consider the patient's habitus when commenting on the size of the spleen. Generally, the spleen is similar in size to the left kidney; however, this must be used with caution.

The spleen should be measured along its length, from the superior-medial tip to the inferolateral aspect. A measurement of 5–12 cm is generally considered normal, although this is subject to variation in shape and the plane of measurement used. A small spleen is of doubtful clinical significance.[2]

Splenomegaly

Enlargement of the spleen is a highly non-specific sign associated with numerous conditions, the most common being infection, portal hypertension, hematological disorders, and neoplastic conditions (Box 5.1).

Measuring the length of the spleen is an adequate indicator of size for most purposes and provides a useful baseline for monitoring changes in disease status which is reproducible by the operator in subsequent scans and comparable to measurements obtained in cross-sectional imaging. Ultrasound is often the modality of choice in monitoring the spleen size because of lack of radiation and good operator reproducibility. A measurement of greater than 12 cm would be considered enlarged in most adults; however, as previously discussed, body size and type can impact the "normal" splenic size range. As the spleen enlarges, it extends downwards and medially. Its inferior margin becomes rounded (Figs. 5.1D–E, 5.2A), and it may extend below the left kidney and into the pelvis.

Although the cause of splenomegaly may not be obvious on ultrasound, the causes can be narrowed down by considering the clinical picture and by identifying other relevant appearances in the abdomen. For example, splenomegaly because of portal hypertension is frequently accompanied by other associated pathologic conditions such as cirrhotic liver changes, varices (Fig. 5.2B), or ascites. In cases of portal hypertension, it is important to assess the splenic vasculature to assess for varices at the hilum.

Splenic Anatomical Variants

Congenital anomalies of the spleen include persistent lobulation, accessory spleen (splenunculi), polysplenia, asplenia (absent), and wandering spleen. In a healthy individual, these anomalies can be seen in isolation or form part of an associated syndrome.

In the normal spleen, the borders are smooth and regular; however, in rare cases, the diaphragmatic surface of the spleen may appear lobulated or even completely septated. This appearance may give rise to diagnostic uncertainty, and Doppler may help establish the vascular supply and differentiate this from other masses in the LUQ or from scarring or infarction in the spleen.

The spleen may lie in an ectopic position, in the left flank or pelvis, or posterior to the left kidney. The ectopic (or wandering) spleen is situated on a long pedicle, allowing it to migrate within the abdomen. The significance of this rare condition is that the pedicle may twist, causing the patient to present acutely with pain from splenic torsion. Ultrasound demonstrates the enlarged, hypoechoic organ in the abdomen, with the absence of the spleen in its normal position.

Splenunculi

A small accessory spleen or splenunculus are common findings identified in around 10%-40% of the population at autopsy.[3] They can be located anywhere in the abdomen, but the splenic hilum is the most common location, with around 80% found at this location.[4] It is important to differentiate these from other pathologic conditions such as enlarged lymph nodes or possible adrenal nodule. It is not uncommon for splenic tissue

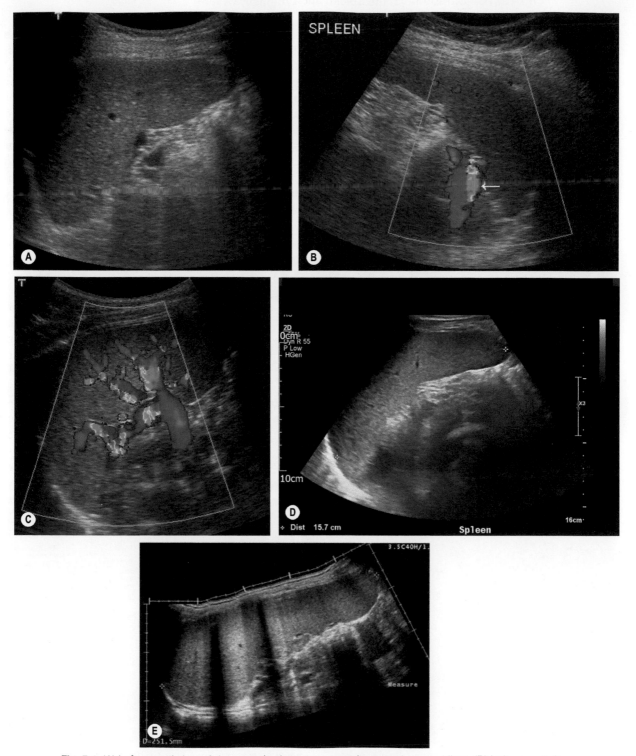

Fig. 5.1 (A) Left coronal view of the normal spleen demonstrating vessels at the hilum. (B) Left coronal view of the normal spleen at the hilum. The splenic artery (arrow) lies alongside the vein. The pulse repetition frequency (PRF) is set for the lower venous velocity, so the artery demonstrates "aliasing." (C) By increasing the Doppler sensitivity (decreasing the PRF), the perfusion within the spleen is demonstrated. (D) Diffusely enlarged spleen, with measurement. (E) An enlarged spleen can be displayed more fully using an extended field of view, allowing measurement of the length (25 cm). Shadowing from the ribs is evident.

BOX 5.1   Examples of Causes of Splenomegaly

- Portal hypertension
- Acute or chronic systemic infection – e.g., hepatitis, acquired immunodeficiency syndrome, infectious mononucleosis, sepsis
- Hemolytic anemia, sickle cell disease, thalassemia, pernicious anemia, spherocytosis
- Malignancy – leukemia, Hodgkin's and non-Hodgkin's lymphoma, myeloproliferative disorders
- Immunological diseases

to be found within the pancreatic tail, which can lead to diagnostic uncertainty, and in some cases, imaging such as positron emission tomography (PET) may be useful.[4]

Splenunculi are typically small, well-defined ectopic nodules of splenic tissue and, therefore, are of similar ultrasound echotexture to the spleen (Fig. 5.2C–D) and rarely exceed 2 cm in diameter. Occasionally the vessels supplying the splenunculus can be seen using color Doppler, and in equivocal findings, contrast ultrasound can be used. Splenunculi enlarge under the same circumstances as those which cause splenomegaly and may also hypertrophy in post-splenectomy patients.

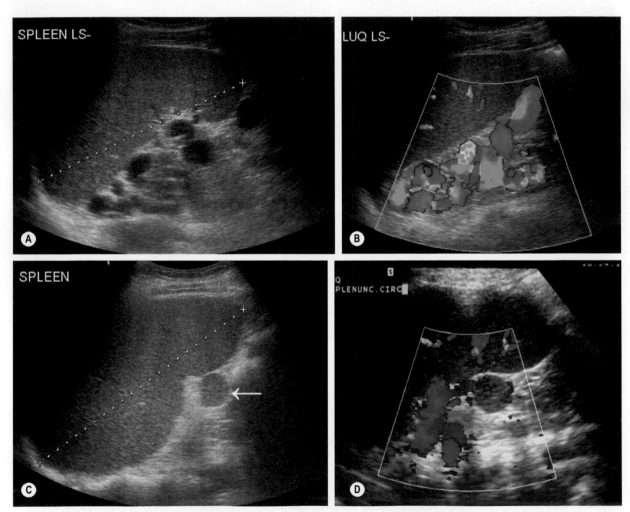

Fig. 5.2 (A) Splenomegaly in portal hypertension. The inferior splenic margin is blunted, descending below and medial to the left kidney. Varices are present around the hilum. (B) Varices, in the form of a splenorenal shunt, in portal hypertension. (C) A splenunculus (arrow) at the hilum of a mildly enlarged spleen. (D) The circulation of the splenunculus derives from the main splenic artery and drains into the main splenic vein.

Polysplenia is the presence of two or more spleens rather than one "normal" spleen and can be linked to syndromes which can result in other abnormalities of the organs of the abdomen. In about 20% of cases of polysplenia syndrome, there is a link with situs inversus abdomonis.[5]

Pitfalls in Scanning the Spleen

- In hepatomegaly, the left lobe of the liver may extend across the abdomen to the LUQ, displacing the spleen. This can give the appearance of a homogeneous, intrasplenic "mass" when the spleen is viewed coronally. A transverse scan at the epigastrium should demonstrate the extent of left hepatic enlargement and confirm its relationship to the spleen.
- Splenunculi may be mistaken for enlarged lymph nodes at the splenic hilum. Color Doppler can confirm that the vascular drainage and supply are shared by the spleen.
- The normal tail of the pancreas may mimic a perisplenic mass.
- A left adrenal mass, or upper pole renal mass, may indent the spleen, making it difficult to establish its origin.

MALIGNANT SPLENIC DISEASE

Lymphoproliferative Disorders

These are malignant hematologic conditions, comprising Hodgkin's and non-Hodgkin's lymphoma, leukemia, and myeloma.

Lymphoma is the most common malignant disease affecting the spleen (Fig. 5.3). Malignant cells can infiltrate the spleen, lymph nodes, bone marrow, and thymus and can also involve the liver, gastrointestinal tract, kidney, and other organs. Approximately 3% of malignant diseases are lymphomas. However, a primary splenic lymphoma is rare, constituting 2% of all lymphomas and 1% of all non-Hodgkin's lymphomas.[6] A primary splenic lymphoma diagnosis is made when the lymphoma is contained within the spleen with no distant spread or only spread to the lymph nodes within the hilar region. Biopsy under ultrasound guidance can be performed and is considered a relatively safe procedure.

Splenic involvement because of malignant infiltration may be found in 30%–40% of patients with Hodgkin's disease and 10%–40% of patients with non-Hodgkin's in the initial stages of the disease.[7]

Lymphoma is also associated with acquired immunodeficiency syndrome (AIDS), and infection with human immunodeficiency virus (HIV) has given rise to a broad spectrum of lymphomatous conditions, which may be demonstrated on ultrasound and computed tomography (CT).[8] These include masses in the liver, spleen, kidneys, adrenal gland, bowel, and other retroperitoneal and nodal masses. In addition, the increased use of immunosuppression in transplant patients and the increased survival in this group have also been the cause of an increased incidence of immunodeficiency-related lymphoma known as post-transplantation lymphoproliferative disorder (PTLD) (Fig. 5.3E).

Clinical Features and Management

Patients may present with a range of non-specific symptoms, which include painless lymph node enlargement particularly in the neck, armpit, and groin; anemia; general fatigue; weight loss; fever; sweating, including night sweats; and infections associated with decreased immunity. If the disease has spread to other organs, these may produce symptoms related to the organs in question. Prognosis depends upon the type of the disease, which must be determined histologically, and its stage.

Diagnosis is usually by biopsy of the lymph node or mass, and ultrasound is useful in guiding this procedure. In some cases, the excision of an affected node can be useful for diagnosis and treatment planning. CT is most frequently used for staging purposes and is superior to ultrasound in demonstrating lymphadenopathy, especially lymph nodes deeper within the abdomen, although ultrasound can be useful in helping to characterize focal lesions and detect renal obstruction.[9] FDG-PET is increasingly useful in staging with a high diagnostic accuracy for identifying residual or recurrent tumor,[10] and it can also help predict the patient's response to therapy.

Depending on the type of lymphoma, chemotherapy regimens may be successful and if not curative, can cause remission for lengthy periods. High-grade types of lymphoma are particularly aggressive, with a poor survival rate.

Ultrasound Appearances

Patients may present with a varied and broad spectrum of appearances in lymphoma (Fig. 5.3). In many cases, the spleen is not enlarged and shows no acoustic abnormality.[11]

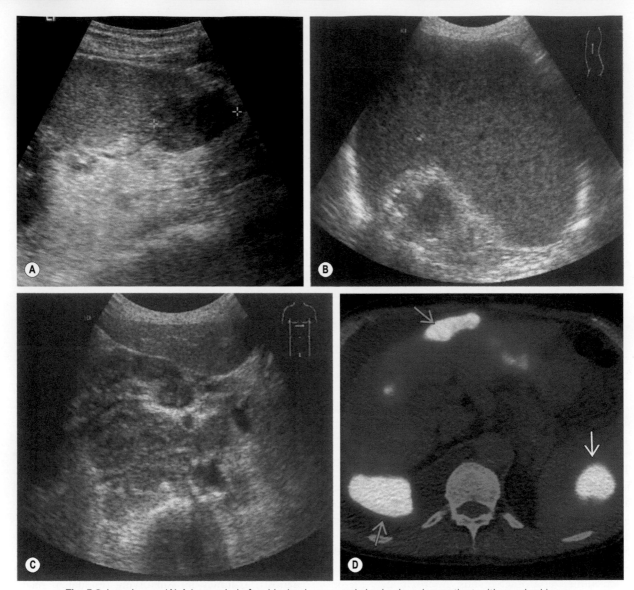

Fig. 5.3 Lymphoma: (A) A hypoechoic focal lesion in a normal-sized spleen in a patient with acquired immunodeficiency syndrome is suspicious for lymphoma. (B) Enlarged, coarse-textured spleen containing multiple tiny lymphomatous lesions. (C) Extensive lymphadenopathy in the epigastric region. (D) Fluorodeoxyglucose-positron emission tomography/computed tomography fusion image shows intense metabolic activity of the splenic lesion. Histology revealed large B-cell lymphoma.

Continued

Lymphoma may produce a diffuse splenic enlargement with normal, hypo-, or hyperechogenicity. In patients with hematological conditions, it is important to consider splenic volume as a way to show the progression of disease.

Although lymphoma usually has a diffuse effect on the spleen, focal lesions may also be present. They tend to be hypoechoic and hypovascular and may be single or multiple. In larger lesions, the margins may be ill-defined, and the echo contents vary from almost anechoic to heterogeneous, often with increased through transmission. In such cases, they may be similar in appearance to cysts. However, the well defined capsule is absent

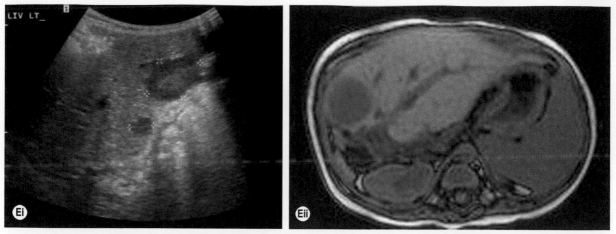

Fig. 5.3, cont'd (E) Post-transplantation lymphoproliferative disorder (PTLD): (Ei) hypoechoic focal lesions in a liver transplant; and (Eii) Magnetic resonance imaging of another case of PTLD. (Source: (5.3d) Diagnostic Ultrasound: Abdomen & Pelvis, 2016.)

in lymphoma, which has a more indistinct margin.[12] Smaller lesions may be hyperechoic or mixed. Tiny lymphomatous foci may affect the entire spleen, making it appear coarse in texture.

Lymphadenopathy may be present elsewhere in the abdomen. If other organs, such as the kidney or liver, are affected, the appearances of mass lesions vary but are commonly hypoechoic or of mixed echo pattern.

A differential diagnosis of metastases should be considered in the presence of multiple solid hypoechoic splenic lesions, but most cases are because of lymphoma. In patients who are immunocompromised and at risk from PTLD, the main differential diagnosis with multiple hepatic or splenic lesions would be abscesses, as both PTLD and abscess may have similar acoustic characteristics.

Leukemia

Leukemia (literally meaning "white blood," from the Greek) is characterized by an increased number of malignant white blood cells. Unlike lymphoma, which affects the lymphatic system, leukemia affects circulation. There are two main types: myeloid and lymphoid, which can be either acute or chronic. The bone marrow becomes infiltrated with malignant cells, which cause the blood to have increasing levels of immature blood cells.

Patients present with fatigue, anemia, recurrent infections, and a tendency to bleed internally. The patient's inability to overcome infections may eventually lead to death.

Chemotherapy is successful in curing acute lymphoblastic leukemia in approximately half the patients and may induce remission in others. The long term prognosis is poor for other types of leukemia, although patients may survive for ten years or more with the slow-growing chronic lymphocytic leukemia.

Leukemia produces diffuse splenic enlargement but rarely with any change in echogenicity. Abdominal lymphadenopathy may also be present.

Metastases

Metastatic deposits occur in the spleen relatively rarely than in the liver but are rarely isolated to the spleen and are generally because of more widespread disease. Autopsy reports an incidence of around 10%, although a proportion of these are microscopic and not amenable to radiological imaging.

The most commonly found splenic metastases on ultrasound are from lymphoma but may occur with any primary cancer. Intrasplenic metastases are more likely in later stage disease and favor pulmonary, osteosarcomas, soft tissue sarcomas, and renal cell carcinoma. Breast and ovarian cancers can also metastasize to the spleen, and melanoma must be considered, even when the disease is distant.

As with liver metastases, the ultrasound appearances vary enormously, ranging from hypo- to hyperechogenic or of a mixed pattern (Fig. 5.4). They may be

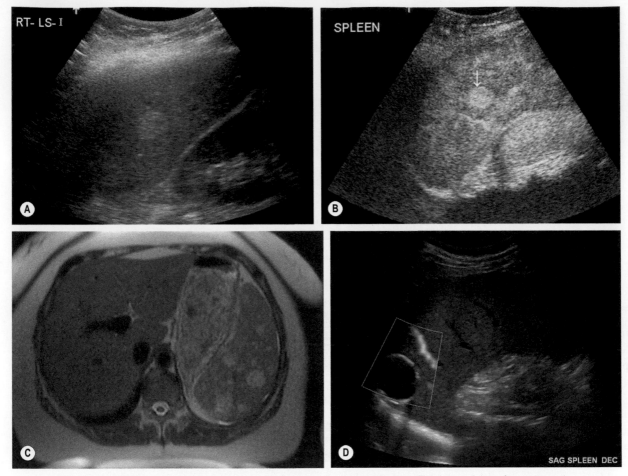

Fig. 5.4 (A) Solitary hyperechoic splenic lesion in a patient with melanoma. This is suspicious for metastasis. (B) Contrast-enhanced ultrasound demonstrates the arterial vascularity in the metastasis and several other lesions. (C) Magnetic resonance imaging confirms splenic metastases. (D) Splenic pseudocyst. (Source: 5.4(d) Fundamentals of Emergency Ultrasound, 2020.)

solitary, multiple, or diffusely infiltrative, giving a coarse echo pattern. Metastases are usually solid in appearance. When cystic components are seen, this could indicate central necrosis or that the primary tumor is mucinous in nature (e.g., ovarian carcinoma).[13]

BENIGN SPLENIC CONDITIONS

Focal lesions within the spleen are rare and are usually incidental findings when examining another organ.

Many benign focal lesions that occur in the spleen are of similar nature and ultrasound appearances to those in the liver.

Cysts

Splenic cysts have a relatively low incidence but are nevertheless the most common benign mass found in the spleen (Fig. 5.4D). Typically, cysts are rounded, with a thin wall with no internal echoes and posterior enhancement; occasionally thin septations may be seen, and also debris because of hemorrhage. Splenic cysts may occasionally be associated with autosomal dominant polycystic disease.

Other causes of cystic lesions in the spleen include post-traumatic cysts (liquefied hematoma) and hydatid cysts (*Echinococcus granulosus* parasite). Non-parasitic cysts are subdivided into congenital (e.g., Dermoid and epidermoid) and neoplastic cysts.[13]

As with hepatic cysts, hemorrhage may occur, causing LUQ pain. To avoid rupture, large cysts may be resected.

Abscess

Splenic abscesses usually result from bloodborne bacterial infection but can also be because of amoebic infection or post-traumatic or fungal infection. Patients with splenomegaly resulting from typhoid fever, malaria, and sickle cell disease are particularly predisposed to the formation of multiple pyogenic abscesses in the spleen.

Splenic abscesses are also particularly associated with immunosuppression, AIDS, and high-dose chemotherapy. Such patients become susceptible to invasive fungal infections, which can cause multifocal microabscesses in the liver and spleen.[14] Patients present, as might be expected, with LUQ pain and fever.

The ultrasound appearances are similar to liver abscesses; they may be single or multiple, hyperechoic, and homogeneous in the early stages, progressing to complex, fluid-filled structures with increased through transmission (Fig. 5.5A–B).

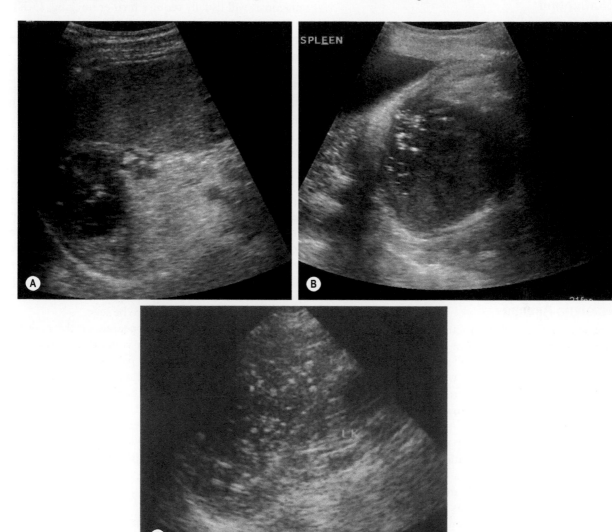

Fig. 5.5 (A) Large splenic abscess in an immunosuppressed patient following hepatic transplantation. (B) Large splenic abscess resulting from an infected hematoma. Note the left pleural effusion. (C) Multiple granulomas throughout the spleen.

Splenic abscesses are frequently hypoechoic, and it may not be possible to differentiate abscess from lymphoma or metastases on ultrasound appearances alone. This applies both in cases of large solitary abscesses and in multifocal microabscesses. They may also contain gas, posing difficulties for diagnosis as the area may be mistaken for overlying bowel.

As with liver abscesses, percutaneous drainage with antibiotic therapy is the management of choice for solitary abscesses.

Calcification

Calcification may occur in the wall of old, inactive abscess cavities, forming granulomatous deposits. Calcification is often found secondary to changes of the splenic tissue because of tuberculosis (TB) and other infective processes. Other conditions causing calcification within the spleen include HIV, histoplasmosis, *Pneumocystis carinii*, and *Mycobacterium avium-intracellulare*.[13] Calcification is also associated with post-traumatic injury and may be seen around the wall of an old, resolving post-traumatic hematoma.

Conditions that predispose to the deposition of calcium in tissues, such as renal failure requiring dialysis, are also a source of splenic calcification.

Ultrasound findings include multiple hyperechoic lesions throughout the splenic tissue, some of which may display acoustic shadowing (Fig. 5.5C) and is sometimes referred to as "spotty spleen."

Hemolytic Anemia

Increased red blood cell destruction, or *hemolysis*, occurs under two circumstances: when there is an abnormality of the red cells – as in sickle cell anemia, thalassemia, or hereditary spherocytosis – or when a destructive process is at work, such as infection or autoimmune conditions. Fragile red cells are destroyed by the spleen, which becomes enlarged (Fig. 5.6A).

Sickle cell anemia is most prevalent in the black American and African populations. Progression of the disease leads to repeated infarcts in various organs, including the spleen, which may eventually become shrunken and fibrosed. Patients have (non-obstructive) jaundice because the increased destruction of red blood cells releases excessive amounts of bilirubin into the blood.

VASCULAR ABNORMALITIES OF THE SPLEEN

A range of vascular neoplasms may occur in the spleen, most of which are relatively rare.[15] These include hemangiomas (see above), lymphangioma, and the (malignant) angiosarcoma. A hamartoma is a rare hypervascular lesion that is found in the spleen and often appears as a solid lesion with cystic or necrotic areas and possible small areas of calcification. These lesions may be demonstrated on ultrasound, but a definitive diagnosis will usually require further imaging, such as magnetic resonance imaging (MRI), and splenectomy may be performed in cases of a mass with atypical features.

Hemangioma

Benign hemangioma rarely occurs in the spleen. As in the liver, it is usually found as an incidental lesion on ultrasound. Multiple hemangiomata are rare and are usually seen as a solitary lesion. There are two types of hemangioma. The more common "capillary" hemangioma is well defined and hyperechoic compared to the splenic tissue. Color Doppler can be used, but machine settings will need to be altered to adequately demonstrate the low velocity flow; contrast-enhanced ultrasound (CEUS) can help view the blood supply of these lesions. A cavernous hemangioma may have a more atypical appearance on ultrasound, appearing more hypoechoic or of mixed echogenicity; partial calcification, and cystic components may also be seen.

Due to the variation in appearances, the presence of a hemangioma can give a conundrum, especially when found incidentally. The patient's clinical history must be taken into consideration; differential diagnoses would include metastases, hematopoiesis, and lymphoma, and in these cases, CEUS, MRI, and CT may be required to aid diagnosis. In cases with a low clinical suspicion of malignancy, such lesions may be followed up with ultrasound and tend to remain stable in size (Fig. 5.6B).

Splenic Infarction

Splenic infarction is most commonly associated with sickle cell anemia, hematological malignancies, thrombophilia, and emboli because of endocarditis. It has also

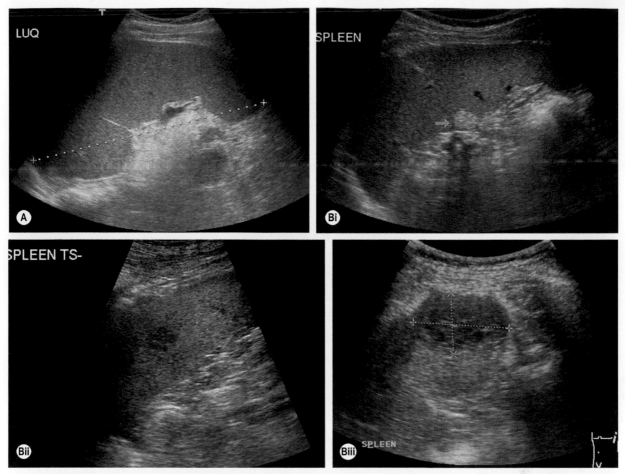

Fig. 5.6 (A) Splenomegaly in hereditary spherocytosis. (B) Splenic hemangiomas: (Bi) a small well-defined hyperechoic hemangioma near the splenic hilum; (Bii) a solitary, hypoechoic splenic hemangioma; and (Biii) a large complex splenic hemangioma.

been reported more recently as a complication of hepatocellular carcinoma embolization.[16] It usually results from thrombosis of one or more of the splenic artery branches. Because the spleen is supplied by both the splenic and gastric arteries, infarction tends to be segmental rather than global. Patients may present with LUQ pain, but not invariably.

Initially, the area of infarction is hypoechoic and usually wedge-shaped, solitary, and extending to the periphery of the spleen (Fig. 5.7). In the acute phase of infarction, B-mode ultrasound is not often useful, only identifying 50% of infarctions resulting in a high false-negative rate. The lesion may decrease in time and gradually fibrose, becoming hyperechoic. If the infarction is large, it may demonstrate reduced Doppler perfusion when compared to the normal splenic tissue, and CEUS may be particularly helpful in outlining the area of non-perfusion, allowing a definitive diagnosis and is represented as a triangular or slightly rounded area with the base extending to the splenic capsule. In rare cases of total splenic infarction (Fig. 5.7D), because of occlusion of the proximal main splenic artery, gray-scale sonographic appearances may be normal in the early stages.

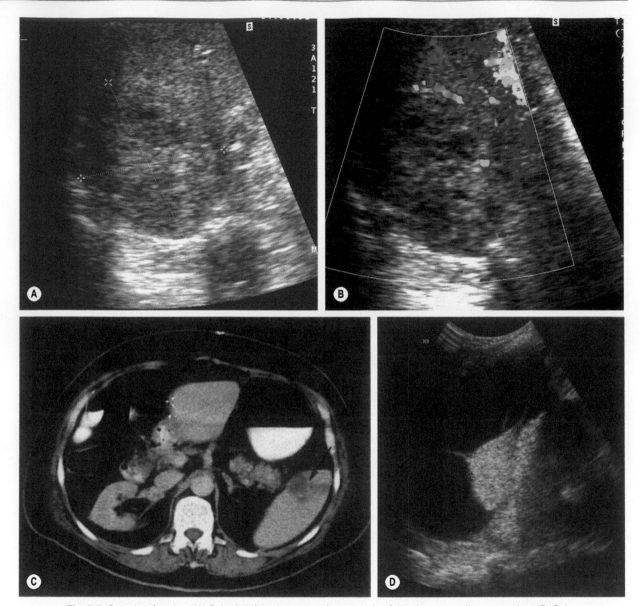

Fig. 5.7 Splenic infarction. (A) Splenic infarct because of an embolus following recent liver resection. (B) Color Doppler of the same patient demonstrates a lack of perfusion in the infarcted area. (C) Computed tomography scan of a splenic infarct. (D) Complete splenic infarction. The spleen is small and hyperechoic. Considerable free fluid is present.

Splenic Vein Thrombosis

This is frequently accompanied by portal vein thrombosis and results from the same disorders. The most common of these are pancreatitis and tumor thrombus. Color and spectral Doppler are an invaluable aid to the diagnosis, particularly when the thrombus is fresh and therefore echo-poor. Contrast agents may be administered if doubt exists over vessel patency. Splenic vein occlusion causes splenomegaly, and varices may be identified around the splenic hilum.

Splenic Artery Aneurysm

Although rare, splenic artery aneurysms are the third most common abdominal aneurysm, with aneurysms of the aorta and iliac arteries having greater incidence.[17] On ultrasound, a cystic lesion may be seen around the splenic hilum, and color Doppler can often identify whether this is a vascular structure or whether this is a cystic lesion, such as pancreatic pseudocysts.

Splenic artery aneurysms are usually asymptomatic and are associated with pregnancy or liver disease with portal hypertension. It is only clinically significant if over 2 cm in diameter when the risk of rupture and fatal hemorrhage is present. Surgical resection and ligation was once the treatment of choice. However, now with growing acceptance for treating arterial aneurysms by endovascular methods, the emergence of endovascular ablative therapy has now become an option, although there is still not much evidence on the long term efficacy of this method.

Pseudoaneurysm

Pseudoaneurysm in the spleen occurs in a minority of cases following splenic trauma or in the context of chronic pancreatitis. An echo-free or "cystic" area may be observed, which demonstrates flow on color Doppler. To distinguish between a "true" aneurysm and pseudoaneurysm, the following features should be present in a true aneurysm: focal arterial disruption and inflammation at the location of an irregular vessel wall.[17]

Splenic Trauma

The presence of free fluid in the abdomen of a trauma victim as part of a FAST (focused abdominal sonography in trauma) scan should alert the sonographer to the strong possibility of organ injury following blunt abdominal injury. However, visualization of the laceration may be difficult to visualize on ultrasound, especially in the acute phase. A frank area of hemorrhage, easily identifiable on ultrasound, may not develop until later. The Royal College of Radiologists is clear that FAST scanning should not delay the transfer to CT and should be used as a triage tool in prioritizing patients, rather than as an alternative to CT.[18]

CT should be performed as the first imaging step in patients with blunt trauma, as it can also detect laceration to the gastrointestinal tract and other extra-visceral injury as well as assess the blood supply within the spleen (Fig. 5.8).

Iatrogenic splenic trauma has been known because of the 'blind' insertion of a drain in the case of left pleural

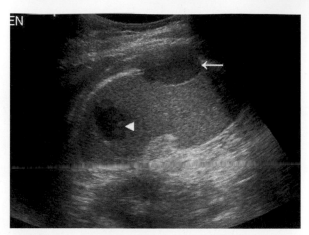

Fig. 5.8 A subcapsular hematoma in the spleen (arrow) following injury, with blood surrounding the spleen and a left pleural effusion. Another hematoma is seen superior to this (arrowhead).

effusion. Thankfully, the guidance from the British Thoracic Society and the National Patient Safety Agency to perform such procedures under ultrasound guidance, following proper training, has reduced such incidents.

Lymphatic System

The lymphatic system is made up of a network of open-ended, low-pressure vessels, lymph nodes, and organs occluding the spleen but also other organs such as the tonsils and thymus, and these provide the route of return of interstitial fluid back into the circulatory system and also to fight infection.

As lymphatic drainage is by one-directional flow back toward the heart, it is necessary to consider this when looking for spread from a known malignancy. Lymphatic circulation from the visceral organs will drain into the nodes between the lungs and around the intestines, and so this is often where the first evidence of malignant spread is seen. This lymphatic drainage will continue either along the right lymphatic duct or the thoracic duct (left side) and then enter the bloodstream via the subclavian veins in the neck, Palpable lymphadenopathy in the supraclavicular fossa may be identified in patients with a malignancy and there is evidence of metastatic spread via the lymphatic system (Fig. 5.9A–B).

Normal lymph nodes are difficult to demonstrate on ultrasound, but in certain areas, such as at the porta hepatis, normal lymph nodes can be demonstrated using a suitable acoustic window, such as the liver (Fig. 5.9C), particularly in young and/or thin patients.

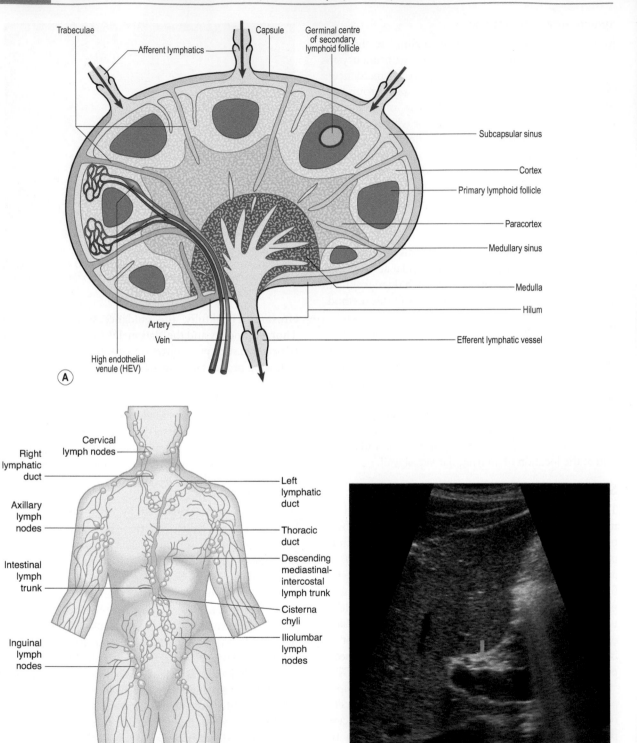

Fig. 5.9 (A) Structure of a lymph node. (B) Anatomic pathways and lymph node groups of the lymphatic system. (C) Normal lymph nodes can be demonstrated at the porta in slim patients.

Continued

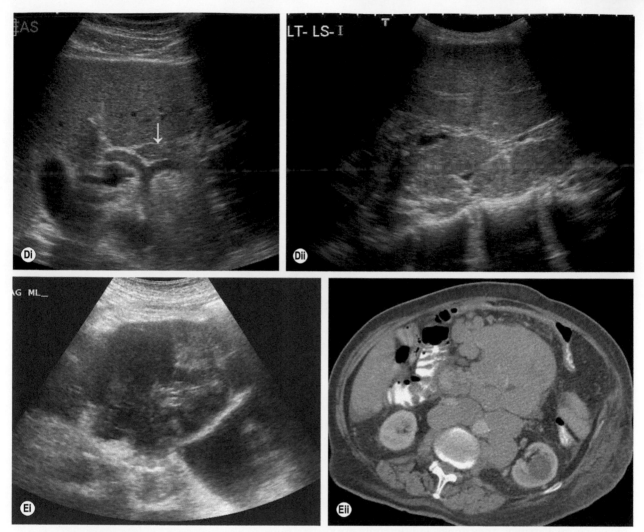

Fig. 5.9, cont'd (Di) Small lymph node (arrow) at the coeliac axis, typical of the findings in hepatitis C. (Dii) Lymphadenopathy in the epigastrium, posterior to the left lobe of the liver. (Ei) Large complex lymphomatous mass in the abdomen, superior to the bladder. (Eii) Computed tomography (CT) of the same case demonstrating extensive small bowel mesenteric node masses.

Continued

A normal lymph node is "bean" shaped and has a smooth, well defined capsule. Because of the tendency of abnormal nodes to be rounder in shape, lymph nodes should be measured at the narrowest point (short axis diameter). Although there can be some variation, a short axis measurement of greater than 10 mm would be considered abnormal. Reactive nodes can sometimes have a more lobular outline and can also be enlarged; clinical context is often useful in these cases. On ultrasound, the cortex of the normal lymph node is mildly hypoechoic with a hyperechoic central hilum which contains the lymphatic vessels and blood supply. This may be clearly seen in superficial nodes, but in deeper positions, the resolution may not be adequate. In these cases, the size and shape of the nodes will be the most important factors to determine abnormality. The search for lymphadenopathy should include the para-aortic and para-caval regions, the splanchnic vessels and epigastric regions, and the renal hilar (Fig. 5.9D–F). Ultrasound has a low sensitivity for demonstrating

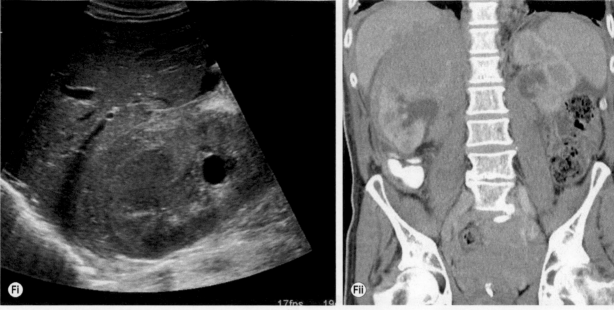

Fig. 5.9, cont'd (Fi) Lymphoma has invaded the right kidney. (Fii) CT confirms the right kidney invasion and obstructive retroperitoneal lymphadenopathy. (Source: 5.9 (a,b): Gray's Anatomy: The Anatomical Basis of Clinical Practice , Forty Second edition, 2021; Sabiston Textbook of Surgery: The Biological Basis of Modern Surgical Practice , Twenty First Edition, 2022.)

lymphadenopathy in the retroperitoneum, as bowel contents frequently obscure the relevant areas. CT and MRI can better define the extent of lymphadenopathy, particularly in the pelvis. PET is now commonly used to look for widespread lymphadenopathy.

The presence of lymphadenopathy is highly non-specific, being associated with a wide range of conditions, including malignancy, infections, and inflammatory disorders. Benign lymphadenopathy is commonly seen in conjunction with hepatitis and other inflammatory disorders such as pancreatitis, cholangitis, and colitis.[19]

Enlarged nodes are most often hypoechoic, rounded, or oval in shape and well defined in some cases infiltrating into adjacent structures or may combine to form large, lobulated masses. Nodes must be differentiated from other masses (such as gastrointestinal tract or other inflammatory masses), and Doppler is helpful here. Larger nodes display color or power Doppler radiating from a central hilum.

Lymphadenopathy occasionally causes obstructive jaundice because of compression of the common bile duct near the porta hepatis or venous thrombosis because of compression of the adjacent vein.

Lymphangioma

These are uncommon congenital malformations of the lymphatic system, which are usually diagnosed in the neonatal period or on prenatal sonography. They are predominantly cystic, frequently septated, and may be large (Fig. 5.10). They can compress adjacent organs and vessels, and their severity depends largely upon their

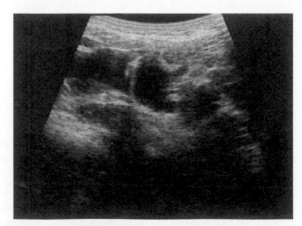

Fig. 5.10 Lymphangioma. This large, septated cystic mass was present in the chest wall of this two-year-old girl.

location. They are most common in the neck (cystic hygroma) but can be found in various locations, including the abdomen,[20] and are occasionally found in adults after a long asymptomatic period.

REFERENCES

1. Hosey RG, Mattacola CG, Jagger S. Ultrasound. *Br J Sports Med.* 2006;40(3):251–254.
2. Chow KU, Luxembourg B, Seifried E, Bonig H. Spleen size is significantly influenced by body height and sex: establishment of normal values for spleen size at US with a cohort of 1200 healthy individuals. *Radiol.* 2016;279:306–313.
3. Preeti T, Fulmali DG, Bakane BC, Chimkumar VK. Accessory splenic tissue: a cadaveric study. *Int J Med Res Prof.* 2018;4:261–263.
4. Bhogal R, Wotherspoon A, Zerize I, Khan A. Pancreatic tail splenunclus: case report and review of literature. *Int J Surg Case Reo.* 2019;57:36–38.
5. Rasool F, Mirza B. Polysplenia syndrome associated with situs inversus abdominis and type I jejunal atresia. *ASPS J Case Rep.* 2011;2(2):18.
6. Ingle S, Hinge C. Primary splenic lymphoma. current diagnostic trends. *World J Clin Cases.* Second Edition. London: Royal College of Radiologists; 2016;4(12):385–389.
7. Frampas E. Lymphomas: basic points that radiologists should know. *Diag Intervent Imaging.* 2013;94(2):131–144.
8. Townsend R, Laing F, Jeffrey B, Bottles K. Abdominal lymphoma in AIDS. Evaluation with ultrasound. *Radiol.* 1989;171:719–724.
9. Leite N, Kased N, Hanna R, et al. Cross-sectional imaging of extranodal involvement in abdominopelvic lymphoproliferative malignancies. *Radiographics.* 2007;27:1613–1634.
10. Jhanwar Y, Straus D. The role of PET in lymphoma. *J Nucl Med.* 2006;47:1326–1334.
11. Siniluoto T, Paivansalo M, Alavaikko M. Ultrasonography of spleen and liver in staging Hodgkin's disease. *Eur J Radiol.* 1991;13:181–186.
12. Ishida H, Konno K, Naganuma H, et al. Splenic lymphoma: differentiation from splenic cysts with ultrasonography. *Abdom Imaging.* 2001;26:529–532.
13. Benter T, Kluhs L. Sonography of the spleen. *J Ultrasound Med.* 2011;30:1281–1293.
14. Gorg C, Weide R, Schwerk WB, et al. Ultrasound evaluation of hepatic and splenic microabscesses in the immunocompromised patient: sonographic patterns, differential diagnosis and follow-up. *J Clin Ultrasound.* 1994;22:525–529.
15. Abbott RM, Levy AD, Aguilera NS, et al. From the archives of the AFIP: primary vascular neoplasms of the spleen: radiologic-pathologic correlation. *Radiographics.* 2004;24:1137–1163.
16. Caremani M, Occhini U, Tacconi D, Lapini L, Accorsi AL, Mazzarelli C. Focal splenic lesions: US findings. *J Ultrasound.* 2013;16(2):65–74.
17. O'Lakin R, Vashyap VS. The contemporary management of splenic artery aneurysms. *J Vasc Surg.* 2011;53(4):958–965.
18. Royal College of Radiologists. Standards of practice and guidance for trauma radiology in severely injured patients. 2011;3(11):3.
19. Gimondo P, Mirk P, Messina G, Pizzi C. Abdominal lymphadenopathy in benign diseases: sonographic detection and clinical significance. *J Ultrasound Med.* 1996;15:353–359.
20. Schmidt M. Intra-abdominal lymphangioma. *Kans Med.* 1995;93:149–150.

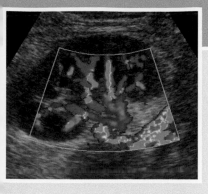

6

Ultrasound of the Renal Tract

Nicola J. Davidson

CHAPTER OUTLINE

The Normal Renal Tract, 186
Ultrasound Technique, 186
Normal Ultrasound Appearances of the
    Kidneys and Urinary Bladder, 186
    Measurements, 188
    Hemodynamics, 189
Assessment of Renal Function, 189
Renal Anatomical Variants, 189
Duplex Kidney, 189
Ectopic Kidneys, 192
Horseshoe Kidneys, 192
Extrarenal Pelvis, 192
Hypertrophied Column of Bertin, 192
Renal Humps, 192
Renal Cysts and Cystic Disease, 193
Cysts, 193
    Ultrasound Appearances, 193
Autosomal Dominant Polycystic
    Kidney Disease, 194
    Ultrasound Appearances, 194
Von Hippel–Lindau Disease, 194
Tuberose Sclerosis (TS), 195
Acquired Cystic Disease, 195
Multicystic Dysplastic Kidney, 196
Benign Focal Renal Tumors, 196
Angiomyolipoma (AML), 196
Adenoma, 196
Malignant Renal Tract Masses, 196
Imaging and Management of Malignant Renal
    Masses, 196
Renal Cell Carcinoma, 197
    Ultrasound Appearances, 197

Transitional Cell Carcinoma, 197
    Ultrasound Appearances, 197
Lymphoma, 199
Metastases, 199
Von Hippel–Lindau Disease, 201
**Pelvicalyceal System Dilatation and Obstructive
Uropathy, 201**
Physiological Dilatation, 201
Obstructive Uropathy, 201
Further Management of Renal Obstruction, 202
Pyonephrosis, 202
    Non-Dilated Renal Obstruction, 204
    Vesicoureteric Junction, 207
Non-Obstructive Hydronephrosis, 207
    Reflux, 207
    Post-Obstructive Dilatation, 207
Renal Tract Calcificaton/Renal Tract Stones, 207
    Ultrasound Appearances, 207
Staghorn Calculi, 209
Nephrocalcinosis, 209
    Ultrasound Appearances, 209
Hyperparathyroidism, 209
Hematuria, 210
    Nutcracker Syndrome, 211
Renal Tract Inflammation and Infection, 211
Pyelonephritis, 211
    Acute Pyelonephritis, 211
    Chronic Pyelonephritis, 211
    Bladder Diverticula, 212
    Focal Pyelonephritis, 212
    Renal Abscess, 213
    Xanthogranulomatous Pyelonephritis, 213

Diffuse Renal Disease and Renal Failure, 214
　Acute/Chronic Kidney Injury (AKI), 214
　Glomerulonephritis, 214
　Medullary Sponge Kidney, 214
　Amyloid, 215
Renal Vascular Pathologic Conditions, 216
　Renal Artery Stenosis (RAS), 216
Renal Trauma, 216
Renal Transplants, 217
　Normal Anatomy, 217
　Normal Ultrasound Appearances, 217
　Postoperative Complications, 217
　Renal Transplant Dilatation, 219
　Rejection, 219
　　Ultrasound Appearances, 219

　　Fluid Collections Associated with
　　　Transplantation, 221
　Vascular Complications, 223
　　Vascular Occlusion, 223
　　Renal Artery Stenosis, 223
　　Renal Vein Thrombosis, 224
　　Pseudoaneurysms and AV Fistulae, 225
　Infection, 226
　Acute Tubular Necrosis, 226
　Cyclosporin Nephrotoxicity, 227
　Renal Transplant Dysfunction and Doppler
　　Correlation, 227
References, 227

THE NORMAL RENAL TRACT

Ultrasound Technique

The kidneys are positioned in the retroperitoneum, on either side of the vertebral column between the level of T12 and L3. The right kidney is usually slightly lower than the left because of the position of the liver, and the upper poles of both kidneys are more posterior than the lower poles. Due to the oblique position, it is often necessary to scan from various angles to ensure the entire kidney is seen. Bowel gas and rib shadowing can also cause poor visualization, and in these situations, it may be necessary to rotate the patient to move the bowel or encourage the patient, if possible, to raise an arm above their head to lift the ribs out of view.

Start by obtaining a longitudinal section of the kidney. Place the probe in the mid axillary line with the upper part of the probe angled more posteriorly, roughly similar to the angle of the ribs. Once the kidney is seen, twist the probe to extend the length of the kidney to ensure both poles are visualized taking care not to foreshorten the kidney. Once in a true longitudinal position, sweep through the kidney making sure to scan beyond the borders of the kidney; the probe can then be rotated to 90 degrees and scanned fully in the transverse section. This will provide the operator confidence that the full kidney has been seen and that extrinsic pathologic conditions have not been missed.

The right kidney is readily demonstrated through the right lobe of the liver, which acts as an acoustic window. Generally, a subcostal approach displays the (more anterior) lower pole to best effect, while an intercostal approach is best for demonstrating the upper pole (Fig. 6.1). The left kidney (LK) lies posterior to the stomach and splenic flexure, making visualization difficult because of the bowel overlying the kidney. The spleen can be used as an acoustic window to the upper pole by scanning coronally, from the patient's left side, with the patient supine or decubitus (left side raised) but, unless the spleen is enlarged, the lower pole must usually be imaged from the left side posteriorly. Coronal sections of both kidneys are particularly useful as they display the renal pelvicalyceal system and its relationship to the renal hilum (Fig. 6.1C). This section demonstrates the main blood vessels and ureter (if dilated). As with any other organ, the kidneys must be examined in both longitudinal and transverse (axial) planes, and the operator must be flexible in their approach to obtain the necessary results.

The bladder should be filled and examined to complete the renal tract scan. An excessively full bladder may cause temporary mild dilatation of the pelvicalyceal system (PCS), which will return to normal following micturition.

Normal Ultrasound Appearances of the Kidneys and Urinary Bladder

The cortex of the normal kidney is slightly hypoechoic when compared to the adjacent liver parenchyma, although this is age dependent. In young people, it may be

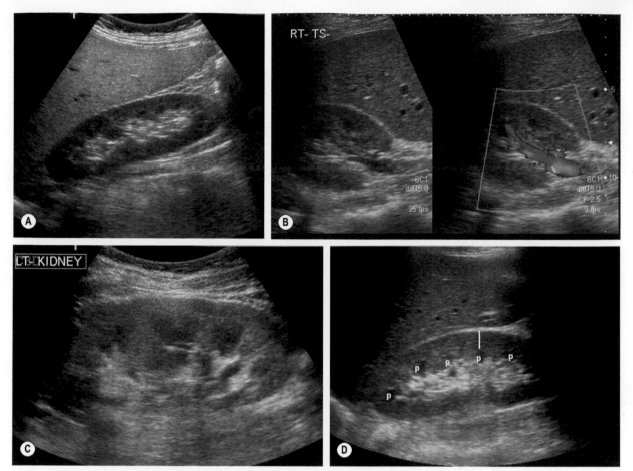

Fig. 6.1 (A) Sagittal section through the normal right kidney (RK), using the liver as an acoustic window. The central echoes from the renal sinus are hyperechoic because of the fat content. The hypoechoic, triangular, medullary pyramids are demonstrated in a regular arrangement around the sinus. The cortex is of similar echogenicity to the liver. (B) Transverse section through the hilum of the RK. Color Doppler shows flow in the main renal vein and artery. (C) LK in coronal section. The renal hilum is seen furthest from the transducer. (Compare this with the sagittal section of the RK in which cortex is seen all the way around the PCS.) (D) Pyramids (p) are arranged regularly around the pelvicalyceal system. The renal cortical thickness is represented by the white line.

of similar echogenicity, and in the elderly, it is not unusual for it to be more hyperechoic and thinner. The medullary pyramids are seen as regularly spaced, hypoechoic (not echo-free) triangular structures between the cortex and the renal sinus (Fig. 6.1D). The tiny reflective structures often seen at the margins of the pyramids are echoes from the arcuate arteries which branch around the pyramids.

The renal sinus containing the pelvicalyceal system is hyperechoic because of the sinus fat that surrounds the vessels. The main renal artery and vein can be read-

ily demonstrated at the renal hilum and should not be confused with a mild degree of pelvicalyceal dilatation. Color Doppler can help differentiate.

The kidney develops in the fetus from several lobes that fuse together. Occasionally the traces of these lobes can be seen on the surface of the kidney, forming *fetal lobulations* (Fig. 6.2A); these may persist into adulthood. The issue for the sonographer is being able to recognize these as normal variations, as distinct from a renal mass or renal scarring.

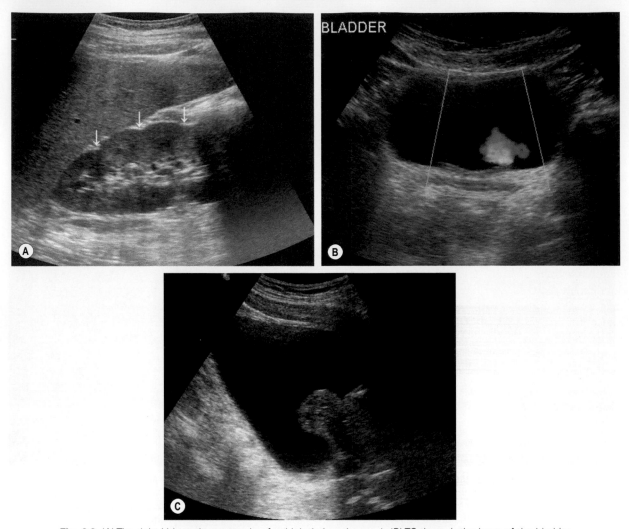

Fig. 6.2 (A) The right kidney demonstrating fetal lobulations (arrows). (B) TS through the base of the bladder, demonstrating a left ureteric jet. (C) An enlarged prostate indents the bladder. It is sometimes easy to confuse this with a bladder mass. This may be associated with incomplete emptying and/or retention. A post-micturition scan is useful in estimating residual volume.

When the bladder is distended with urine, the walls are thin, regular, and hyperechoic. The walls may appear thickened or trabeculated if the bladder is insufficiently distended, making it difficult to exclude a bladder lesion. The ureteric orifices can be demonstrated in a transverse section at the bladder base. Ureteric jets can easily be demonstrated with color Doppler at this point and normally occur between 1.5 and 12.4 times per min (a mean of 5.4 jets per min) from each side (Fig. 6.2B).[1]

Measurements

The normal adult kidney measures between 9 cm and 12 cm in length and should be routinely recorded in the report as part of the protocol. There is also evidence to suggest that renal size decreases in age once 60 years is reached;[2] this ensures that any variance outside of normal parameters can be compared to previous imaging, rather than seen in isolation. Obtaining the maximum renal length may involve an intercostal scan with rib shadowing over the central portion of the kidney or trying to obtain an alternative position. A subcostal section, which foreshortens the kidney, often underestimates the length, and it is more accurate to measure a coronal or posterior longitudinal section with the beam perpendicular to the renal axis.

The cortical thickness of the kidney is generally taken as the distance between the capsule and the margin of the medullary pyramid (Fig. 6.1D) and normally measures 10 mm or more.[2] Evaluation of the cortex thickness is generally a good indicator of renal function, with a reduced cortex being linked to poorer eGFR.[3] Cortical thickness will vary between individuals and within individual kidneys and tends to decrease with age.

The most common method of measuring bladder volume with 2D ultrasound is a prolate ellipsoid method. The ellipsoid requires the operator to firstly identify the transverse, anteroposterior, and superoinferior diameter lengths of the bladder from 2D ultrasound images and then calculates volume based on a mathematical formula that is inbuilt into the software of the ultrasound machine.[4] If the software is unavailable, the bladder volume can be estimated by multiplying the three measurements obtained by 0.56.

TIP BOX

Bladder volume (mLs) =

(Transverse × Anteroposterior × Superoinferior) × 0.56

Bladder volume can also be assessed with a 3D ultrasound probe, in which all of the measurements can be obtained while scanning in one plane. Studies show that although a 3D technique may underestimate the bladder volume, it is still an acceptable method of assessment, especially in a clinic or treatment setting.[5]

Hemodynamics

The vascular tree of the kidney can be effectively demonstrated with color Doppler (Fig 6.3). By manipulating the system sensitivity and using a low pulse repetition frequency, small vessels can be demonstrated at the periphery of the kidney.

Demonstration of the extrarenal main artery and vein with color Doppler is most successful in the coronal or axial section by identifying the renal hilum and tracing the artery back to the aorta or the vein to the inferior vena cava (IVC). The best Doppler signals, i.e., the highest Doppler shift frequencies, are obtained when the direction of the vessel is parallel to the beam and taken on suspended respiration. The left renal vein (LRV) is readily demonstrated between the superior mesenteric artery (SMA) and aorta by scanning just below the body of the pancreas in the transverse section. The origins of the renal arteries may be seen arising from the aorta in a coronal section (Fig. 6.3D).

The normal adult renal vasculature is of low resistance with a fast, almost vertical systolic upstroke and continuous forward end diastolic flow (EDF). Resistance generally increases with age.[6] The more peripheral arteries are of lower velocity with weaker Doppler signals and are less pulsatile than the main renal artery at the hilum.

ASSESSMENT OF RENAL FUNCTION

Blood and urine tests can be useful indicators of pathologic conditions. The request to perform ultrasound is frequently triggered by biochemical results outside of the normal range.

Raised serum levels of urea and creatinine are associated with a reduction in renal function. However, any damage is usually quite severe before this becomes apparent. The creatinine clearance rate estimates the amount of creatinine excreted over 24 h and is a guide to the glomerular filtration rate (GFR) (normal GFR 100–120 mL/min). A poor rate of clearance (mL/min) is indicative of renal failure.

Blood in the urine is a potentially serious sign that should prompt investigation with ultrasound. Frank hematuria may be a sign of renal tract malignancy. Microscopic hematuria may reflect inflammation, infection, calculi, or malignancy. The urine can be easily examined for protein, glucose, acetone, and pH using chemically impregnated strips.

RENAL ANATOMICAL VARIANTS

Duplex Kidney

This term is used to describe a spectrum of possible appearances from two separate kidneys with separate collecting systems and duplex ureters to a more simple division of the pelvicalyceal system at the renal hilum (Fig. 6.4A). The latter is more difficult to recognize on ultrasound, but the two moieties of the pelvicalyceal system are separated by a zone of the normal renal cortex, which invaginates the kidney – a *hypertrophied column of Bertin* (see below).

Duplex kidney is the most common congenital renal abnormality with an incidence of 0.8% and is more

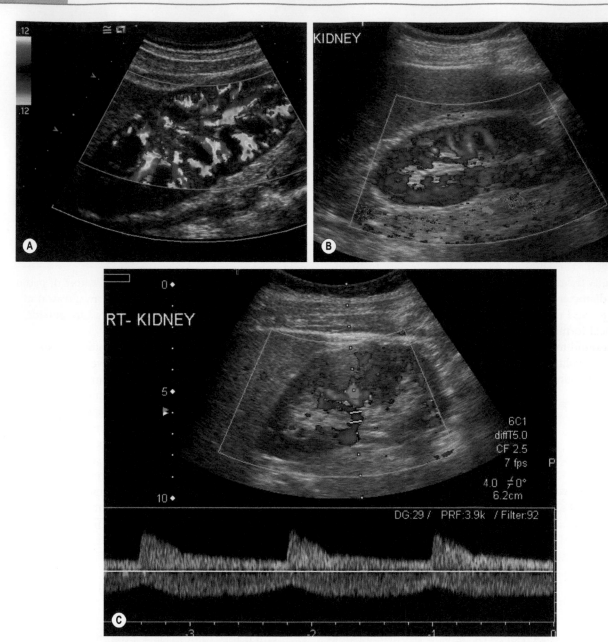

Fig. 6.3 (A) Color Doppler of the right kidney demonstrating normal intrarenal perfusion throughout the kidney. (B) Power Doppler demonstrating renal perfusion. (C) The waveform from the main renal artery at the hilum of the kidney is of low resistance with good end diastolic flow. The spectrum from the adjacent vein can be seen below the baseline.

Continued

common in women than men.[7] It may be associated with reflux, ectopic ureteric orifice, or ureterocele and may predispose the patient to infection or obstruction. However, patients may be asymptomatic, and a duplex system is identified incidentally. The main issue for the sonographer here is that one moiety may be mistaken on ultrasound for the entire kidney, especially if bowel gas overlies part of the kidney, and the operator must ensure that both renal poles are properly demonstrated.

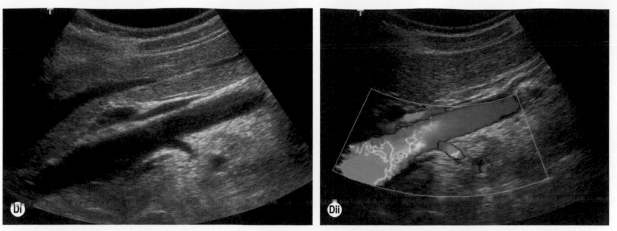

Fig. 6.3, cont'd (Di) Coronal section through the aorta taken from the patient's right side showing the origin of the left renal artery (LRA). (Dii) The LRA appears in blue as it is flowing away from the transducer.

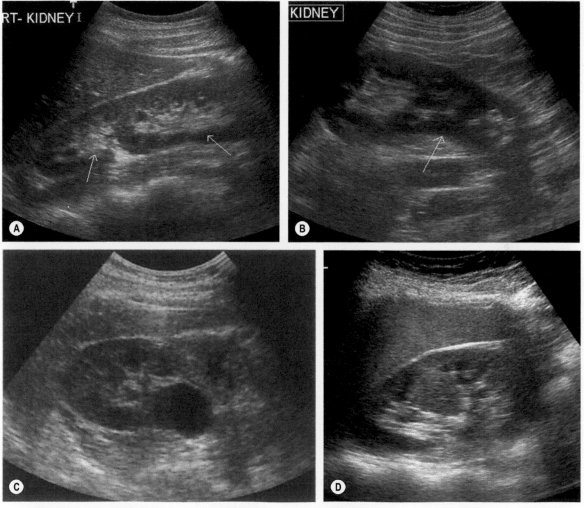

Fig. 6.4 (A) Duplex kidney showing two separate intrarenal collecting systems (arrows). (B) TS through the abdomen demonstrating the fused lower poles of the horseshoe kidney (arrow) anterior to the spine. (C) TS through the right kidney demonstrating a baggy extrarenal pelvis. The pelvicalyceal system remains undilated, and this should not be confused with hydronephrosis. (D) Hypertrophied column of Bertin.

Continued

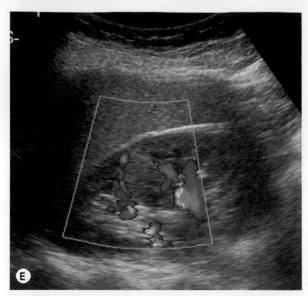

Fig. 6.4, cont'd (E) Color Doppler of the hypertrophied column reveals regular, normal interlobar vessels (as opposed to the irregularly distributed, increased flow through a renal cell carcinoma).

The main renal artery and vein may also be duplicated, which can occasionally be identified using color or power Doppler.

Ectopic Kidneys

An ectopic kidney is atypically positioned within the abdominal, lumbar, or pelvic regions because of incorrect migration during fetal development. During the "migration," it rotates inwards so that the renal hilum faces medially. A failure of this mechanism causes the kidney to fall short of its normal position, remaining in the pelvis, i.e., a pelvic kidney. Usually, it lies on the correct side. However, occasionally it can cross to the other side, lying inferior to its normally placed partner – *crossed renal ectopia*. Frequently it may fuse with the lower pole of the other kidney, *crossed fused renal ectopia*, resulting in what appears to be a very long, unilateral organ.

The incidence of ectopic kidneys in the clinical setting is 1:12,000. However, it can be seen in as many as 1:900 cases at post mortem, which shows that many are asymptomatic. Problems usually occur when the kidney is malrotated, leading to obstruction and stone formation.[8]

Horseshoe Kidneys

In the horseshoe kidney, the kidneys lie on each side of the abdomen, but their lower poles are fused by a connecting band of renal tissue, or *isthmus*, which lies

anterior to the aorta and IVC (Fig. 6.4B). The kidneys tend to be rotated and lie with their lower poles medially.

It may be difficult to visualize the isthmus because of bowel gas anterior to it. However, a horseshoe kidney should always be suspected when the operator cannot confidently identify the lower poles of the kidneys or when the lower pole seems unusually anterior and medial.

When the isthmus can be seen, it is important not to confuse it with other abdominal masses, such as lymphadenopathy.

Although a horseshoe kidney is the most common fusion defect of the kidney, the incidence is only around 0.01%–0.25%.

Extrarenal Pelvis

Not infrequently, the renal pelvis projects outside the kidney, medial to the renal sinus. This is best seen in a transverse section through the renal hilum. It is frequently "baggy" containing anechoic urine, which is prominently demonstrated on the ultrasound scan (Fig. 6.4C). The importance of recognizing the extrarenal pelvis lies in not confusing it with dilatation of the PCS or with a parapelvic cyst or collection.

Hypertrophied Column of Bertin

The septum of Bertin is an invagination of the renal cortex down to the renal sinus. It occurs at the junctions of original fetal lobulations and is present in duplex systems (see above), dividing the two moieties. Particularly prominent, hypertrophied columns of Bertin may mimic a renal tumor. It is usually possible to distinguish between the two as the column of Bertin does not affect the renal outline and has the same acoustic characteristics as the adjacent cortex (Fig. 6.4D–E).

> **TIP BOX**
>
> Color or power Doppler are helpful in revealing the normal, regular vascular pattern in a hypertrophied column of Bertin (as opposed to the chaotic and increased blood flow pattern of malignant renal tumors).

Renal Humps

These are areas of the renal cortex, which form a bulge in the renal outline. Like the hypertrophied column of Bertin, a hump may mimic a renal mass. Careful scanning can usually solve the dilemma as the cortex remains constant in thickness. The most usual manifestation is the dromedary or *splenic hump* on the LK, which is a flattening of the upper pole with a lateral prominence just below the margin of the spleen.

RENAL CYSTS AND CYSTIC DISEASE

Cysts

Simple cysts are a common finding in the general population, with the incidence increasing with age. Most cysts are asymptomatic and may be solitary or multiple. Most cysts are found within the renal cortex or extending beyond the renal capsule. A parapelvic cyst (within the renal pelvis) may be difficult to distinguish from pelvicalyceal dilatation, a calyceal diverticulum, or an extrarenal pelvis, and careful scanning is required to differentiate. Occasionally cysts can hemorrhage, causing pain. Large cysts, particularly of the lower pole, may be palpable, prompting a request for an ultrasound scan.

Ultrasound Appearances

Like cysts in any other organ, to be considered "simple," they must display three basic characteristics – anechoic; a thin, well-defined capsule; and exhibit posterior enhancement. It can be difficult to appreciate the posterior enhancement if the hyperechoic perirenal fat lies distal to the cyst; scanning from a different angle (Fig. 6.5) is

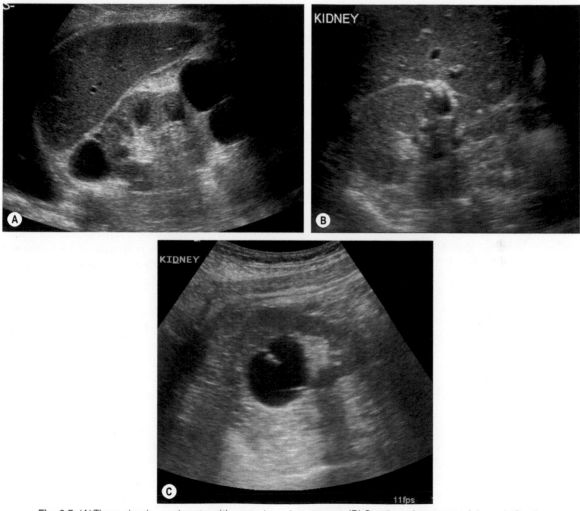

Fig. 6.5 (A) Three simple renal cysts with posterior enhancement. (B) Small renal cyst, containing calcification following episodes of infection. This remained stable on follow-up. (C) cyst with a thin septum and nodule of calcification on the wall. No contrast enhancement was demonstrated, and the cyst remained stable.

helpful. Hemorrhage or infection can give rise to low-level echoes within a cyst, and there may also be calcification of the cyst wall.

While a solitary, simple cyst can almost certainly be ignored, cysts with more complex acoustic characteristics may require further investigation, e.g., CT. A calcified wall may be associated with malignancy. Increasingly small renal cysts are incidentally discovered on ultrasound because of improved technology, and they are by no means always simple. In 1989, Bosniak proposed a classification of cysts to be used with CT to differentiate benign from malignant lesions[9]; although this has stood the test of time, it has recently been updated to try and reflect the differences seen in interpretation in different reporters (Table 6.1).[10] Since then, the image quality with 2D ultrasound has improved significantly, and evaluating complex cysts has become more common. 2D ultrasound could still provide the same levels of accuracy as CT/MRI when used to assess minimally complex

cysts.[11] With the wider use of contrast-enhanced ultrasound (CEUS), many studies have compared CT/MRI and CEUS and found that they show similar results when classifying renal cysts.[12]

These lesions can now be successfully characterized into the Bosniak classification using CEUS (Table 6.1).[13] CEUS can differentiate the vascularized solid components of complex renal masses at least as well as CT and can also be used to monitor lesions, thereby reducing the radiation dose from CT.

Autosomal Dominant Polycystic Kidney Disease

Autosomal dominant polycystic kidney disease (ADPKD) is the most common genetically linked renal disorder, and it is associated with progressive renal failure. A renal transplant offers a successful "cure" for many patients. Adult polycystic kidney disease (APKD) demonstrates a spectrum of severity, with some patients having renal failure in early life and others achieving a normal life span with no appreciable symptoms. In about 50% of cases, cysts are also present in the liver; they are also found in the spleen and pancreas in a small proportion of patients.

Ultrasound screening for APKD is performed in families with a positive history, as patients may then be monitored and treated for hypertension. A negative scan does not entirely exclude disease, especially in the pediatric group, and multiple examinations may need to be performed over the years.

Autosomal recessive polycystic kidney disease is often diagnosed prenatally or in young children (see pediatric chapter for more information).

Ultrasound Appearances

The disease is always bilateral, causing progressively enlarging kidneys with multiple cysts of various sizes, many having irregular margins (Fig. 6.6). There may be little or no demonstrable normal renal tissue, and the kidneys may become so large that they visibly distend the abdomen.

APKD predisposes the patient to urinary tract infections, stones, and cyst hemorrhage. The liver, spleen, and pancreas should also be examined on ultrasound for associated cysts.

Von Hippel–Lindau Disease

Von Hippel–Lindau disease (VHL) is an inherited autosomal dominant disease that affects the central nervous

Class	Bosniak Classification
TABLE 6.1	**Bosniak Classification (2019)**
I	Hairline-thin wall; water attenuation; no septa, calcifications, or solid components; nonenhancing
II	Two types:
	Few thin septa with or without perceived (not measurable) enhancement; fine calcification or a short segment of slightly thickened calcification in the wall or septa
	Homogeneously high-attenuating masses ≤3 cm that are sharply marginated and do not enhance
IIF	Two types:
	Minimally thickened or more than a few thin septa with or without perceived (nor measurable) enhancement that may have thick or nodular calcification
	Intrarenal nonenhancing hyperattenuating, renal masses >3 cm
III	Thickened or irregular walls or septa with measurable enhancement
IV	Soft-tissue components (ie, nodule[s]) with measurable enhancement

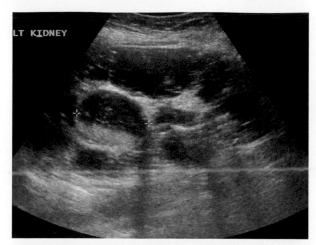

Fig. 6.6 Autosomal dominant ("adult") polycystic disease. Numerous cysts of varying sizes are seen within the renal bed. No discernable renal architecture is apparent. A cyst containing debris, i.e., hemorrhage (calipers), is present.

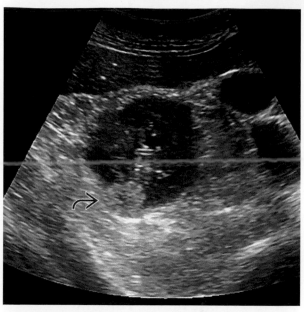

Fig. 6.7 Ultrasound shows a 1.3 cm uniform, highly echogenic lesion consistent with an angiomyolipoma. (Source: ExpertDDX: Abdomen & Pelvis, Second Edition, 2017.)

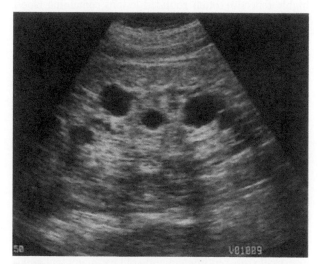

Fig. 6.8 In acquired kidney disease, the kidney can become shrunken with multiple cysts, which may contain hemorrhage or become infected.

system and retina with haemangioblastomas. Renal disease may present later, with cysts occurring in approximately 60%–70% of sufferers. Because there is a recognized association with renal adenocarcinoma in up to 45% of patients, ultrasound is useful in screening patients with the disease.

Tuberose Sclerosis (TS)

TS is a rare multisystem disorder with a wide spectrum of possible presentations. Up to 75% of patients may develop multiple renal cysts and/or multiple angiomyolipomas (AMLs).[14] Rarely, renal cell carcinoma may occur, although it is thought that the occurrence is similar to that of the general population. However, renal cell carcinoma (RCC) tends to occur at a younger age in patients with TS (Fig. 6.7).

Acquired Cystic Disease

This condition tends to affect patients on long term dialysis who may already have shrunken, end-stage kidneys. Its frequency increases with the duration of dialysis (Fig. 6.8).

Multiple cysts form in the kidneys, which may, like ADPKD, hemorrhage or become infected. The disease tends to be more severe the longer the patient has been on dialysis. The proliferative changes which cause acquired cystic disease also give rise to small adenomata, and the ultrasound appearances may be a combination of cysts and solid, hypoechoic nodules. In particular, acquired cystic disease has the potential for malignancy.[15,16] Therefore, it is prudent to screen native kidneys, even after renal transplantation has been performed.

Multicystic Dysplastic Kidney

Multicystic dysplastic kidney (MCDK) is a congenital malformation of the kidney in which the renal tissue is completely replaced by cysts. It is frequently diagnosed prenatally (although it is naturally a lethal condition if bilateral). Most MCDKs shrink with age, although a minority (around 10%) are stable or increase in size. By adulthood, the MCDK be so small that it is difficult to detect and may be mistaken for an absent kidney. Contralateral renal hypertrophy is often present.

MCDK can be associated with contralateral pelvic ureteric junction obstruction, which is also frequently diagnosed in utero. It is thought that MCDK occurs because of severe, early renal obstruction during development in utero. Obstructed calyces become blocked off, forming numerous cysts which do not connect.

BENIGN FOCAL RENAL TUMORS

Angiomyolipoma (AML)

These are usually solitary, asymptomatic lesions found incidentally on the scan. They tend to be well-defined and highly reflective, often rounded lesions containing blood vessels, muscle tissue, and fat. They are usually asymptomatic, although the larger lesions can hemorrhage, causing hematuria and pain. AMLs are also associated with TS when they are often multiple and bilateral (Fig. 6.7). Because the contrast between the hypoechoic renal parenchyma and the hyperechoic AML is so great, very small lesions in the order of a few millimeters can be recognized on ultrasound.

An AML may cause a diagnostic dilemma, particularly in patients presenting with hematuria. They tend to be smaller and more echogenic than RCCs and sometimes demonstrate shadowing, which is not normally seen in small carcinomas[17] or could be mistaken for calculi. In these situations, the clinical context must also be considered: is the patient young with no other medical history, an older patient, or one with known cancer? Where lesions are small (sub-centimeter) and solitary, many will advocate an interval ultrasound in the first instance.[18] As angiomyolipoma tends to be slow growing, it is reassuring to see no or minimal interval growth change. When doubt persists, CT is usually able to differentiate in these cases by identifying the fat content of the lesion, and understanding of MRI is also important as this has shown to be better at identifying lesions with lower fat content.[19]

Adenoma

Renal adenoma is usually a small, well-defined hyperechoic lesion, similar in appearance to the AML. It is felt that adenomas are frequently early manifestations of renal carcinoma as distinct from a benign lesion,[20,21] and the two may be histologically indistinguishable.

Renal adenomas are often found in association with an RCC in the same or contralateral kidney,[22] although these are radiologically indistinguishable from metastases. The management of patients with these masses is uncertain because of the controversy surrounding the distinction between adenomas and small RCCs. Most incidentally discovered, small (less than 3 cm) parenchymal renal masses are slow growing and may safely be monitored with CT or ultrasound, particularly in the elderly.[23]

There are a number of other benign renal tumors, including leiomyoma, haemangioma, fibroma, oncocytoma, and lymphangioma. Ultrasound including CEUS is usually unable to characterize these, and CT may help evaluate the kidney further.[20]

MALIGNANT RENAL TRACT MASSES

Imaging and Management of Malignant Renal Masses

Ultrasound is the first-line of investigation in patients with hematuria. It is highly sensitive in detecting renal masses over 2.5 cm in diameter and readily differentiates them from renal cysts. However, small masses may be missed with ultrasound, as they are frequently isoechoic (in 86% of cases); CT is more sensitive in small lesion detection.

Renal malignancy is not infrequently detected incidentally on ultrasound. Such lesions tend to be small (<4 cm) and isolated, with a good prognosis. Surveillance with ultrasound is an option in older patients or those with comorbidities, as many small lesions in older patients are stable in size.

There is now a range of treatment options for renal malignancy; in addition to nephrectomy, which is still the treatment of choice in most centers, it is possible to offer minimally invasive techniques, such as laparoscopic removal, nephron-preserving partial nephrectomy, or percutaneous ablation (CT or ultrasound-guided). CEUS may be used to guide percutaneous ablation for small renal tumors and is useful in demonstrating tumor devascularization post-ablation or to monitor ablated tumors for signs of recurrence (see below and also Fig. 6.10).[24]

> **TIP BOX**
>
> It can be difficult to determine if a renal mass is malignant or benign. Things to consider:
> Examine the blood vessels; are vessels displaced around the mass or able to pass through unimpeded? If they pass through, a malignant mass is unlikely.
> Is the mass contained within the kidney, or does it distort the renal capsule? An exophytic lesion which disrupts the renal border is more likely to be malignant.
> Assess in a minimum of two planes. This is useful in those cases where a hypertrophied column of Bertin can mimic a solid mass.

Renal Cell Carcinoma

Adenocarcinoma is the most common type of renal malignancy (referred to as RCC), occurring less commonly in the bladder and ureter.

Ultrasound Appearances

The RCC is a heterogeneous mass that often enlarges and deforms the shape of the kidney (Fig. 6.9). The mass may contain areas of cystic degeneration and/or calcification. It can spread into the ipsilateral renal vein and IVC. The increasing use of ultrasound and its improved quality has led to an increase in the detection of small tumors, often in asymptomatic patients. Around 50% of all RCCs diagnosed fall into this category.[25]

Color Doppler reveals a disorganized and increased blood flow pattern in larger masses with high velocities from the arteriovenous (AV) shunts within the carcinoma. CEUS may demonstrate a variety of contrast uptake patterns, with heterogeneous uptake or hyper-enhancement in the sinusoidal phase.[26] CEUS is also helpful in identifying residual tissue after tumors have been ablated (Fig. 6.10). In equivocal cases, PET-CT may be used to stage and plan treatment; however, it needs to be recognized that around 50% of RCCs may not be fluorodeoxyglucose (FDG) avid and that the tracer is excreted into the urinary tract.[27]

> **TIP BOX**
>
> Smaller RCCs can be hyperechoic and may be confused with benign angiomyolipoma. The latter has well-defined borders while a RCC is ill-defined: differentiation may not be possible on all occasions – biopsy or interval scan may be required.

Transitional Cell Carcinoma

Transitional cell carcinoma (TCC) is the most common bladder tumor, occurring less frequently in the collecting system of the kidney and the ureter. It usually presents with hematuria while still small. It is best diagnosed with cystoscopy. Small tumors in the renal collecting system are difficult to detect on ultrasound unless there is proximal dilatation. Depending on its location, it may cause hydronephrosis, particularly if it is situated in the ureter (rare) or at the vesicoureteric junction (VUJ). The exact position and extent of the tumor are best demonstrated with CT urography.

TCCs in the renal pelvis account for approximately 10% of renal tumors. Spread to the contralateral collecting system is a recognized risk,[28] and patients are regularly monitored following treatment.

Ultrasound Appearances

The TCC is typically a relatively hyperechoic, solid mass distending the renal sinus (Fig. 6.11A). Some pelvicalyceal dilatation is not unusual. The TCC is less likely to distort the renal outline (compared with RCC) and so is more easily missed by the unwary operator. A TCC can mimic a hypertrophied column of Bertin (see above); CT may differentiate in cases of doubt.

Once large, they invade the surrounding renal parenchyma and become indistinguishable from RCC on ultrasound. They frequently spread to the bladder, and the entire renal tract must be carefully examined.

The role of ultrasound here is usually limited to that of the first-line investigation in hematuria, particularly as the ureters are not well demonstrated. CT urography has higher sensitivity, especially in demonstrating ureteric lesions.

TCCs are potentially easier to see in the bladder as they are surrounded by urine (Fig. 6.11B). Invasion of the bladder wall can be identified on ultrasound in the larger ones, but biopsy is necessary to formally determine the level of invasion.

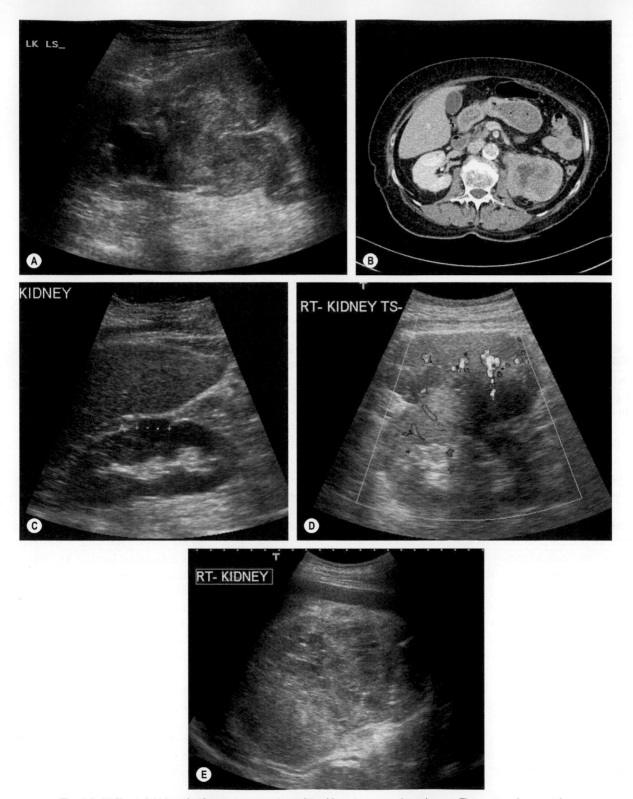

Fig. 6.9 (A) The left kidney is almost completely replaced by a large renal carcinoma. The ureter also contains tumor thrombus. (B) Computed tomography of the case in (A). (C) A small renal cell carcinoma (RCC; calipers) discovered incidentally during an abdominal ultrasound. (D) Color Doppler of an exophytic RCC reveals disorganized, multidirectional blood flow. (E) Large RCC completely replacing the right kidney.

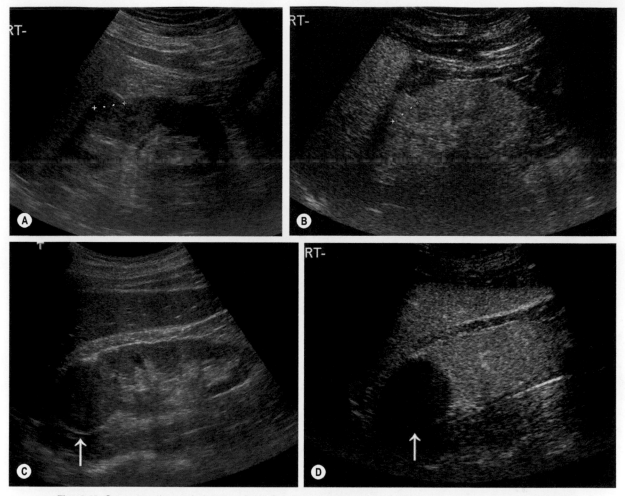

Fig. 6.10 Contrast-enhanced ultrasound: (A) Small renal cell carcinoma (RCC; calipers) pre-contrast. (B) The lesion in (A) is hypervascular and takes up contrast throughout. (C) Another small RCC post-ablation (arrow) before contrast. (D) The lesion in (C) is avascular following successful ablation. Note the normal contrast uptake in the background kidney.

Lymphoma

Renal involvement of non-Hodgkin's or Hodgkin's lymphoma is not uncommon and depends upon the stage of the disease. The ultrasound appearances are highly variable and range from solitary to multiple masses, usually hypoechoic but sometimes anechoic, hyperechoic, or mixed (Fig. 6.11C–D).

The masses may have increased through the transmission of sound and may mimic complex fluid lesions such as hematoma or abscess. The clinical history should help to differentiate these cases. Occasionally diffuse enlargement may occur secondary to diffuse infiltration.

Metastases

Renal metastases from a distant primary are usually only found in cases of widespread metastatic disease and are frequently multiple. In such cases, the primary diagnosis is usually already known, and other abdominal metastases, such as liver deposits and/or lymphadenopathy, are commonly seen on ultrasound.

Rarely, a single metastasis is seen in the kidney without other evidence of metastatic spread making the diagnosis difficult (as the question arises of whether this could be a primary or secondary lesion). In cases where the primary tumor site is unknown, PET-CT can often be used to try and identify the location.

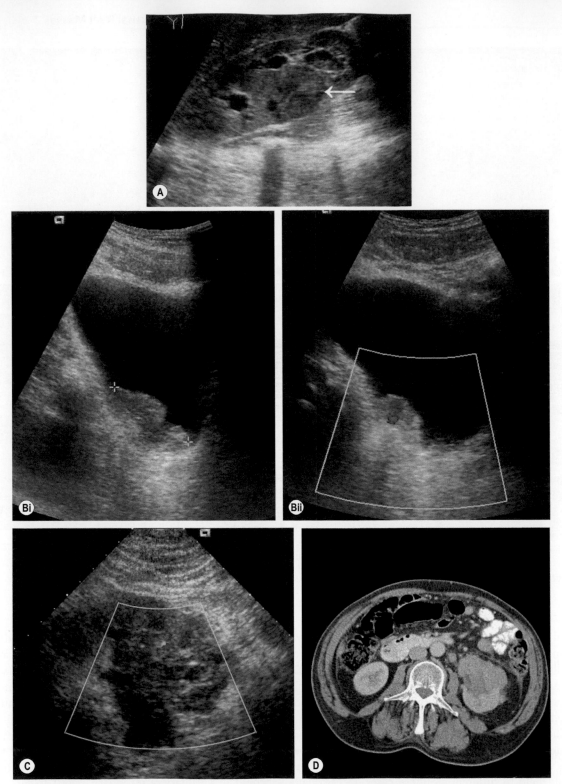

Fig. 6.11 (A) A transitional cell carcinoma (TCC; arrow) in the right kidney. The changes are more subtle than those of renal cell carcinoma, and the renal outline remains intact. (Bi) TCC in the bladder at the right vesico-ureteric junction (calipers). (Bii) Another TCC demonstrates arterial flow and is immobile on repositioning the patient, distinguishing it from a blood clot. (C) Renal lymphoma: hypoechoic, poorly perfused mass distending the left kidney. (D) Computed tomography of the case in (C).

Von Hippel–Lindau Disease

VHL is a comparatively rare autosomal dominant multi-system disorder which is associated with the development of tumors, both benign and malignant. Retinal and CNS haemangioblastomas, pancreatic cysts and tumors, and pheochromocytomas are among the varied possible spectrum of disease. RCC is one of the most common causes of death in these patients,[29] and screening with ultrasound is advocated in some centers. Where early detection of RCC occurs, timely treatment options are available, and patient morbidity and mortality are reduced.

PELVICALYCEAL SYSTEM DILATATION AND OBSTRUCTIVE UROPATHY

Not all pelvicalyceal system dilatation is pathological or obstructive; there can be dilatation without physiological obstruction. Conversely, not all obstructive uropathy necessarily results in pelvicalyceal system dilatation.

Physiological Dilatation

Mild dilatation of the renal collecting system is a common finding, most commonly being secondary to an over-distended bladder. Following micturition, the collecting system decompresses and returns to normal. An external renal pelvis (see above) is a non-obstructive "baggy" dilatation of the pelvis and can be regarded as a normal variant. The intrarenal collecting system is normal in this situation (Fig. 6.4C).

Pregnancy is another common cause of mild pelvicalyceal dilatation, more frequently on the right, particularly in the second and third trimesters. This is thought to be due partly to pressure on the ureters from the advancing pregnancy and partly hormonal. It is, however, wrong to assume that the kidney is not obstructed just because the patient is pregnant. If symptomatic, the suspicion of obstruction in a dilated system is increased, particularly if echoes are present in the pelvicalyceal system.

Obstructive Uropathy

Causes of renal obstruction vary (Table 6.2), but the most common is because of stone obstruction, either in the pelvic ureteric junction, ureter, or VUJ. Most patients with obstructive uropathy will often present with loin pain, fever, and hematuria with evidence of raised creatinine on blood analysis. Renal obstruction, particularly if long standing, can irreversibly damage the kidney

TABLE 6.2 Causes of Renal Tract Obstruction	
Intrinsic Factors	
Stones	Accompanied by renal colic. May be situated anywhere along the renal tract
Tumor	In the bladder, pelvicalyceal system or ureter
Blood clot	From infection or trauma
Papillary necrosis	Sloughed papillae can travel down the ureter, causing obstruction
Infective Processes	
Stricture	Caused by chronic, repeated infection
Fungal balls	Rare
Congenital	
Idiopathic pelvic ureteric junction obstruction	Usually unilateral; pelvicalyceal system dilatation only
Posterior urethral valves	Entire renal tract dilatation. Frequently diagnosed antenatally
Ureterocele	Unilateral hydronephrosis with hydroureter
Outflow Obstruction	
Prostate enlargement	Benign or malignant
Urethral stricture	May be iatrogenic, congenital, or as a result of infection. Accompanied by disturbed micturition

Continued

TABLE 6.2 Causes of Renal Tract Obstruction—cont'd	
Extrinsic Pelvic Mass	
Cervical carcinoma	Proximity to the ureters causes obstruction
Endometriosis	Endometriotic lesions adhere to the peritoneal and/or ureteric surfaces, causing compression
Others: lymphadenopathy, inflammatory bowel masses, gynecological masses, bulky fibroid uterus, gravid uterus in pregnancy	Always scan the kidneys to exclude obstruction when a pelvic mass is present
Iatrogenic	
Post-surgical procedure	Ligation of ureters in gynecological procedures
Trauma	Can cause a stricture of the ureter or can cause the renal tract to be blocked by a blood clot from damage to the kidney

or kidneys, leading to renal failure. If diagnosed early enough, renal function can be preserved, and therefore ultrasound plays an important role as one of the first-line investigations in patients with loin pain, renal colic, or micturition disorders. CT urogram is the imaging modality of choice when an acute obstruction is suspected, as the ureters are clearly demonstrated, unlike ultrasound, and tiny stones are confidently demonstrated (Fig. 6.12B). CT is advocated by the National Institute for Health and Care Excellence (NICE) guidance in cases of renal colic in adults; patients where pregnancy may be a risk may opt for ultrasound in first instance.

In most cases, urinary tract obstruction causes dilatation of the collecting system proximal to the site of obstruction (Fig. 6.12). Hydronephrosis may be bilateral or unilateral. Whether or not it involves the ureter(s) depends on the cause and site of the obstructing lesion.

Dilatation of the collecting system may be localized. Sometimes only one moiety of the kidney may be obstructed by a stone or tumor, while the rest of the kidney remains normal. In a duplex kidney, dilatation of the upper pole moiety is a common occurrence because of a ureterocele at the VUJ.

It is often difficult to quantify the severity of the obstruction within a written report as this is often subjective; the use of the descriptive terms mild, moderate and severe are used in conjunction with grading systems 0-IV.

It is quite common to see a trace of fluid within the collecting system, especially with the high resolution of newer ultrasound machines, if the patient is thin or the bladder has recently been distended (6.12H) and

this is considered physiological, often reducing or disappearing post-micturition. Mild hydronephrosis will often demonstrate distention of the collecting system, but the normal shape of the calyces can still be seen. Moderate hydronephrosis will see an enlargement of the renal pelvis and extension of the fluid into the medullary pyramids, which will give a more rounded appearance, and fluid will be distending the renal pelvis. In this situation, it is still possible to see normal renal tissue peripherally although this may appear to be thinner than normal. Severe hydronephrosis will see gross distension of the collecting system. Individual pyramids that lose their shape may seem "ballooned" or they may not be visualized at all, being replaced with a large fluid filled structure. The normal renal tissue will appear reduced or, in some cases, no longer visible (Fig. 6.13).

FURTHER MANAGEMENT OF RENAL OBSTRUCTION

Pyonephrosis

Pyonephrosis is a urological emergency. An obstructed kidney is prone to become infected. High fever and loin pain can suggest obstructive pyonephrosis. Pus or pus cells may also be detected in the urine. The reasons for pyohydronephrosis can be varied and include calculi and external compression from a mass or tumor.

Low-level echoes/debris can be seen within the dilated PCS on ultrasound, which may represent pus

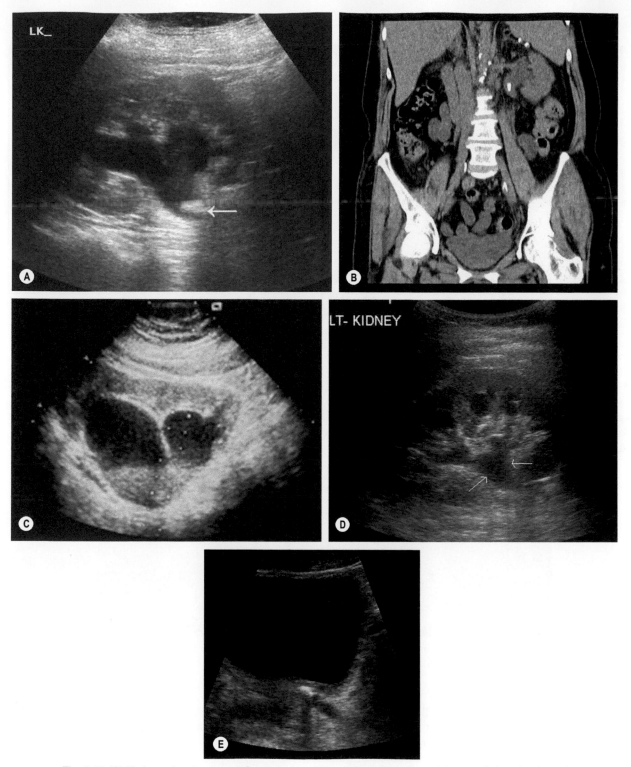

Fig. 6.12 (A) Hydronephrosis of the left kidney, secondary to a stone in the pelvic ureteric junction (arrow). (B) Computed tomography urography of the same case demonstrating left vesicoureteric junction (VUJ) stone. (C) Hydronephrosis of the lower moiety of a duplex kidney containing debris within the dilated pelvicalyceal system prior to percutaneous nephrostomy. (D) Mild dilatation of the left pelvicalyceal system (arrows) heralds obstruction. (E) A stone in the left VUJ, with acoustic shadowing, is the cause of the obstruction in case (D).

Continued

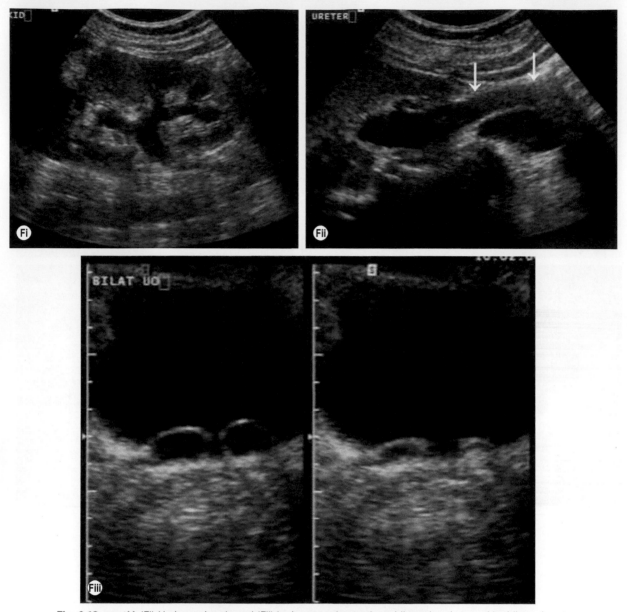

Fig. 6.12, cont'd (Fi) Hydronephrosis and (Fii) hydroureter (arrows) are bilateral and caused by bilateral ureteroceles (Fiii), seen at the VUJ.

Continued

(Fig. 6.14B). Blood in the collecting system (Hemohydronephrosis) can have a similar appearance and may be because of infection of a tumor. It is not possible with ultrasound to differentiate between blood or pus. Clinical history should help differentiate pyo- from simple hydronephrosis (Fig. 6.14). Percutaneous drainage by ultrasound or fluoroscopically guided nephrostomy is usually necessary, partly as diagnostic confirmation and partly as a therapeutic procedure.

Non-Dilated Renal Obstruction

The finding of a non-dilated PCS on ultrasound does not exclude obstruction in a patient with symptoms of renal colic. Obstruction may occasionally be present

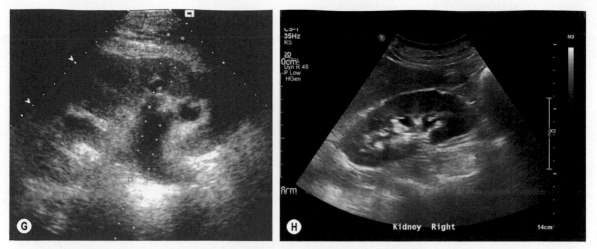

Fig. 6.12, cont'd (G) A dilated kidney about to undergo percutaneous nephrostomy under ultrasound guidance; the needle guide is lined up to enter the dilated collecting system. (H) The right kidney in a thin patient showing a normal kidney containing a trace fluid. This will often resolve post-micturition.

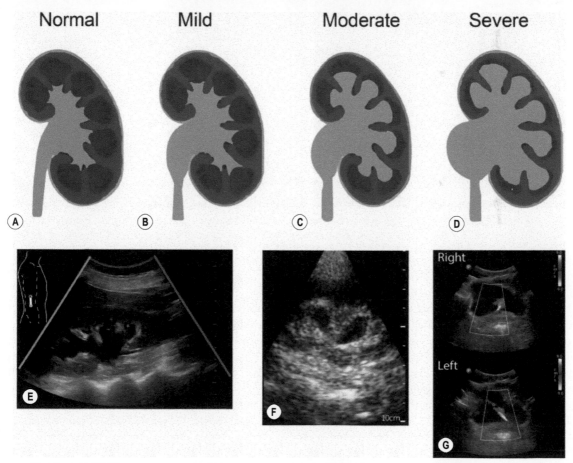

Fig. 6.13 (A–D) Diagrams illustrating the progression of hydronephrosis from mild (mild renal pelvis dilation) to moderate (dilatation of major calyces) to severe (dilatation of minor calyces). (E) Moderate hydronephrosis. (F) The presence of cysts in the renal medulla sometimes can be mistaken for a calyceal dilatation. (G) The permeability of the ureters can be demonstrated by the direct visualization of ureteric jet in the bladder using a transverse view and color Doppler. (Source: YJCAN, ISSN: 1053-0770, 2019.)

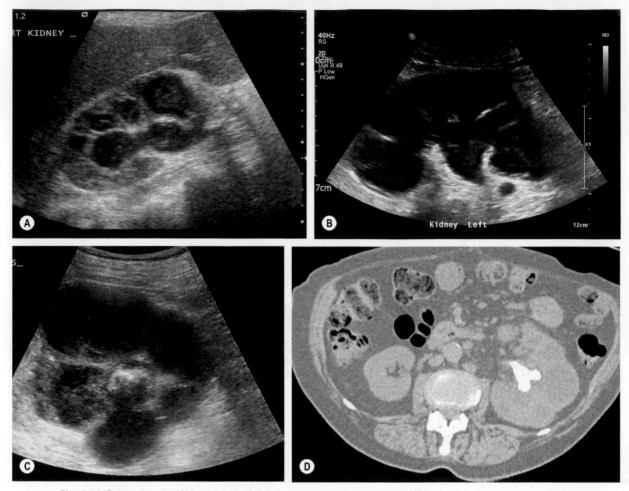

Fig. 6.14 Pyonephrosis: (A) Low-level echoes from pus can be seen in the dilated pelvicalyceal system. (Note that absence of echoes does not exclude pyonephrosis.) (B) Grossly dilated kidney with low-level echoes within the collecting system suggestive of pus. (C) This obstructed kidney contains a large central staghorn calculus. The echoes within the pelvicalyceal system represent pus. (D) Computed tomography of the case in (B), demonstrating the staghorn calculus and pyonephrosis.

in the acute stages before renal dilatation is apparent. Spectral Doppler is useful in diagnosing acute, early renal obstruction before pelvicalyceal dilatation develops because of the associated increase in blood flow resistance in the affected kidney (Fig. 6.14). This causes an increase in the resistance and pulsatility indices (RI and PI) on the obstructed side because of a reduction in diastolic flow.

A raised RI in itself is a non-specific finding, not necessarily indicating obstruction; it is known to be age-related or can be associated with extrinsic compression of the kidney (for example, by a fluid collection or mass [Table 6.3]) or with some chronic renal diseases or vascular disorders. This can be overcome by analyzing Doppler spectra from both kidneys and evaluating any difference between the two sides. A marked *difference* in RI between the kidneys in a patient with renal colic points toward obstruction of the kidney with the higher resistance.[30,31] A difference in RIs of greater than six is highly suspicious of obstruction in a patient with renal colic; a reduction in the RI on the affected side can be observed when the obstruction has been relieved or after the renal PCS has become dilated.

This effect often does not persist once the kidney dilates, presumably because the intrarenal pressure is relieved, which emphasizes the use of Doppler in acute cases before dilatation has become established.[32] Because of the vagaries of the stage of obstruction and renal pressure, the interpretation of RI should be made cautiously.

TABLE 6.3 Differential Diagnoses for Fluid-Filled Renal Masses

Solitary lesions	Simple cyst
	Infected or hemorrhagic cyst
	Hydatid cyst (rare)
Complex fluid lesions	Hematoma
	Abscess
	Lymphoma
	Necrotic primary or secondary tumor
	Tuberculosis
Pelvicalyceal system dilatation	Obstructive or non-obstructive causes
	Xanthogranulomatous pyelonephritis
Multiple cystic lesions	Polycystic or acquired cystic disease
	Multiple abscesses

Vesicoureteric Junction

The normal ureters may be identified on ultrasound as they enter the bladder. Jets of urine emerge into the bladder at these points and can be demonstrated with color Doppler (Fig. 6.2B). An absent or reduced number of jets may indicate obstruction on that side. Again, this finding should be interpreted cautiously; ureteric jet analysis is not a useful test of renal obstruction. Careful scanning at the VUJs can identify significant anomalies:

- Reflux can be seen to dilate the ureter intermittently (see below).
- A ureterocele may be diagnosed as it dilates with the passage of urine; it may not be obvious until the operator has watched carefully for a few minutes.
- Stones may become lodged at the VUJ, causing proximal dilatation.

Non-Obstructive Hydronephrosis

Not all renal dilatation results from an obstructive process, and the kidney may frequently be dilated for other reasons.

Reflux

This is the most common cause of non-obstructive renal dilatation and is usually diagnosed in children (see Chapter 9). Reflux is associated with recurrent urinary tract infections (UTIs) and can result in reflux nephropathy, in which the renal parenchyma is irretrievably damaged. Reflux can be distinguished from other causes of renal dilatation by observing the dilatation of the ureters at the bladder base because of the retrograde passage of urine.

Post-Obstructive Dilatation

If a kidney has been obstructed for some time, this can often persist even once the cause for obstruction is no longer present, because of the collecting system having a "baggy" appearance because of long standing distension.

RENAL TRACT CALCIFICATON/RENAL TRACT STONES

Renal calculi are a common finding on ultrasound. They may be an incidental discovery in an asymptomatic patient; alternatively, they may be present in patients with acute renal colic and complete or partial obstruction of the ipsilateral renal tract. They may cause hematuria and can also be associated with UTIs. The composition of calculi can vary. The common types include:

- *Calcium stones* – are the most common type and are frequently associated with patients who have abnormal calcium metabolism.
- *Struvite (triple phosphate) stones* – have a different composition of salts and are associated with UTIs. They may form large, staghorn calculi (see below).
- *Uric acid stones* – are rare and tend to be associated with gout.
- *Cystine stones* – are the rarest of all and result from a disorder of amino acid metabolism, cystinuria.

Ultrasound Appearances

Most renal calculi are calcified foci located in the collecting system of the kidney. Careful scanning with modern equipment can identify up to 88% of these. However, sensitivity is decreased in calculi of less than 3 mm in size.[33] Most stones are highly reflective structures that display distal shadowing (Fig. 6.15). However, the shadowing may be difficult to demonstrate because of the proximity of hyperechoic sinus echoes distal to the stone or because of the relatively small size of the stone compared to the beamwidth. Many newer ultrasound machines will have presets that allow imaging optimization, which may include compounding. As the ultrasound beam is angled in different directions, this can affect the ability to cast an acoustic shadow. If specifically looking for stones, ensure this feature is switched off.

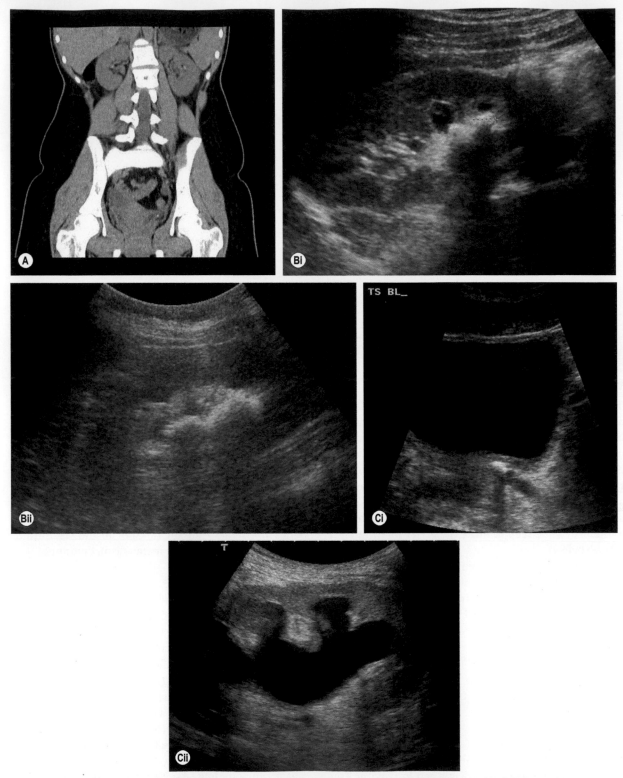

Fig. 6.15 (A) Computed tomography confirms a tiny stone in the left vesicoureteric junction (VUJ), causing the obstruction before dilatation becomes apparent. (Bi) Two calculi within the pelvicalyceal system of the right kidney cast distal acoustic shadows. (Bii) A staghorn calculus fills the collecting system of the kidney. (Ci) A stone in the left VUJ with posterior shadowing, causing left hydronephrosis (Cii).

Continued

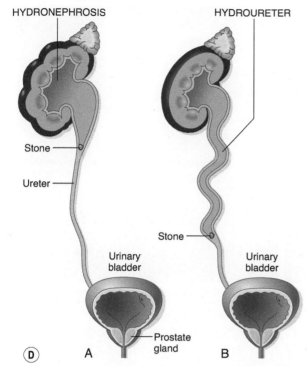

HYDRONEPHROSIS

HYDROURETER

Stone

Ureter

Stone

Urinary
bladder

Urinary
bladder

Prostate
gland

(D)   A   B

Fig. 6.15, cont'd (D) A, Hydronephrosis caused by a stone (obstruction) in the proximal part of a ureter. B, Hydroureter with hydronephrosis caused by a stone in the distal part of the ureter. (Source: [6.15D] The Language of Medicine, Twelfth Edition, 2021).

Differentiation of stones from sinus fat and reflective vessel walls is dependent on careful technique and optimal use of the equipment. Tiny stones must be within the focal zone of the beam to be demonstrated clearly. A high-frequency is also necessary to maximize the chances of seeing small stones. Clearly, the identification of large calculi is usually straightforward. However, for many of the reasons above, identification of small calculi can be difficult, especially in a patient with pain. Both false-positive and false-negative studies are well recognized. NICE guidance now suggests low-dose, non-contrast CT in patients with suspected renal colic within 24 h of onset of symptoms, with ultrasound suggested for pregnant people and younger patients (Figs. 6.12B, 6.14C).[34]

However, ultrasound still has a major role not just in calculus detection but in identifying the secondary effects, i.e., hydronephrosis, and where necessary, guiding renal drainage.

Staghorn Calculi

These large calculi are so-called because they occupy a significant proportion of the collecting system (Fig. 6.15), giving the appearance of a staghorn on X-ray. On ultrasound, they cast a dense shadow from the pelvicalyceal system, which may obscure any associated dilatation and can, in small, atrophied kidneys, be misinterpreted as shadowing from bowel gas. Because of the lobulated shape of the calculus, it may appear as several separate calculi on ultrasound. Therefore, a coronal section may be more successful in confirming a staghorn calculus than a sagittal section.

Nephrocalcinosis

This term is used to describe the deposition of calcium in the renal parenchyma. It is most often related to the medullary pyramids but may also affect the cortex, sparing the pyramids. It is frequently associated with medullary sponge kidney (see below). It may also be seen in papillary necrosis, in patients with disorders of calcium metabolism, e.g., hyperparathyroidism, and in renal tubular acidosis, sarcoidosis, and metastatic disease.

Ultrasound Appearances

Nephrocalcinosis is usually bilateral but may affect one kidney and can be present in some or all of the pyramids. A regular arrangement of hyperechoic pyramids is seen, which may shadow if large calcific foci are present, but not if the foci are numerous and tiny, as they are smaller than the beamwidth (Fig. 6.16).

Cortical nephrocalcinosis is less common and may occur with acute cortical necrosis, chronic conditions such as glomerulonephritis and hypercalcemia and sickle cell disease, and AIDS-related infection.

Hyperparathyroidism

The (normally) four parathyroid glands in the neck regulate calcium metabolism in the body. Patients with *primary hyperparathyroidism* (because of an adenoma or hyperplasia of one or more of the parathyroid glands) have hypercalcemia, making them prone to nephrocalcinosis or stones in the kidneys.

Secondary hyperparathyroidism is associated with chronic renal failure. Hypocalcemia, which results from chronic renal failure, induces compensatory hyperplasia of the parathyroid glands. There is a

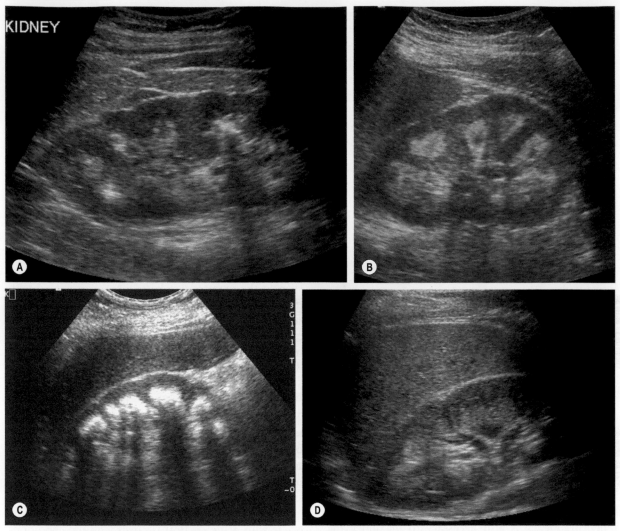

Fig. 6.16 Nephrocalcinosis: (A) Deposits of calcium within the renal pyramids are too small to cast an acoustic shadow. A larger, frank stone at the lower pole, however, casts a shadow. (B) Hyperechoic, non-shadowing renal pyramids in nephrocalcinosis. (C) Calcification in the renal pyramids with strong acoustic shadowing. (D) Medullary sponge kidney, with hyperechoic renal pyramids.

high incidence of hyperparathyroidism secondary to chronic renal failure in patients on dialysis.

Hematuria

Hematuria is defined as blood in the urine and can be described a microscopic (non-visible) or macroscopic (visible). There are many causes of blood in the urine, including infection, calculi, and intrinsic renal disease (see Box 6.1), but a thorough investigation is required because of the possibility of malignancy being the cause. In the United Kingdom, around 10,000 renal cancers and 10,000 bladder cancers are diagnosed each year,[35] and the most common symptom of these is hematuria. Macroscopic hematuria should be presumed because of malignancy until proven otherwise. It is important to rule out infection as a possible cause in primary care. Most referrals are now within a two-week wait one-stop setting, which incorporates both

BOX 6.1   Causes of Hematuria

- Urinary tract infection
- Stones
- Neoplasm (renal cell or transitional cell carcinoma in the kidney, ureter, or bladder)
- Prostatic pathologic conditions (benign hypertrophy or carcinoma)
- Renal cyst hemorrhage
- Papillary necrosis
- Glomerulonephritis
- Trauma
- Tuberculosis
- Renal infarct

ultrasound and cystoscopy. The ultrasound examination should include an assessment of the kidneys, ureters if they can be seen, and the urinary bladder. A thorough assessment should be undertaken to identify potential causes of hematuria, including renal stones and renal or bladder masses.

Nutcracker Syndrome

This occurs when there is compression of the LRV, usually between the aorta and SMA, which can cause left flank pain, proteinuria, and hematuria. The hematuria is caused by the increased pressure within the kidney, which may cause varices which in time, can rupture. Occasionally, left-sided varicocele can also be present because of the drainage of the left gonadal vein into the LRV being affected, or pelvic varices may be seen. While CT and, to a lesser extent, MRI can be used to identify this condition, the evidence suggests ultrasound is ideally placed to assess this. Color and spectral Doppler can identify areas of high velocity because of stenosis caused by compression. Also, as ultrasound is a dynamic procedure, this can be used to re-assess with the patient in different positions if the compression is posture related.

More uncommon causes of nutcracker syndrome include aortic aneurysm, retroperitoneal fibrosis, late-stage pregnancy, and pancreatic pathologic conditions.

RENAL TRACT INFLAMMATION AND INFECTION

The most common UTIs are bacterial in origin, with viral and fungal infections being comparatively rare. The diagnosis is made by urine analysis after the patient presents with symptoms of dysuria, hematuria, and/or suprapubic or renal angle pain. The origin of the infection may be via the bloodstream (hematogenous) or the urethra (ascending).

Ultrasound is often requested, particularly in children, to identify any unsuspected renal pathologic conditions which may be associated with the infection, e.g., a duplex collecting system and pelvic kidney.

Common conditions which may be identified on ultrasound include renal cystic diseases, calculi, obstructive uropathy, reflux, and anatomical variants. Infection may be either acute or chronic. Ultrasound signs of acute renal infection may be absent altogether, and this is the most common scenario as the subtler signs of interstitial nephritis are not usually demonstrable on ultrasound. The infection may be confined to the bladder, called *cystitis*, in which case low-level echoes and/or hyperechoic debris may be identified or may have progressed to the kidneys. Scarring and/or cortical thinning may be present in cases of repeated infections (see "Chronic Pyelonephritis" below).

Pyelonephritis
Acute Pyelonephritis

Acute inflammation of the kidney rarely results in any ultrasound abnormality. Occasionally the kidney may be enlarged and hypoechoic. The contrast between the kidney and the hepatic or splenic parenchyma is increased because of edema, but the ultrasound changes are generally subtle. Tenderness when scanning over the affected kidney is common, and it is good to include this clinical correlation within the report. Other possible ultrasound findings include congenital anomalies, hydronephrosis, stones, and a loss of the hyperechoic sinus fat echoes, because of edema, and loss of corticomedullary differentiation.[36]

Chronic Pyelonephritis

This chronic inflammatory state is usually the result of frequent previous inflammatory/infective episodes. The kidney may be small and often has focal scarring present. Scar tissue has the appearance of a hyperechoic, linear lesion that affects the smooth renal outline and crosses the renal cortex. The cortex can appear focally thinner (Fig. 6.17A). Do not confuse focal scarring with fetal lobulation, the latter being smooth, thin, continuous with the capsule, and forming an indentation between the pyramids.

The renal cortex is frequently thin and scarred in chronic pyelonephritis and may appear abnormally hyperechoic. Overall the kidneys may be reduced in length.

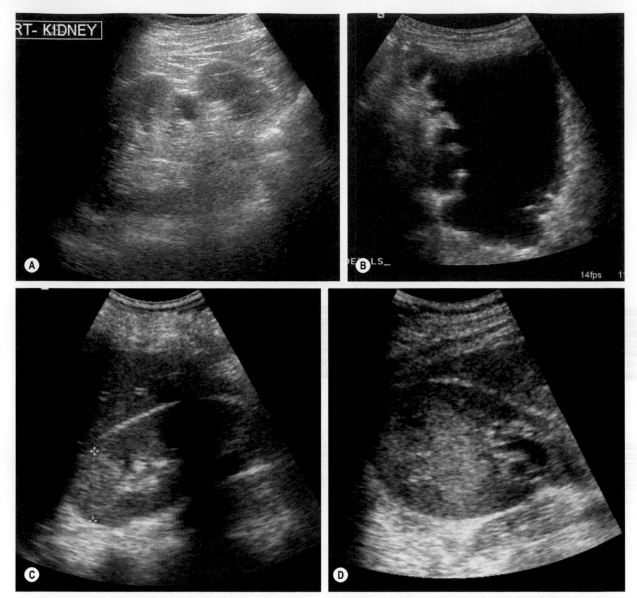

Fig. 6.17 (A) Cortical scar tissue, demonstrating a focal area of cortical thinning, following repeated episodes of urinary tract infection. (B) Numerous bladder diverticulae in chronic infection. (C) Focal pyelonephritis (calipers). This subtle area of altered echogenicity in the kidney corresponds to the patient's pain. (D) Another case of focal inflammation in an enlarged right kidney with an area of increased echogenicity.

Continued

Bladder Diverticula

Repeated infections can cause the bladder wall to thicken and become trabeculated. In such cases, a bladder diverticulum may form, making treatment of subsequent infections particularly difficult. The diverticulum may harbor debris or stones and may fail to empty properly, often enlarging as the urine refluxes into it when the patient micturates, so it is important to always perform a post-micturition assessment (Fig. 6.17B).

Focal Pyelonephritis

The presence of acute infection within the kidney may progress in focal regions of the renal parenchyma. This phenomenon is particularly associated with

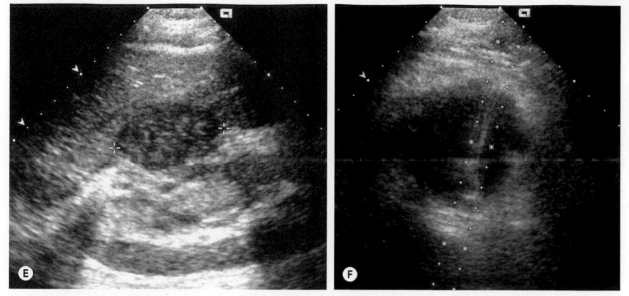

Fig. 6.17, cont'd (E) Focal renal infection (calipers) is developing into a renal abscess. Note the posterior acoustic enhancement. (F) The abscess in (E) undergoes ultrasound-guided drainage before antibiotic therapy.

diabetes. The ultrasonic changes are subtle, as in diffuse pyelonephritis, but it is possible to detect a slight change in echogenicity when it is surrounded by normal-looking parenchyma.

Focal pyelonephritis (sometimes called focal or lobar nephronia) may be either hypo- or hyperechoic compared with normal renal tissue. Depending on the size of the lesion, it may cause a mass effect, mimicking a renal tumor. The outline of the kidney is preserved, however (Fig. 6.17C).

The patient presents with fever and tenderness on the affected side and frequently has a history of UTI. A focal renal mass under these circumstances is highly suggestive of focal pyelonephritis and is also well demonstrated on CT.[37] It usually responds to antibiotic therapy, and the resolution of the lesion can be monitored with ultrasound scans.

Renal Abscess

A renal abscess is generally a progression of focal inflammation within the kidney (Fig. 6.17E). The area liquefies and may enlarge to form a complex mass with distal acoustic enhancement. Low-level echoes from pus may fill the abscess cavity, giving it the appearance of increased echogenicity, but it may also be hypoechoic. The margins of the abscess may be ill-defined at first but may develop a more obvious capsule as the lesion becomes established

(Fig. 6.17D–F); the capsule often has an easily identifiable thick rim. Flow may be seen in the inflammatory capsule with color Doppler but not in the liquefied center.

A renal abscess may mimic a lymphoma as both may be hypoechoic on ultrasound, and both may have either single or multiple foci. The abscess may be intrarenal, subcapsular, or perirenal. Frequently, drainage under ultrasound guidance is the preferred treatment; gradual resolution of the abscess can also be monitored with ultrasound.

Xanthogranulomatous Pyelonephritis

This condition (which gets its name from the yellow color of the kidney) results from chronic recurrent bacterial infection. It is most frequently associated with renal dilatation and obstruction by calculi (usually a staghorn calculus) in the pelvicalyceal system or possibly because of previous surgery or adhesions which cause fibrosis.

The kidney becomes chronically infected, and the calyces enlarge and become filled with infected debris. The cortex may be eroded and thin (Fig. 6.18).

On ultrasound, these appearances are similar to pyonephrosis, although pyonephrosis is generally associated with more acute pain and fever, whereas xanthogranulomatous pyelonephritis is associated with lower grade, chronic pain. The kidney may be

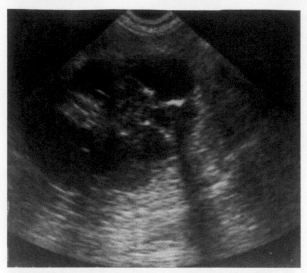

Fig. 6.18 Xanthogranulomatous pyelonephritis. Numerous stones have obstructed the pelvicalyceal system, which contains debris. The renal cortex is thin, and the architecture of the kidney is difficult to recognize.

enlarged with strong reflection and shadowing from a staghorn calculus. The dilated collecting system contains inflammatory debris.

DIFFUSE RENAL DISEASE AND RENAL FAILURE

Most diffuse medical renal conditions have non-specific appearances on ultrasound, and the kidneys often appear normal in the early stages of the disease. Renal failure may be acute or chronic, and its causes are numerous. If acute, an increase in overall renal size may be observed, and there may be a diffuse alteration in the renal echogenicity. However, this can be either hypo- or hyperechoic compared to normal. Either increased or decreased corticomedullary differentiation may also be observed (Fig. 6.19). Although ultrasound is successful in detecting renal parenchymal disease, the acoustic changes are not specific, and the cause must usually be diagnosed histologically, and ultrasound is invaluable in directing the biopsy procedure.

Acute/Chronic Kidney Injury (AKI)

AKI, previously known as acute renal failure, is a common history provided on a clinical ultrasound request and indicates that the kidneys have stopped working, from a minor loss of function to complete renal failure. The first role of ultrasound should be to assess for ob-

struction as a cause but also allow the opportunity to assess the structure of the kidneys. Each kidney should be assessed for size and cortical thickness, and the cortex can be assessed against the echotexture of the surrounding organs (liver and spleen) and the differentiation between the cortex and the medulla of the kidney. If there is previous imaging, it can help to identify whether the appearances are new or long-standing and could indicate acute-on-chronic renal disease. In cases of chronic renal failure, the kidney can often be small with a reduced corticomedullary differentiation. The end-stage kidney can be quite tiny and hyperechoic and may be difficult to differentiate from the surrounding tissues (Fig. 6.19C). Depending on the cause, either one, but generally both, of the kidneys are affected. If the kidneys are enlarged, color Doppler can be used to assess the renal veins to check for patency. The urinary bladder can be assessed. However, fluid loading the patient to obtain a full bladder should be avoided, and as many patients may also be catheterized, this may not be possible.

Glomerulonephritis

Glomerulonephritis is an inflammatory condition that affects the glomeruli of the kidney. It may be either acute or chronic and frequently follows prolonged infection.

Patients may present in acute renal failure, with oliguria or anuria, or with features of nephrotic syndrome such as edema, proteinuria, and hypoalbuminemia. Depending on the cause, acute renal failure may be reversible or may progress to chronic renal failure requiring dialysis. Glomerulonephritis can be caused by numerous mechanisms:

- *Immunologic mechanisms* – e.g., in systemic lupus erythematosus or AIDS.
- *Metabolic disorders* – e.g., diabetes.
- *Circulatory disturbances* – e.g., atherosclerosis or disseminated intravascular coagulation.

As with acute tubular necrosis, the ultrasound appearances are non-specific. In the acute stages, the kidneys may be slightly enlarged; changes in the echogenicity of the cortex may be observed. In the chronic stages, the kidneys shrink, become hyperechoic, lose cortical thickness, and have increased corticomedullary differentiation.

Medullary Sponge Kidney

In medullary sponge kidney, the distal tubules, which lie in the medullary pyramids, dilate. This may be because of a developmental anomaly, but this is uncertain. In itself,

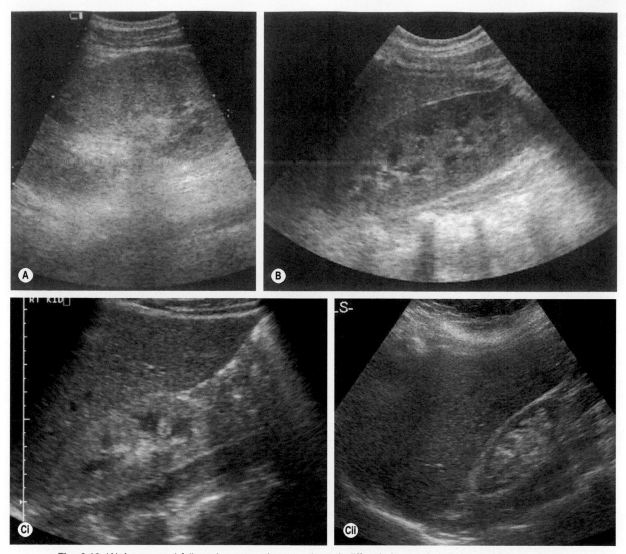

Fig. 6.19 (A) Acute renal failure demonstrating an enlarged, diffusely hyperechoic kidney with loss of corticomedullary differentiation. (B) Acute renal failure in paracetamol overdose. The kidney is large (16 cm) and hyperechoic with increased corticomedullary differentiation. (C) Chronic renal failure. (Ci) The kidney is small and hyperechoic compared with the adjacent liver. (Cii) Another example of chronic renal failure, with a small kidney in which the cortex is of similar echogenicity to the liver but very thin.

it is usually asymptomatic and therefore rarely seen on ultrasound. However, the condition is prone to nephrocalcinosis, particularly at the outer edges of the pyramids and stone formation (see above), which may cause pain and hematuria. Involvement is usually bilateral but may be unilateral or segmental. On ultrasound, the kidneys tend to be normal in size, and the pyramids may be hyperechoic regardless of the presence of nephrocalcinosis.

Other possible ultrasound findings include possible nephrocalcinosis (Fig. 6.16), stones, and the results of stone obstruction and/or chronic infection if present.

Amyloid

In amyloid disease, excess protein is deposited in the renal parenchyma, predominantly the cortex. This causes proteinuria and may progress to nephrotic syndrome (edema, proteinuria, and hypoalbumin-emia). Amyloidosis can cause acute renal failure and is particularly associated with long-standing rheumatoid arthritis.

Ultrasound findings are non-specific. As with other diffuse renal diseases, the acute stage may cause renal enlargement, and the parenchyma tends to be diffusely hyperechoic. By the time the chronic stage of the disease has been reached, the kidneys become shrunken and hyperechoic in keeping with all end-stage appearances.

RENAL VASCULAR PATHOLOGIC CONDITIONS

Renal Artery Stenosis (RAS)

Stenosis of the renal artery is because of arteriosclerotic disease in the vast majority of patients or fibromuscular dysplasia of the arterial wall in the younger patient. RAS may cause hypertension and may eventually cause renal failure. It is frequently bilateral and is responsible for up to 15% of patients who require long term dialysis. It is associated with aortic aneurysm or neurofibromatosis or can be traumatic in origin. Ultrasound is commonly used in assessing the renal artery transplant patients; however,

CT and MRI are considered to be the superior imaging modality for other clinical situations, such as hypertensive patients. Ultrasound screening should not be considered unless other imaging modalities are unsuitable (Fig. 6.20).

RENAL TRAUMA

A direct injury can rupture the kidney. This will result in blood and/or urine leaking out into the perinephric space to form a urinoma or hematoma. The main renal vessels may also be damaged, causing a lack of perfusion. Trauma resulting in hematuria and suspected renal damage is usually imaged with CT as a first-line. This has the advantage of demonstrating a range of possible injuries to all the abdominal viscera.

The role of ultrasound in such cases is more usually reserved for guiding drainage of subsequent fluid collections such as urinoma or infected hematoma. The insertion of a drain carries a risk of infection and is therefore limited to infected collections in symptomatic patients. Patients who cannot attend a CT department (for example, unstable patients in intensive care) may benefit from a careful bedside ultrasound scan to identify free fluid and organ damage.

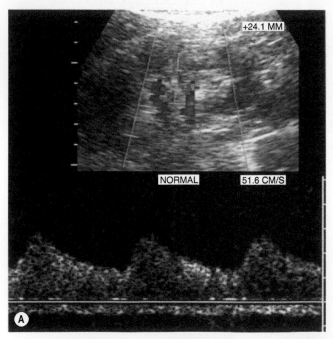

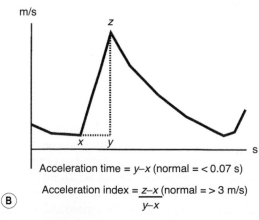

Acceleration time = $y - x$ (normal = < 0.07 s)

Acceleration index = $\dfrac{z - x}{y - x}$ (normal = > 3 m/s)

Fig. 6.20 Renal artery stenosis. (A) The kidney is small, with subjectively reduced perfusion on color Doppler. (B) The spectrum displays the parvus tardus pattern with a delayed systolic upstroke.

RENAL TRANSPLANTS

Although there are several treatment choices for patients with renal failure, including peritoneal and hemodialysis, undoubtedly the treatment of choice is renal transplantation. From the very early days of Carrel's experimental attempts at transplantation in the 1900s resulting in the Nobel Prize of 1912,[38] to the non-immunosuppressed allografting of the 1950s, the more successful and encouraging outcome of twin-to-twin transplants,[39] a better understanding of tissue rejection and the introduction of azathioprine and steroid in 1963,[41] and more specifically cyclosporin A by Calne in the 1970s,[40] all have contributed immensely to slow but positive progress in this field. Improvements in surgical technique; newer, more effective, and less toxic anti-rejection therapy; the routine use of ultrasound in the 1970s and then Doppler a decade later; and the development of interventional radiology have all combined to make this the successful operation with successful clinical outcomes we now take so much for granted.

Although many different imaging modalities are available, ultrasound is still the single most useful investigation in the postoperative monitoring of the transplant, especially as it can be taken to the patient's bedside for assessment and is well tolerated by the patient.

Normal Anatomy

Most renal transplants are *heterotopic*; that is, they are placed in addition to the diseased, native kidneys, which remain *in situ*. The transplanted organ is usually positioned in the iliac fossa anterior to the psoas and iliacus muscles. It lies outside the peritoneal cavity.

Within the United Kingdom, most transplanted kidneys are cadaveric and are harvested with their main vessels intact, which are then anastomosed to the recipient iliac artery and vein. Increasingly, live donors are supplementing the transplant program, although this accounts for less than 25% of all transplants performed,[41] and ultrasound is useful in both donor (in confirming normality prior to donation) and recipient.

Normal Ultrasound Appearances

The transplanted kidney is particularly amenable to ultrasound because its position relatively near to the skin surface allows a high-frequency transducer, 5–6 MHz, to be used for better detail.

The ultrasonic appearances of the transplanted kidney are the same as would be expected for a native kidney, allowing for a higher resolution. The transplant kidney should be assessed in the same way as the native organ, i.e., in two planes. Features to be observed include:

- *Morphological appearances*: this should include an assessment of the relative echogenicity of the cortex, medulla, and renal sinus and corticomedullary differentiation. Focal or diffuse changes in echogenicity may be observed but are non-specific findings associated with inflammation, infection, or infarction.
- *Pelvicalyceal system dilatation*: even mild pelvicalyceal dilatation may be significant, as it may represent an early obstructive process. The bladder should be empty before assessing the pelvicalyceal system to eliminate physiological dilatation. Any degree of hydronephrosis should be correlated with the clinical findings and biochemistry – hydronephrosis in isolation is not a reason for nephrostomy.
- *Vascular anatomy*: the main transplant artery and vein are anastomosed to the recipient's external iliac artery and vein respectively and can usually be visualized throughout their length. Assessment with color Doppler to check for patency and direction of blood flow and spectral Doppler should be performed recording the RI and PI (resistance and pulsatility index). Overall global perfusion can be assessed with color or power Doppler, and spectral assessment of the interlobar arteries at the periphery of the kidney should also be assessed with RI measurements recorded (Fig. 6.21). The normal spectral Doppler waveform is a low-resistance waveform with continuous forward EDF. However, the operator needs to be aware of differences in waveform immediately posttransplant and how this may change in subsequent days.
- *Perirenal fluid*: A small amount of free fluid is not unusual postoperatively. This usually resolves spontaneously. Fluid collections around the kidney are a common complication and will be visualized as an encapsulated hypoechoic, mixed echo area surrounding the transplanted kidney or in the pelvis. They may resolve on further scanning; drainage is only performed for good clinical reasons (see below).

Postoperative Complications

Ultrasound has an essential role in assessing the transplant and makes a significant contribution

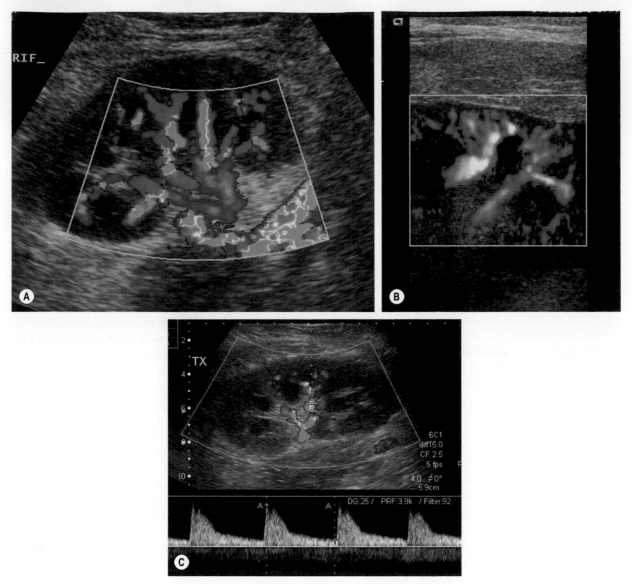

Fig. 6.21 (A) Perfusion within the transplanted kidney is easily displayed. A higher frequency may be used as the kidney is usually superficially situated in the iliac fossa. (B) By using an even higher frequency and power Doppler, tiny vessels can be displayed in the periphery of the transplant kidney. (C) Normal spectrum from the interlobar renal artery, demonstrating good end diastolic flow (low resistance) with a vertical systolic upstroke.

Continued

toward graft survival through the early recognition of postoperative complications.[42] Complications are varied and include acute rejection, ureteric obstruction, vascular occlusions, perirenal fluid collections, renal dysfunction (of various aetiologies), and infection. Drug toxicity from immunosuppressive therapy can also compromise graft function. Finally, in the long term, the original disease for which transplantation was performed may recur.

Complications can be divided into three main categories: immediate postoperative complications and primary and secondary renal dysfunction.

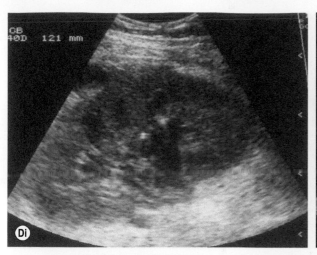 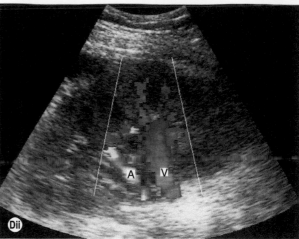

Fig. 6.21, cont'd (Di) Large vessels at the hilum may mimic dilatation; (Dii) color Doppler demonstrates this is the main renal vein.

Immediate:

- Non-perfusion. This is usually the result of an occluded or twisted renal artery; correction is usually surgical
- Hematoma

Primary dysfunction:

- Non-perfusion (arterial occlusion) – total or lobar
- Acute tubular necrosis
- Renal vein thrombosis (Fig. 6.22)
- Obstruction
- Acute or accelerated acute rejection

Secondary dysfunction:

- Acute rejection
- Ciclosporin nephrotoxicity
- Acute tubular necrosis
- Obstruction
- RAS
- Post-biopsy fistula
- Infection
- Chronic rejection

Renal Transplant Dilatation

A mild degree of pelvicalyceal system dilatation is normal postoperatively, because of edema, at the site of the vesicoureteric anastomosis. This phenomenon is usually transient, and serial scans in conjunction with biochemistry (urea, creatinine) are usually all that is required.

More severe dilatation may be indicative of obstruction, especially if the individual calyces are also dilated. A trend of increasing dilatation is a poor prognostic indicator. A ratio between the area of the pelvicalyceal system and the renal outline in two planes, the *dilatation index*, has been found to predict obstruction and differentiate obstructive from non-obstructive dilatation (Fig. 6.23).[43] The degree of dilatation of the pelvicalyceal system correlates well with the severity of obstruction.

Obstruction of the transplant kidney may be because of an ischemic-related stricture at the vesicoureteric anastomosis or may result from a blood clot or infected debris in the ureter. Hematoma or debris within the pelvicalyceal system may appear echogenic but require differentiation from fungal balls. Percutaneous nephrostomy (X-ray and/or ultrasound-guided) is the method of choice to relieve the obstruction.

Rejection

This can be acute or chronic. Furthermore, 10%–30% of transplanted kidneys are acutely rejected; this presents as a decline in renal function, usually within the first three months. Hyperacute rejection, which occurs within hours, is very rare.[41] Ongoing episodes of acute rejection should raise the possibility of non-compliance with therapy. Acute rejection cannot be differentiated on ultrasound from other causes of delayed function, particularly acute tubular necrosis, and therefore biopsy is invariably necessary.

Ultrasound Appearances

These are varied and non-specific. In the majority of cases, the kidney appears normal. However, gray-scale findings can include enlargement because of edema (this change is

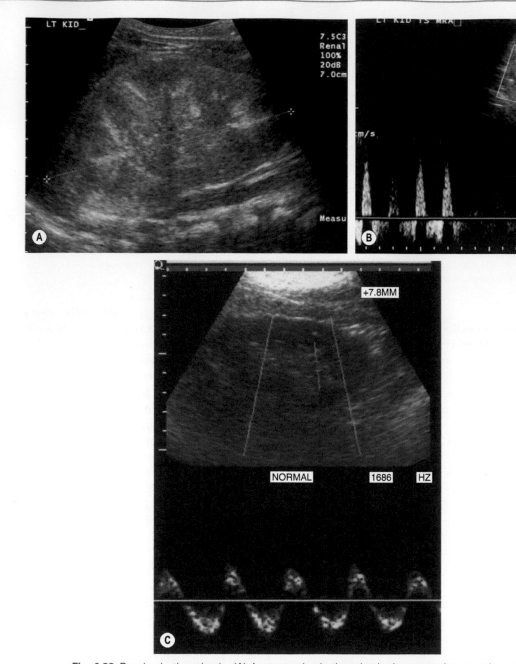

Fig. 6.22 Renal vein thrombosis. (A) Acute renal vein thrombosis demonstrating an enlarged, diffusely hyperechoic kidney. (B) Doppler demonstrates high-resistance bidirectional arterial flow with no venous flow. (C) Small shrunken kidney (6 cm) demonstrating hardly any perfusion, apart from a tiny interlobar artery with bidirectional flow.

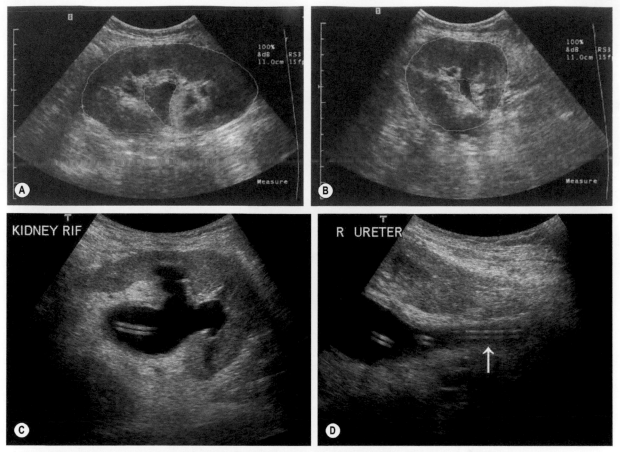

Fig. 6.23 (A) LS and (B) TS of a dilated transplant kidney showing the measurements used to calculate the ratio between the dilated pelvicalyceal system and the kidney. This kidney was dilated but not obstructed. (C) Ureteric stenosis: A dilated transplant kidney with a stent seen in the pelvicalyceal system. (D) The stent is seen in the ureter shortly following its insertion through the stenosis (arrow). The collecting system subsequently returned to normal.

subtle in the early stages and not a reliable ultrasonic indicator), increased corticomedullary differentiation with prominent pyramids, infundibular thickening (thickening of the acute tubular necrosis walls), and decreased fat in the renal sinus (Fig. 6.24). These findings are subjective, non-specific, and limited in the diagnosis of rejection.

In chronic rejection, there may be an overall increase in the echogenicity of the kidney with reduced corticomedullary differentiation. Eventually, the kidney will shrink. The Doppler RI are increased in rejection, but, again, this finding is non-specific (Table 6.4, Fig. 6.24B).[44] In general, the higher the RI, the more likely is the diagnosis of acute rejection. The cause of renal dysfunction is established by ultrasound-guided biopsy.

Fluid Collections Associated with Transplantation

Up to 50% of renal transplants will demonstrate perirenal fluid.[45] The size of the collection should be monitored with ultrasound, as significant growth may require intervention. While it is not possible to classify the collection on the ultrasound appearances alone, the clinical picture, including the time interval following transplantation, can often give a clue.

- *Lymphocele*: the most common perirenal fluid collection, lymphocoeles usually occur several weeks or months after the transplant. They may resolve spontaneously but occasionally require percutaneous drainage if large. They may compress the kidney, causing an increase in vascular resistance on spectral

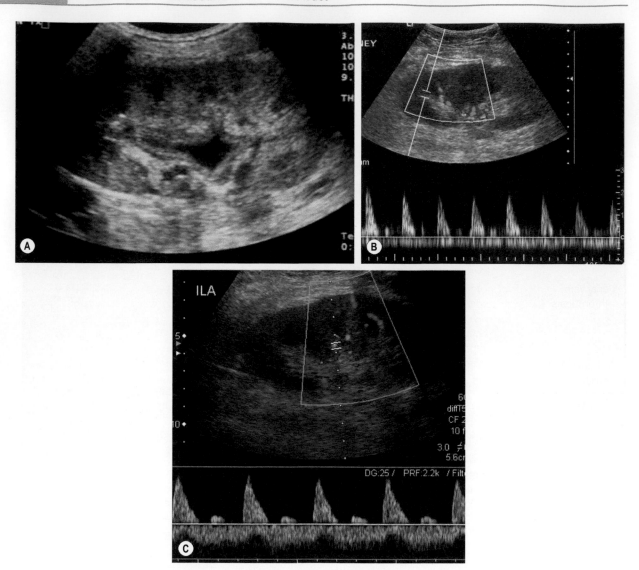

Fig. 6.24 Transplant rejection. (A) Peri-infundibular or mural thickening is present in the pelvicalyceal system. (B) Perfusion is reduced throughout the kidney, and the high-resistance vasculature demonstrates a high Doppler resistive index, with no end diastolic flow (EDF). (C) Another example of high-resistance vasculature in transplant rejection with a pulsatile arterial waveform with no EDF.

Doppler (Fig. 6.25). The collection is anechoic but may contain loculations or septa. If treated, then surgical laparoscopic marsupialization is the treatment of choice.

- *Hematoma*: an immediate postoperative phenomenon, which usually resolves spontaneously. If the hematoma is because of an anastomotic leak at the main artery or vein, it can compress the renal vein,

causing thrombosis in rare cases. On ultrasound, the hematoma can appear hyperechoic and ill-defined in the early stages. As it resolves and liquefies, the margins become more defined, and the center becomes anechoic. Hyperechoic blood clots and strands of fibrin may be seen within the hematoma.

- *Urinoma*: this occurs because of an anastomotic leak in the ureter. Urinomas are uncommon but may

TABLE 6.4 Causes of High-Resistance Doppler (Low End-Diastolic Flow) in Renal Transplants

Acute rejection	Does not occur in the first 48 h
Acute tubular necrosis	Occurs in the first 48 h
Obstruction	Has a relatively slight increase in the resistive index and is accompanied by pelvicalyceal system dilatation
Cyclosporin nephrotoxicity	Has to be prolonged and severe to affect the end diastolic flow and blood levels A late complication of renal transplants
Renal vein thrombosis	Has a characteristic reversed end-diastolic flow pattern. The artery has a low-velocity systolic peak in the early stages. No venous flow identified
Perirenal fluid collections	Compression of the kidney causes an increase in intrarenal pressure

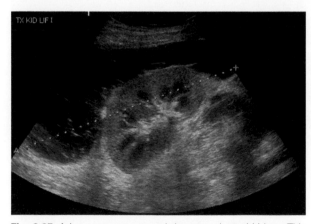

TX KID LIF I

Fig. 6.25 A large seroma around the transplanted kidney. This was drained under ultrasound guidance.

progress to urinary ascites. They occur early following the surgical procedure, unlike lymphoceles.

- *Abscess*: if any of the above fluid collections becomes infected, this leads to an abscess. Hyperechoic debris can be seen in the collection, and this may be treated with ultrasound-guided percutaneous drainage.

Vascular Complications

Vascular Occlusion

Color and spectral Doppler are essential for the diagnosis of postoperative vascular complications. Nonperfusion may be total or lobar (Fig. 6.26). Focal areas of hypoperfusion may be because of edema in focal infection, AV fistula, or severing of an accessory artery during harvesting of the transplant or at the time of implantation causing infarction. Total vascular occlusion is rare but occurs early. Patients may be asymptomatic, and non-perfusion of the transplant may be inadvertently seen on either a routine scan or isotope study. Graft nephrectomy is the most likely outcome. Conversely, the appearance of good renal perfusion throughout the kidney on color or power Doppler does not necessarily indicate normal vascularity, and severe vascular rejection or acute tubular necrosis can be present under such circumstances.[46] Vascular complications may include arterial stenosis or thrombosis, venous stenosis or thrombosis, pseudoaneurysms, and AV fistulae.

Renal Artery Stenosis

This is one of the most common post-transplant vascular complications, affecting up to 10% of transplants. It generally occurs at the site of the anastomosis close to the iliac artery but also along the length of the artery or even affecting the intra-renal branches. The patient may present with severe, difficult-to-control hypertension, graft dysfunction, or both. Alternatively, the patient's renal function may deteriorate following angiotensin-converting enzyme inhibitor therapy, and this is also an indication of a possible underlying RAS.

Careful Doppler examination is now the accepted first-line investigation in the diagnosis of RAS. In most cases, it is possible to trace the artery back to its anastomosis with the iliac artery using color Doppler. If the site of the stenosis is identified, spectral Doppler will demonstrate an increase in peak systolic velocity at the lesion, followed by post-stenotic turbulence (Fig. 6.26B–C). The point of stenosis can be difficult to pinpoint in the main renal artery, especially if the bowel is overlying the vessel.

A delayed systolic rise (the *parvus tardus* waveform) can be identified in the intrarenal spectral Doppler waveforms, as for the native kidney (see above). The diagnosis, however, is primarily made on the peak systolic velocity within the renal artery. A value of <2.5 m/s

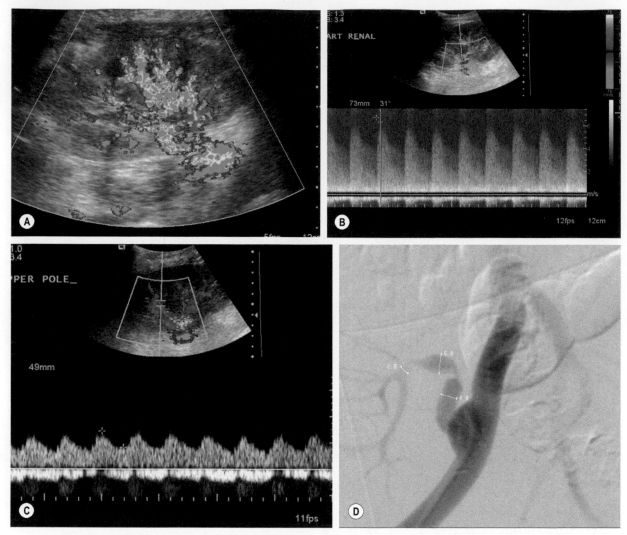

Fig. 6.26 (A) The upper pole of this transplant kidney lacks perfusion (despite reducing the pulse repetition frequency setting) because of infarction. (B) High-velocity jet at the site of magnetic resonance angiography stenosis in a transplant kidney. The patient had increasing, badly controlled hypertension since transplantation. (C) Downstream from arterial stenosis, Doppler displays a tardus parvus pattern of delayed systolic upstroke. (D) Arteriography of the case in (C) demonstrates two stenoses.

is normal, whereas >2.5 m/s constitutes RAS. If the stenosis is severe, it may be difficult to identify color flow in the kidney, and the waveform may be reduced in velocity with a tiny, damped trace in the main vessel.

Stenosis affecting an interlobar artery may result in focal, segmental non-perfusion or ischemia on Doppler ultrasound. In general, contrast angiography is only used to grade and treat stenoses after a positive ultrasound scan or when a high index of clinical suspicion persists, despite a negative ultrasound.

Renal Vein Thrombosis

This is uncommon and usually the result of surgical technique or vein compression. The occlusion may be partial or complete, and the venous Doppler spectrum may therefore be absent (Fig. 6.27). If venous thrombosis is partial, the arterial spectral waveform becomes very pulsatile, with reverse EDF, which in the clinical setting of an oliguric patient with a tender graft in the early postoperative period is highly suspicious for renal vein thrombosis (RVT).

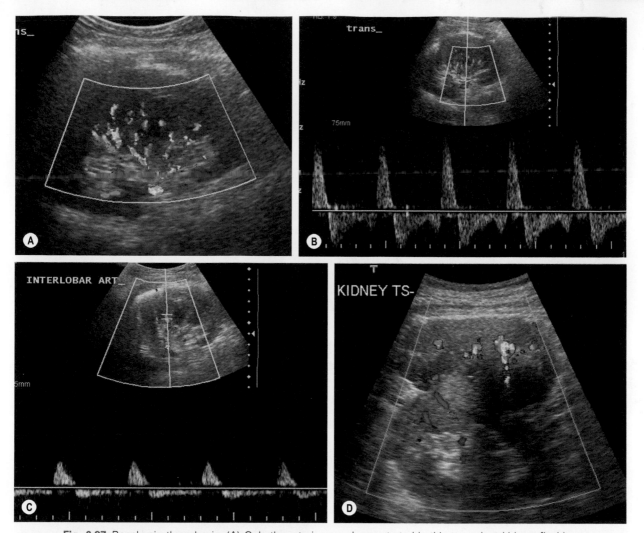

Fig. 6.27 Renal vein thrombosis. (A) Only the arteries are demonstrated in this transplant kidney, flashing alternately red and blue. (B) Doppler of the case in (A) demonstrates reversed flow in the arteries without venous flow. (C–D) Another example of transplant renal vein thrombosis.

During the early stages, when thrombosis is incomplete, venous flow may be seen in the kidney, but the artery is of reduced velocity.[47] The ultrasound findings of RVT may be indistinguishable from severe rejection. However, venous flow is generally unaffected in the latter.

Thrombosis is rare, occurring typically in the immediate postoperative period. It may be associated with a faulty venous anastomosis, secondary to compression of the vein, for example, by a large, peri-venous collection, or the patient may have an increased thrombotic tendency for a number of reasons.

Pseudoaneurysms and AV Fistulae

These may sometimes form as a result of vascular damage during biopsy procedures. They are usually not significant and tend to resolve spontaneously (Fig. 6.28A). An AV fistula follows damage to an artery and vein, showing an irregular knot of vessels on color or power Doppler with a pulsatile venous waveform and high peak- and end-diastolic velocity in the feeding artery. A large draining vein may also be seen.

A pseudoaneurysm results from arterial damage and may appear cystic on the gray-scale image but will demonstrate filling on color Doppler with a pulsatile

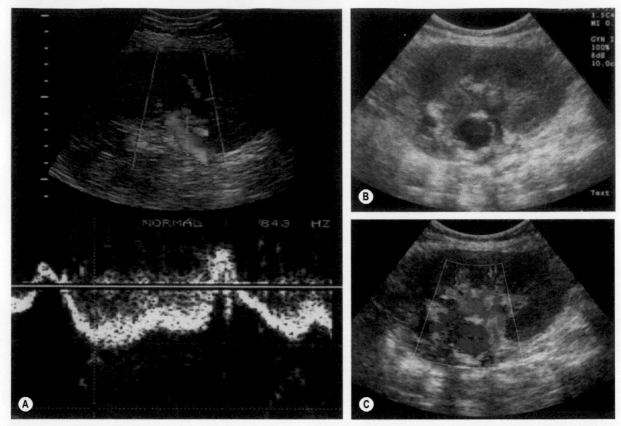

Fig. 6.28 (A) Pulsatile venous waveform is seen as a result of a small arteriovenous fistula following the biopsy procedure. (B) This renal artery aneurysm appears cystic on a gray-scale. (C) Color Doppler demonstrates arterial flow.

flow velocity waveform (Fig. 6.28B–C). A careful, ultrasound-guided biopsy technique helps to avoid such lesions (see Chapter 11).

Infection

This is characterized by swelling of the uroepithelium, especially with fungal infections. Fungal balls may be visible as relatively hyperechoic structures within the pelvicalyceal system (Fig. 6.29).

Acute Tubular Necrosis

Acute tubular necrosis is the most common form of delayed graft function immediately following transplant. It is associated with ischemia after removal from the donor and reperfusion injury. Mild acute tubular necrosis may resolve spontaneously. On ultrasound, it may demonstrate prominent medullary pyramids, with Doppler

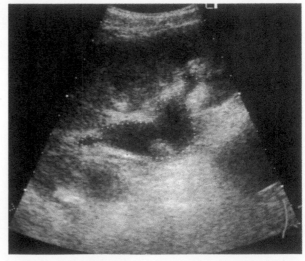

Fig. 6.29 Fungal ball in the dilated pelvicalyceal system.

demonstrating low EDF. Reverse EDF is uncommon but recognized. A biopsy is required for confirmation.

Cyclosporin Nephrotoxicity

The toxic nature of the immunosuppressive regimen requires the dose to be very carefully adjusted. Drug toxicity is a recognized cause of poor renal function and decreased perfusion. There may be increased Doppler resistance, as for acute tubular necrosis, but normally indices remain unaffected. Histology is required to confirm the diagnosis or a clinical improvement following reduction or withdrawal of the immunosuppressive agent.

Renal Transplant Dysfunction and Doppler Correlation

Doppler correlation with the different types of renal graft dysfunction is not possible. However, it is possible to differentiate these situations by taking the clinical picture into account (Table 6.4).

REFERENCES

1. Burge HJ, Middleton WD, McClennan BL, et al. Ureteral jets in healthy subjects and in patients with unilateral ureteral calculi: comparison with color Doppler US. *Radiol.* 1991;180:437–442.
2. Faubel S, Patel NU, Lockhart ME, Cadnapaphornchai MA. Use of ultrasonography in patients with AKI. *CJASN.* 2014;9(2):394.
3. Beland MD, Walle NL, Machan JT, Cronan JJ. Renal cortical thickness measured at ultrasound: is it better than renal length as an indicator of renal function in chronic kidney disease? *AJR Am J Roentgenol.* 2010;195(2):W146–W149.
4. Matsumoto M, Tsutaoka T, Yabunaka K, et al. Development and evaluation of automated ultrasonographic detection of bladder diameter for estimation of bladder urine volume. *PLoS ONE.* 2019;14(9), e0219916.
5. Liang C-C, Wei T-Y, Chang S-D, Hsieh C-C. Bladder volume determination: two-dimensional versus three-dimensional transvaginal ultrasound. *Taiwan J Obstet Gynecol.* 2009;48:258–261.
6. Brkljacic B, Drinkovic I, Delic-Brkljacic D, Hebrang A. Age-related changes of renal vascular resistance in normal native kidneys: colour duplex Doppler ultrasound assessment. *Radiol Oncol.* 1995;29:102–106.
7. Davda S, Vohra A. Adult duplex kidneys: an important differential diagnosis in patients with abdominal cysts. *JRSM Short Rep.* 2013;4(2):13.
8. Bhoil R, Sood D, Singh YP, Nimkar K, Shukla A. An ectopic pelvic kidney. *Pol J Radiol.* 2015;80:425–427.
9. Bosniak M. The current radiological approach to renal cysts. *Radiol.* 1986;158:1–10.
10. Silverman S, Pedrosa I, Ellis JH, et al. Bosniak classification of cystic renal masses, version 2019: an updated proposal and needs assessment. *Radiol.* 2019;292.
11. Destefani MH, Elias J, Trazzi Manzano Serra Negra A, et al. Minimally complex renal cysts: outcomes and ultrasound evaluation compared with contrast-enhanced cross sectional imaging Bosniak classification. *Ultrasound Med Biol.* 2017;43(10):2167–2173.
12. Rübenthaler J, Bogner F, Reiser M, Clevert DA. Contrast-enhanced ultrasound (CEUS) of the kidneys by using the Bosniak classification. *Ultraschall Med.* 2016;37(3):234–251.
13. Ascenti G, Mazziotti S, Zimbaro G, et al. Complex cystic renal masses: characterisation with contrast-enhanced US. *Radiol.* 2007;243:158–165.
14. Umeoka S, Koyama T, Miki Y, et al. Pictorial review of tuberous sclerosis in various organs. *Radiographics.* 2008;28, e32.
15. Heinz-Peer G, Schoder M, Rand T, et al. Prevalence of acquired cystic kidney disease and tumours in native kidneys of renal transplant recipients: a prospective study. *Radiol.* 1995;195:667–671.
16. Levine E. Acquired cystic kidney disease. *Radiol Clin North Am.* 1996;34:947–964.
17. Siegel CL, Middleton WD, Teefey SA, McClennan BL. Angiomyolipoma and renal cell carcinoma: US differentiation. *Radiol.* 1996;198:789–793.
18. Hussain T, Lam V, Farhad M, et al. Can subcentimetre ultrasound detected angiomyolipomas be safely disregarded? *Clin Radiol.* 2020;75(4):287–292.
19. de Silva S, Copping R, Malouf D, Hutton A, Maclean F, Aslan P. Frequency of angiomyolipomas among echogenic nonshadowing renal masses (> 4 mm) found at ultrasound and the utility of MRI for diagnosis. *AJR Am J Roentgenol.* 2017;209(5):1074–1080.
20. Prasad SR, Surabhi VR, Menias CO, et al. Benign renal neoplasms in adults: cross-sectional imaging findings. *AJR Am J Roentgenol.* 2008;190:158–164.
21. Curry NS, Schabel SI, Betsill WL. Small renal neoplasms: diagnostic imaging, pathologic features and clinical course. *Radiol.* 1986;158:113–117.
22. Licht MR. Renal adenoma and oncocytoma. *Semin Urol Oncol.* 1995;13:262–266.
23. Bosniak MA, Birnbaum BA, Krinsky GA, Waisman J. Small renal parenchymal neoplasms: further observations on growth. *Radiol.* 1996;197:589–597.
24. Correas J, Tranquart F, Claudon M. Guidelines for contrast enhanced ultrasound (CEUS). *J Radiol.* 2009;90:123–140.

25. Sánchez-Martín FM, Millán-Rodríguez F, Urdaneta-Pignalosa G, et al. Small renal masses: incidental diagnosis, clinical symptoms, and prognostic factors. *Adv Urol.* 2008;310694.

26. Haendl T, Strobel D, Legal W, et al. Renal cell cancer does not show a typical perfusion pattern in contrast-enhanced ultrasound. *Ultraschall Med.* 2009;30:58–63.

27. The Royal College of Radiologists, Royal College of Physicians of London, Royal College of Physicians and Surgeons of Glasgow, Royal College of Physicians of Edinburgh, British Nuclear Medicine Society and Administration of Radioactive Substances Advisory Committee. Evidence-based indications for the use of PET-CT in the United Kingdom 2016. *Clin Radiol.* 2016;71(7).

28. Browne RF, Meehan CP, Colville J, et al. Transitional cell carcinoma of the upper urinary tract: spectrum of imaging findings. *Radiographics.* 2005;25:1609–1627.

29. Leung RS, Biswas SV, Duncan M, Rankin S. Imaging features of von Hippel-Lindau disease. *Radiographics.* 2008;28:65–79.

30. Rodgers PM, Bates JA, Irving HC. Intrarenal Doppler ultrasound studies in normal and acutely obstructed kidneys. *Br J Radiol.* 1992;65:207–212.

31. Miletic D, Fuckar Z, Sustic A, et al. Resistance and pulsatility indices in acute renal obstruction. *J Clin Ultrasound.* 1998;26:79–84.

32. Hak-JL Seung HK, Yoong KJ, Kyung MY. Doppler sonographic resistive index in obstructed kidneys. *J Ultrasound Med.* 1996;15(9):613–618.

33. Vijayakumar M, Ganpule A, Singh A, Sabnis R, Desai M. Review of techniques for ultrasonic determination of kidney stone size. *Res Rep Urol.* 2018;10:57–61.

34. National Institute for Health Care and Excellence (NICE). *Renal or Ureteric Colic – Acute*; 2020. Available at: https://cks.nice.org.uk/topics/renal-or-ureteric-colic-acute/.

35. National Institute for Health Care and Excellence (NICE). *Urological cancers – recognition and referral*; 2015. Available at: https://cks.nice.org.uk/topics/urological-cancers-recognition-referral/.

36. Craig WD, Wagner BJ. Travis MD. Pyelonephritis: radiologic-pathologic review. *Radiographics.* 2008;28:255–277.

37. Li Y, Zhang Y. Diagnosis and treatment of acute focal bacterial nephritis. *Chinese Med J.* 1996;109:168–172.

38. Hamilton D. Alexis Carrel and the early days of tissue transplantation. *Transplant Rev.* 1987;2:1–15.

39. Murray JE, Merrill JP, Harrison JH. Kidney transplantation between seven pairs of identical twins. *Ann Surg.* 1958;148:343–359.

40. Calne RY, White DJG, Thiru S, et al. Cyclosporin A in patients receiving renal allografts from cadaveric donors. *Lancet.* 1978;ii:1323–1327.

41. He M, Taylor J. Renal transplantation. *BMJ.* 2014;348.

42. Cosgrove DO, Chan KE. Renal transplants: what ultrasound can and cannot do. *Ultrasound Q.* 2008;24:77–87.

43. Kashi SH, Irving HC. Improving the evaluation of renal transplant collecting system dilatation by computerised ultrasound imaging digitisation. *Br J Radiol.* 1993;66:1002–1008.

44. Perella RR, Duerincky AJ, Tessler FN, et al. Evaluation of renal transplant dysfunction by duplex Doppler sonography; a prospective study and review of the literature. *Am J Kidney Dis.* 1990;15:544–550.

45. Tublin ME, Dodd GD. Sonography of renal tranplantation. *Radiol Clin North Am.* 1995;33:447–459.

46. Hilborn MD, Bude RO, Murphy KJ, et al. Renal transplant evaluation with power Doppler sonography. *Br J Radiol.* 1997;70.

47. Witz M, Kantarovsky A, Morag B, Shifin EG. Renal vein occlusion: a review. *J Urol.* 1996;155:1173–1179.

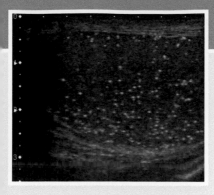

7

Ultrasound of the Testes and Male Pelvis

Simon J. Freeman and Pamela C. Parker

CHAPTER OUTLINE

The Penis and Scrotum, 230
  General Considerations and US Technique, 230
  Chaperones, 231
  Patient Dignity, 232
  Environment, 232
The Scrotum, 232
  Anatomy, 232
  Measurements, 234
  Varicoceles, 235
  Undescended Testes, 235
  Trauma, 236
  Testicular Torsion, 237
  *Torsion of the Epididymal or Testicular
    Appendix, 240*
  Other Causes of Acute Scrotal Pain, 240
  Epididymitis, 240
  Orchitis, 241
  Mumps Orchitis, 241
  Fournier Gangrene, 241
  Palpable Scrotal Masses, 242
  Extra-Testicular Mass, 242
  Scrotal Pearls, 245
  Hydroceles, 245
  Intratesticular Masses, 246
  Microlithiasis, 247
  Benign Intratesticular Masses, 247

Intratesticular Cysts, 248
Epidermoid Cysts, 248
Adrenal Rest Tumors, 248
Sarcoid, 249
Focal Orchitis, 249
Small Intratesticular Masses, 249
Other Tumor-Mimicking Abnormalities, 250
Malignant Intratesticular Masses, 250
Primary Malignant Lesions, 251
Secondary Testicular Tumors, 252
The Penis, 253
  Anatomy, 253
  Palpable Penile Mass, 254
  Peyronie's Disease, 254
  Benign Penile Mass, 255
  Malignant Penile Mass, 255
The Prostate, 255
  Anatomy, 255
  Measurements, 257
  Benign Prostate Disease, 258
  Benign Prostatic Hypertrophy (BPH), 258
  Cysts, 259
  Infection and Prostatitis, 259
  Infertility, 260
  Prostate Cancer, 260
References, 261

THE PENIS AND SCROTUM

General Considerations and US Technique

The superficial position of the penis and scrotal contents lend themselves to be optimally imaged by high-frequency ultrasound. Indeed, ultrasound is the modality of choice, and alternative imaging is rarely required.[1,2,3]

A high-frequency linear transducer should be employed and will be appropriate for the vast majority of examinations. It is advised that a minimum of 12 MHz be used, but with the development of matrix and broad-spectrum transducers, high frequencies can be optimized to produce exquisite imaging. Optimizing pre- and post-processing is required to ensure that the normal testicular echo pattern is one of mid-gray level homogeneity (Fig. 7.1A–C).[4]

A lower frequency transducer may be required for assessment of deep scrotal contents in patients presenting with large hydroceles, scrotal wall thickening, or scrotal hernias; a range of transducers is therefore advocated with the operator being mindful to change technique or transducer to optimize diagnostic imaging in challenging cases and presentations. Color Doppler techniques are widely used in both scrotal and penile ultrasound to assess vascular perfusion; assessment of blood flow characteristics with spectral Doppler is also occasionally indicated in particular clinical circumstances. As with Doppler studies elsewhere in the body, the pulse repetition frequency and gain should be adjusted and optimized to ensure that flow is shown without aliasing or artifact. Modern ultrasound may include microvascular imaging technologies that may permit visualization of very low-velocity blood flow not seen with conventional color Doppler techniques.[5] Contrast-enhanced ultrasound (CEUS) can be utilized to assist with the assessment of the vascularity of testicular and epididymal lesions and can be highly valuable in selected cases. Microbubble resonance is suboptimal at the high ultrasound frequencies used for scrotal imaging, a higher dose of contrast is required than for

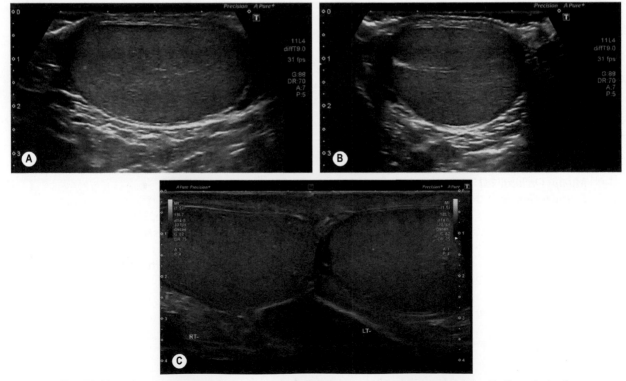

Fig. 7.1 Normal appearances of the right testis in long section (A) and transverse (B) with the rete testis clearly seen as a hyperechoic line in the center of the testis. (C) Comparison of both testes should be made to ensure both are similar in size, texture, and echogenicity.

abdominal applications, and it is frequently necessary to use a lower transducer frequency. Most modern high-end ultrasound systems will have a manufacturer pre-set that has been optimized for small-parts CEUS use, and this will usually be the optimal setting. Guidelines on CEUS use in the scrotum have been produced by the European Federation of Societies for Ultrasound in Medicine and Biology (EFSUMB) (Fig. 7.2A, B).[6]

Ultrasound elastography has also been successfully applied to scrotal evaluation, usually as part of a "multiparametric ultrasound" assessment of testicular masses. Most malignant lesions show high stiffness with both strain and shear wave elastographic techniques (Fig. 7.2C, D).

Chaperones

Imaging of both the penis and scrotum is an intimate examination. The use of chaperones must be considered, and reference to local and national chaperone guidance and employers' policy will be required prior to undertaking this type of examination. Where a chaperone is present, they must be introduced to the patient, and the patient's consent for them to be present must be gained, prior to the examination commencing. If either the practitioner performing the examination or the patient has any concerns, these are to be raised and discussed; if necessary, delay the examination until an appropriate chaperone and support are available.

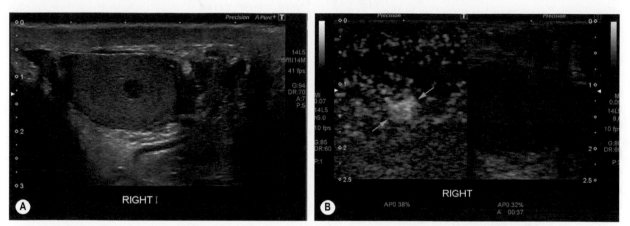

Fig. 7.2A, B Incidentally discovered small echo-poor testicular mass (A). CEUS image showing that the mass is hyper-vascular in the early phase (arrows - B).

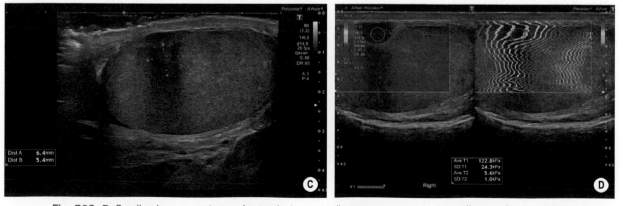

Fig. 7.2C, D Small echo-poor subcapsular testicular mass (between measurement calipers - C). On shear wave elastography, the mass is shown to be much harder than adjacent testicular parenchyma (red color and very calculated high stiffness - 122.8 kPa in comparison to adjacent testicular parenchyma - 5.6 kPa - D).

Patient Dignity

Imaging of the male genital tract can be embarrassing for some patients, and consideration of patient dignity is an essential component of scrotal and penile ultrasound examinations. Clear and concise communication with the patient is required prior to commencing the examination so that it is clear what the examination will involve and what is required of the patient.

While testicular tumors constitute only 1% of all malignant tumors in men, anxiety regarding testicular cancer is common in patients referred for scrotal ultrasound examinations, particularly if they have a palpable scrotal mass. Although the majority of ultrasound findings are benign, patients are usually apprehensive about the scan outcome. Ideally, the patient should be offered a preliminary verbal summary of the scan findings immediately after the examination; this will usually allay any anxieties. When an indeterminate or sinister finding is identified, the patient should be given clear advice regarding the next steps in their management. A local process for immediate or urgent urological review that can be initiated by the ultrasound practitioner is desirable.

Environment

Consideration of suitable surroundings is required for intimate examinations. It is recommended that the examinations be performed in a room with a comfortable temperature and dim lighting. A curtain around the bed can help ensure that privacy and dignity are maintained. Interruptions into the scan room during the procedure should be avoided.

For examination of the scrotum, the patient should be asked to hold their penis up out of the way, usually on the anterior abdominal wall. The scrotum should be gently elevated by the patient, asking them to lie with their legs closed with the thighs acting as support for the scrotum. A tissue roll or an appropriate cover should then be placed over the hands and penis to aid dignity.

TIP BOX

Consideration of gel temperature is required. A cold gel may be uncomfortable, particularly when scanning the acute scrotum.

The patient should be asked to find any palpable lump and hold between two fingers prior to the gel being applied. Once palpated by the patient, this area should be scanned first prior to the rest of the scrotum being examined.

The scanning technique for the penis will be determined by the indication. The penis is usually scanned from the ventral aspect, with the patient holding the penis against the anterior abdominal wall. It is sometimes necessary to scan from the dorsal and lateral aspects. The most common referrals are for penile lumps. As for the scrotum, the patient should be asked to find any palpable lump and hold between two fingers, if possible, prior to the gel being applied. Once palpated by the patient, this area should be scanned first prior to the rest of the penis being examined.

THE SCROTUM

Anatomy[7,8,9]

The scrotum is a pouch of connective and fibrous tissue and smooth muscle; it contains the testes, epididymides, and spermatic cords. Its purpose is to suspend the male reproductive glands outside the peritoneum to ensure they are cooler than the body's core temperature. The testes require a temperature of approximately two degrees below normal body temperature to allow optimum sperm production (Diagram 7.1).

The testes are situated within the abdomen of the developing fetus until the 28th week of gestation, at which point they commence their descent into the scrotum. This is an important consideration when imaging a small neonate.

The testes are surrounded by three layers of connective tissue. The tunica vaginalis is the outer covering of the testes and is a down-growth of the abdominal and pelvic peritoneum. It consists of parietal and visceral layers covering the inner surface of the scrotal wall and tunica albuginea of the testis, respectively. The space between the two layers may become filled with fluid in patients with hydroceles. There is a bare area posterior to the testis in most men, not invested in the tunica vaginalis, attaching the testis directly to the scrotal wall. In approximately 12% of men, the tunica vaginalis may completely surround the testis and epididymis, leaving the testis mobile within the scrotum. This is known as the "bell-clapper deformity" and is a risk factor for torsion of the spermatic cord (Fig. 7.3A).[10]

The tunica albuginea is a fibrous covering surrounding the testes and situated under the visceral tunica

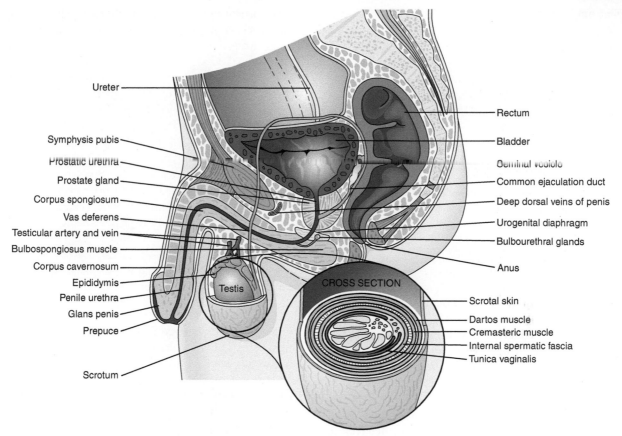

Diagram 7.1 Male genitourinary anatomy, including a cross-section of the scrotum and its layers. (Source: Pathophysiology, Seventh Edition, 2022).

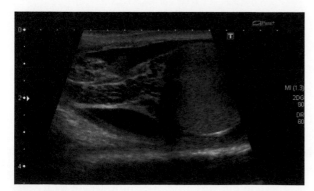

Fig. 7.3A Bell-Clapper testis. In this 27-year-old man presenting with intermittent episodes of scrotal pain, the presence of a hydrocoele shows that the intra-scrotal spermatic cord and the testis are surrounded by fluid, allowing the testis to rotate freely within the scrotum.

vaginalis. It is often visible on ultrasound as a thin echogenic line surrounding the testis. Ingrowths of the tunica albuginea form the mediastinum testis and septa dividing the glandular testicular tissue into lobules. The segmental vasculature and seminiferous tubules can occasionally be discerned, particularly with modern microvascular imaging or when there is dilatation of the efferent ductules. The rete testis is a connection of tubules formed by the terminal parts of the seminiferous tubules; it lies within the mediastinum testis at the testicular hilum. Dilatation of the tubules in the rete testis (tubular dilatation or cystic ectasia of the rete testis) is a benign condition regularly encountered in older men on scrotal ultrasound where multiple small cystic or tubular structures are seen in the mediastinum testis (Fig. 7.3B).

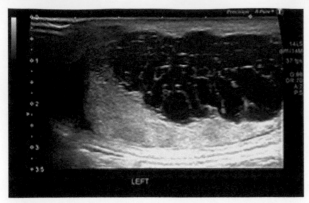

Fig. 7.3B Cystic ectasia of the rete testis. An 85-year-old man with advanced prostate cancer. Ultrasound shows multiple cystic and tubular masses in the testis. This is a florid example of cystic ectasia of the rete testis, likely because of malignant obstruction of the vas deferens.

The third layer is the tunica vasculosa and consists of a network of capillaries supported by delicate connective tissue lying immediately below the tunica albuginea; it cannot be separately resolved by ultrasound. Testicular rupture occurs when the tunica albuginea is breached and usually results in damage to the tunica vasculosa leading to testicular ischemia.

As the testes descend, they take the blood and lymph vessels, nerves, and deferent ducts (vasa deferentia), which, in turn, form the spermatic cord. The blood supply to the testes is predominantly through the testicular arteries arising from the abdominal aorta at the level of the L1/2 vertebrae descending through the retroperitoneum to enter the spermatic cord at the deep inguinal ring. There is an additional anastomotic arterial supply from the cremasteric artery and artery of the ductus deferens. Venous drainage of the testis arises from the pampiniform plexus, a venous plexus around the testis, which then drains into several venous tributaries in the spermatic cord, which combine to form the testicular veins above the inguinal canal. The testicular veins pass cranially to drain into the renal vein on the left side and inferior vena cava on the right side.

A small pedunculated appendage, the appendix testis, extends from the superior surface of the testis in approximately 30% of men. A similar appendix epididymis can also be present. Both are usually only seen with the presence of a co-existing hydrocele (Fig. 7.3C, Fig. 7.3D).

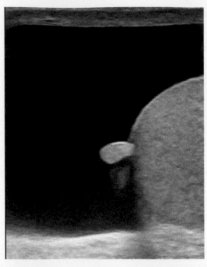

Fig. 7.3C A small appendix testis is clearly seen because of the presence of a small amount of fluid surrounding the testis.

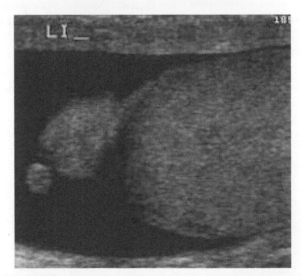

Fig. 7.3D The appendix epididymis is seen in this case because of the presence of fluid. Commonly, appendices of the testes or epididymis are not well seen.

Measurements

The testes are ovoid structures measuring approximately $4 \times 3 \times 3$ cm but vary from 3–5 cm in length to 2–3 cm in width and anteroposterior dimensions. Calculation of testicular volume from ultrasound measurements is often desirable, particularly in men with sub-fertility or with varicoceles; Lambert's formula ($L \times W \times H \times 0.71$)

is the most accurate method; a combined testicular volume of 20–24 mL is associated with normal testicular function.[11] Both testes are usually remarkably similar in size. Caution is required in patients who have had previous undescended testis repair (orchidopexy); this can cause some degree of vascular compromise and may reduce the testicular volume on the affected side. Patient history is invaluable in cases of testicular asymmetry (Fig. 7.4).

The epididymis is sub-divided into the head, body, and tail located above, lateral, and below the testis, respectively. The average epididymal size is approximately 8 mm for the head, 3–4 mm for the body, and 8 mm for the tail, although comparison with the contralateral side is useful. Incidental epididymal changes are a frequent finding in men following vasectomy and include enlargement and cyst formation.[12,13]

Varicoceles

Varicose dilatation of the pampiniform plexus usually begins at puberty.[14] The prevalence of varicoceles is estimated to be 15% but is nearly 35% among men with primary infertility and increases by 10% with each decade of life.[15] In 90% of these, the left side is involved; in 10%, it is bilateral; and in only <1% does this occur unilaterally on the right. This dilatation causes slow venous flow and impaired venous return. Patients with varicoceles often present with a palpable mass and dragging

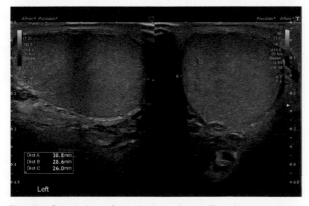

Fig. 7.4 Calculation of testicular volume. The three measurements of testicular size are multiplied by 0.71 to give an estimation of testicular volume (by Lambert's formula – in this case, 20.5 mL). This calculation should be performed by the ultrasound practitioner directly. The automated volume calculation used by most ultrasound systems will not use this formula and will underestimate testicular volume.

scrotal ache on standing or after exercise or present for investigation of infertility.

Varicoceles may be associated with impaired testicular function. Although most men with varicoceles will have normal fertility, it is the most common treatable cause of male infertility.

The cause of impaired venous flow is either because of obstruction of the returning blood or reflux, particularly during periods of increased intrabdominal pressure. Therefore, it is often recommended that the left kidney and retroperitoneum be evaluated upon initial diagnosis of a varicocele to exclude an occult malignancy obstructing the testicular vein. Identification of an unsuspected renal or retroperitoneal tumor in a man with a varicocele is, however, very uncommon, this recommendation does not have a clear evidence base, and the need to extend the examination to the abdomen in all cases has been challenged. However, ultrasound evaluation of the kidneys and retroperitoneum is advised when a varicocele is identified in a child or in adults where the varicocele is of sudden onset, large, or fails to decompress with the patient in the supine position.[15]

Varicoceles are well visualized on fundamental imaging with additional confirmatory interrogation with color Doppler. In equivocal cases, the examination should include an evaluation with the patient standing and performing a Valsalva maneuver – the diagnosis cannot be excluded without this additional information.

Diagnosis of a varicocele requires a maximal venous diameter of 3 mm or more in a pampiniform plexus vein. Venous reflux is the most important finding in infertility as it is believed to be the primary cause of testicular damage. This should be assessed with color and spectral Doppler examination, with the patient standing if necessary. Significant reflux is present when the venous flow is continuously reversed or reflux lasts for more than 2 s during Valsalva (Fig. 7.5A–C).

Large varicoceles may extend into the testes at the hilum, and isolated intratesticular varicoceles may also occur. These can be differentiated from intratesticular cysts and rete testis cystic ectasia by their tubular shape and the presence of flow on Doppler assessment.

Undescended Testes

Cryptorchidism is a term that is commonly used with undescended testes, but strictly this term should describe only abdominal tests; those in the inguinal canal

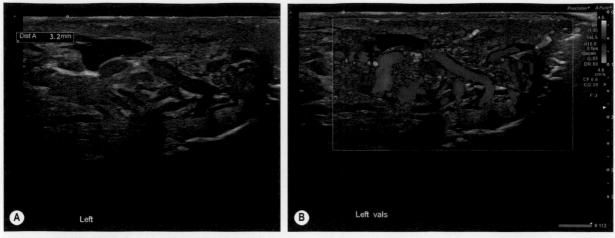

Fig. 7.5A, B A 36-year-old man referred for ultrasound assessment of sub-fertility. The grayscale image shows significant dilatation of left pampiniform plexus veins with the patient supine and at rest (>3 mm) (A). On Valsalva, venous reflux is seen on the color Doppler image (blue color) (B).

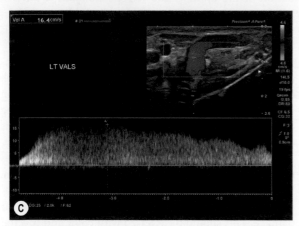

Fig. 7.5C Spectral Doppler trace of a dilated pampiniform plexus vein in a patient with a varicocele. Venous reflux during Valsalva lasts for more than 2 s indicating significant reflux.

should be termed incompletely descended. Those found in other positions, such as the thigh, are ectopic testes.

Approximately 3% of term and 20% of preterm male babies will have undescended testes. However, only 1% of male infants will have persistent undescended testes by One year of age. Orchidopexy (testicular repositioning and fixation) is ideally performed prior to five years of age and at the latest by puberty to avoid fertility issues and atrophy of the testes associated with this condition. Undescended testis also significantly increases the risk of development of testicular germ cell tumor and

is present in approximately 10% of cases of testicular cancer. There is some evidence that orchidopexy prior to puberty may reduce this risk with the additional benefit that moving the testis to the scrotum will make for easier tumor detection.[16]

Ultrasound is superior to clinical examination for identifying incompletely descended testes in the inguinal canal; the testis will often be small, and identification of the mediastinum testis is required to differentiate the testis from a lymph node or remnant of the gubernaculum testis. A retractile testis may be found in younger boys where the testis moves from the scrotum to the inguinal canal because of cremasteric muscle contraction, and this can usually be diagnosed by clinical examination (Fig. 7.6A, B).

True cryptorchidism within the abdomen or pelvis is rarely identified by ultrasound, and MRI or diagnostic laparoscopy are more accurate (Fig. 7.6C).

Trauma

Testicular injuries are uncommon because of the mobility of the testis in the scrotum and the strength of the tunica albuginea. The majority of cases are because of blunt trauma and are often sporting injuries. Scrotal trauma often results in a swollen, tender scrotum, hindering a valuable clinical examination that is unreliable in predicting injury severity. Gentle scrotal ultrasound is usually well-tolerated and provides useful information to triage patients into operative or conservative management. There is a spectrum of injuries ranging from

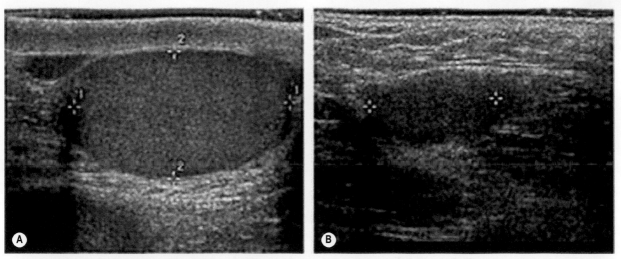

Fig. 7.6A, B The right testis in this 14-year-old boy is seen within the inguinal testes canal (B). It is smaller and more hypoechoic than the normal left testis (A).

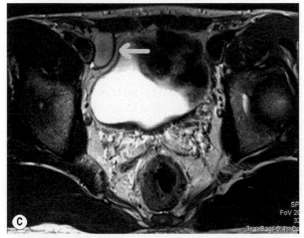

Fig. 7.6C MRI cryptorchidism demonstrates the position of the right testis high in the inguinal canal.

can be difficult to identify directly on ultrasound, particularly where there is no hydrocoele/hematocele. An abnormal contour of the testis, because of extrusion of testicular tissue through the tunical defect, is the most valuable ultrasound predictor and has high accuracy for rupture diagnosis (Fig. 7.6D, E).

In all cases of testicular injury, testicular perfusion should be assessed with color Doppler techniques to identify areas of non-perfusion; where there is complete or significant non-perfusion surgical exploration will also frequently be required. CEUS may also be helpful to demonstrate avascular areas and better delineate fracture lines and hematomas.

Testicular tumors will sometimes present following minor scrotal trauma. Any focal abnormality assumed to represent a traumatic hematoma should undergo a follow-up ultrasound to confirm resolution and ensure that there is no underlying mass.

Testicular Torsion

Testicular torsion is a surgical emergency.[17] Intervention should not be delayed by imaging. Where there is a high clinical suspicion, immediate surgical exploration is required as the possibility of testicular salvage depends on the time to detorsion; the best outcomes occur when surgery is performed within 6–8 h, but surgery may still be valuable up to 24h from the time of onset.

Imaging should only be considered when the clinical diagnosis is uncertain; the main differential diagnosis

hematocele to intra- or extra-testicular hematomas, testicular laceration, testicular rupture, or, very rarely, testicular dislocation.

Common findings are swelling of the scrotal wall, hematoma, and occasional hematocele. These do not usually require surgical intervention unless there is a large hematoma compromising testicular perfusion. Testicular rupture is a surgical emergency as an early repair usually allows the testis to be preserved; delayed diagnosis often results in orchidectomy. Rupture occurs when the tunica albuginea is breached; however, this

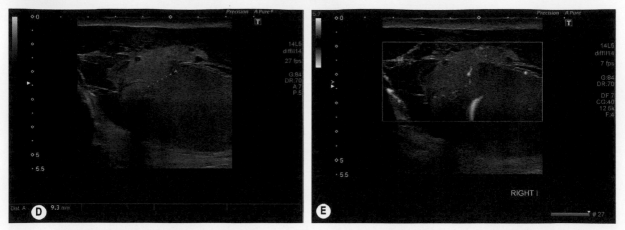

Fig. 7.6D, E A 46-year-old man with acute scrotal pain following a fall from a bike. The grayscale image shows a breach in the tunica albuginea (between measurement calipers) with extrusion of testicular parenchyma through the defect (D). The color Doppler image shows perfusion of the testis and extruded tissue (E).

is epididymo-orchitis, torsion of the appendix testes, or appendix epididymis. Imaging may be valuable in these cases to avoid unnecessary surgery. A clinical assessment tool (TWIST score) has been proposed for assessing the possibility of torsion in patients aged less than 18.[18]

Torsion of the spermatic cord has a bimodal distribution. Neonatal torsion occurs prenatally or within 30 days of delivery. It is usually a clinical diagnosis, and the testis is usually not salvageable unless the torsion occurs after birth. In this situation, the testis and tunica twist around the spermatic cord at the level of the external inguinal ring (extravaginal/supravaginal torsion). More commonly, torsion of the spermatic cord occurs within the tunica vaginalis (intravaginal torsion). The bell-clapper deformity is the most common predisposing cause. This type of torsion usually occurs in adolescents and young adults; however, it may occur at any age, and torsion should be considered in an acute presentation with severe unilateral scrotal pain and swelling, even in older men.

TIP BOX

Torsion can be difficult to diagnose on fundamental and Doppler imaging, and ultrasound may give misleading information to the unwary. B-mode imaging will usually show normal testicular appearances. Where testicular changes are present, this often indicates infarction and hemorrhage and irreversible damage that is non-salvageable.

The absence of discernible blood flow within a testis (where flow is visible on the contralateral normal side) is highly predictive of testicular torsion. However, the presence of blood flow does not exclude torsion, and blood flow may still be detectible in approximately a quarter of patients with torsion. Reduced flow compared to the asymptomatic side or increased intratesticular vascular resistance on spectral Doppler examination of intratesticular arteries is a suspicious feature of incomplete torsion.[19] In small preadolescent boys, microvascular imaging may be required to detect flow in small vessels not seen with traditional Doppler techniques. Ultrasound examination of the spermatic cord results in the highest levels of diagnostic accuracy but is dependent on the experience of the examiner. The presence of the "whirlpool sign" where the twist of the cord is directly identified is a highly specific sign of torsion but is not always visible. More commonly, a pseudomass of redundant edematous spermatic cord and epididymis will be seen, usually above the testis (torsion knot).[20] Normal or increased blood flow (because of rebound hyperemia) may be seen in patients with intermittent torsion where spontaneous detorsion has occurred prior to the ultrasound study; this can be impossible to differentiate from epididymo-orchitis (Fig. 7.7).

The ultrasound practitioner should be aware that testicular torsion can also cause epididymal swelling and hydrocele formation, mimicking epididymo-orchitis. However, in this situation, epididymal blood flow will

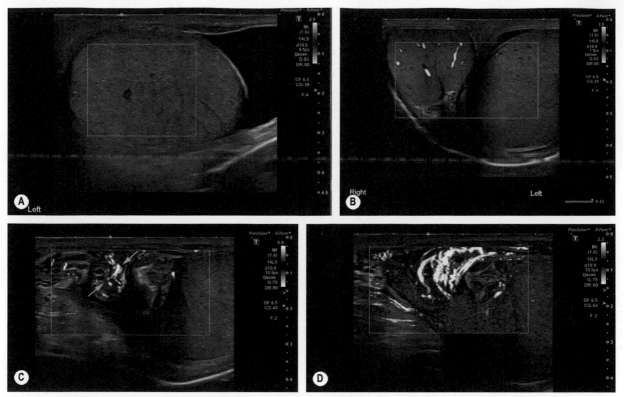

Fig. 7.7 Torsion of the spermatic cord. A 28-year-old man with sudden onset of acute scrotal pain. Power Doppler shows no evidence of left testicular perfusion. There is a reactive hydrocoele and evidence of edema of the testicular parenchyma (A). Perfusion is clearly visible in the normal right testis on a transverse image of both testes (B). Examination of the spermatic cord shows a coiled configuration of the vessels (whirlpool sign - arrows - C). In another case, both a whirlpool sign and torsion knot (pseudomass because of redundant spermatic cord and epididymis above the testis) are seen (D).

be low or absent, unlike the hyperemia usually seen in acute infective epididymitis.

A missed torsion is a term used in cases of torsion that have not been diagnosed or treated for 48 h or more. The testis is enlarged, either homogenously hypoechoic or of a mixed echo pattern and centrally avascular. There is often a hyperechoic rim around the periphery of the testes, with a rim of blood flow seen around the testicular margin. The epididymis will usually be enlarged, and frequently a reactive hydrocoele will be present. The testis will almost always be non-viable, and if orchidectomy is not undertaken over time, this will lead to a small atrophic testis lacking in perfusion and function (Fig. 7.8A, B).

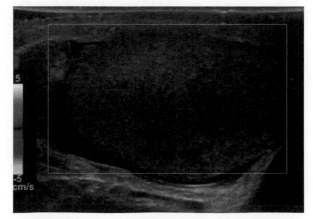

Fig. 7.8A An undiagnosed torsion of 48 h or more becomes enlarged and, in this case, homogenously hypoechoic.

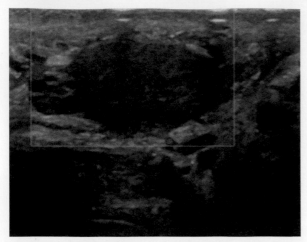

Fig. 7.8B As time progresses, the testis becomes atrophic in a case of a missed torsion.

Torsion of the Epididymal or Testicular Appendix

The testicular appendix is a remnant of the Wolffian duct. It is a projection of tissue from the upper pole of the testis. The epididymal appendix is a remnant of the Müllerian duct and arises from the head of the epididymis. The appendices are usually only seen with the presence- of a co-existing hydrocoele. Either may tort, which is a common cause of acute pain in boys. The diagnosis is usually made clinically, and no treatment or intervention is required. Ultrasound may be valuable to exclude other causes of acute pain and avoid unnecessary surgery (Fig. 7.8C).

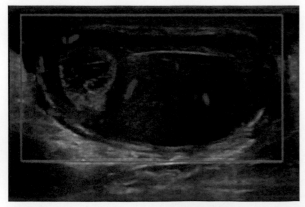

Fig. 7.8C Torsion of the appendix is demonstrated as an enlarged area adjacent to the testis or epididymis with absent blood flow.

Hydatids of Morgagni may be seen as cystic structures within the epididymal appendix but are most likely described as cysts. The hydatids of Morgagni can tort within the epididymis, causing a rounded mass with a cystic center. Surrounding tissues may be edematous and hyperemic in the acute phase.

Other Causes of Acute Scrotal Pain

Except for spermatic cord or appendiceal torsion, acute scrotal pain is most commonly caused by epididymo-orchitis. A differential diagnosis of acute scrotal pain includes appendicitis which may rarely present with scrotal pain mimicking torsion. Diagnosis can be made by extending the examination into the lower abdomen and considering appendicitis as a differential diagnosis. Other uncommon causes of the acute scrotum include incarcerated or strangulated inguinal hernia, acute segmental testicular infarction, and Henoch-Schoenlein purpura (systemic vasculitis usually occurring in children).

Epididymitis

The most common cause of epididymitis in young men is a sexually transmitted disease and in older men, a urinary tract infection. Catheterization is a common precursor. Repetitive trauma, including cycling and exercise, is also a predisposing cause for this common condition.

Appearances may vary greatly, but the most common ultrasound finding is of an enlarged hyperemic epididymis. This may be focal or diffuse depending upon the duration and severity of the infection/inflammation at the time of the examination. The epididymal tail is most likely affected, and only in severe cases will the whole epididymis be inflamed. There can be a variable reactive hydrocele (Fig. 7.9A, B).

Doppler assessment of the epididymis is invaluable, and care needs to be taken to assess the whole structure. In severe cases, or where antibiotics are ineffective, abscesses may form, particularly in the tail. Swelling and edema usually resolve rapidly with appropriate antibiotic treatment, although palpable hard areas may remain, which are often difficult to visualize on subsequent imagining, despite the patient feeling these "lumps." A scan to assess normality is reassuring in these cases. Interval scans are also indicated where there is a poor response to antibiotic treatment to exclude

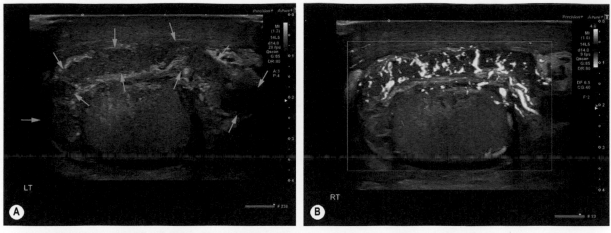

Fig. 7.9A, B Acute epididymitis. On grayscale images, the epididymis is diffusely thickened (arrows) with thickening of the scrotal wall and a small reactive hydrocoele (A). On color Doppler imaging, the epididymis shows marked diffuse hypervascularity (B).

developments of complications such as an abscess or pyocele formation.

Occasionally the spermatic cord can be affected; this is termed funiculitis. The cord has a similar appearance to the epididymis when affected. The scrotal wall should be assessed in severe cases to exclude the presence of a scrotal wall abscess, particularly in cases of significant scrotal wall edema.

Orchitis

Orchitis is usually a sequela of epididymitis and rarely occurs in isolation. Orchitis may occur post-trauma or post-surgery (including post vas ligation/vasectomy). Mumps is a cause of isolated orchitis.

Comparison with the non-affected testes is essential to aid diagnosis. The affected testis is likely to be enlarged and have a diffuse change in echo pattern with a hypoechoic appearance. A reactive hydrocele may be present.

Perfusion should be assessed with Doppler. The affected testis may be hyperaemic, but the vessel pattern should not be disturbed or affected; there should be no evidence of mass effect in orchitis. Focal orchitis may occur and be more severe, sometimes complicated by areas of venous infarction, necrosis, and abscess formation. It is sometimes difficult to distinguish between focal/diffuse orchitis and a discreet tumor. Therefore,

a repeat scan in the non-acute phase, for instance, six weeks later, is strongly advised to confirm resolution or identify a persistent and, therefore, significant mass (Fig. 7.10A–D).

Mumps Orchitis

Mumps causes a diffuse homogeneous or patchy hypoechoic pattern but does not cause focal orchitis. The diagnosis should be clinically apparent, although difficult where orchitis occurs in the absence of parotitis. Epididymitis is usually not present. Infarcts may occur in the acute phase, and atrophy can be a long-term complication.

Fournier Gangrene

Fournier's gangrene is a rare but life-threatening disease. It is an infective necrotizing fasciitis of the perineal, genital, or perianal regions. Although originally thought to be an idiopathic process, Fournier's gangrene has been shown to have a predilection for patients with diabetes and long term alcohol misuse, immunocompromised patients, and following perianal sepsis or surgery.

Diagnosis is clinical and is a medical emergency. Early surgical debridement of necrotic tissues and antibiotics are fundamental in the treatment of Fournier's gangrene. Despite advanced management, mortality is still high and averages 20%–30%.

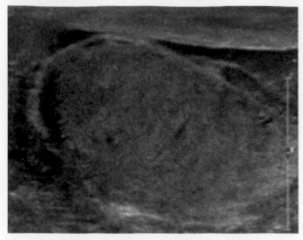

Fig. 7.10A The testis becomes enlarged and edematous on B-mode imaging.

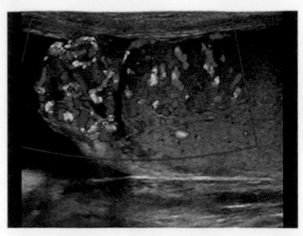

Fig. 7.10B Assessment of the perfusion of the testis with color Doppler will demonstrate hyperaemic flow in the testis and commonly epididymis, compared to the normal contralateral side.

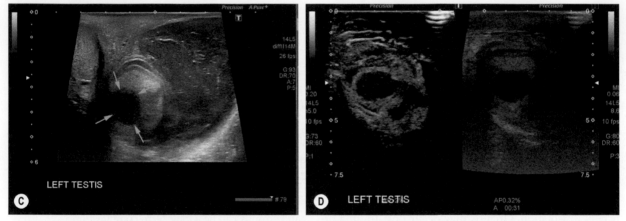

Fig. 7.10C, D Testicular abscesses in complicated epididymo-orchitis. Grayscale image showing a large septated hydrocoele containing low-level internal echoes suspicious of a pyocoele. There is a low echogenicity mass within the testis (arrows - D). On CEUS, the mass shows a vascular rim but no internal flow consistent with a testicular abscess (E). Follow-up of this lesion would be indicated to ensure resolution.

In the early stage, ultrasound will show marked edema and shadowing from gas within the affected tissue. While ultrasound does not add value in the later stages, an early scan, where Fournier's gangrene is a high clinical concern, may provide the diagnosis before it is clinically apparent (Fig. 7.11A, B).[21,22]

Palpable Scrotal Masses

Masses within the scrotum are differentiated between extra- and intratesticular masses. The majority of extra-testicular masses are benign. Ultrasound is highly accurate in differentiating between intra- and extra-testicular masses and is a useful test to confirm the clinical findings and to provide reassurance to the patient when the mass is confirmed to be extra-testicular.

Extra-Testicular Mass

The majority of extra-testicular masses are cysts and sperm granulomas.[23] Benign tumors are uncommon, and malignant lesions (sarcomas or mesotheliomas) are rare.

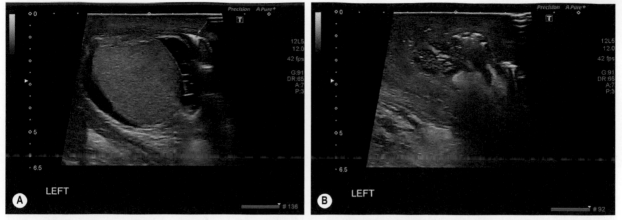

Fig. 7.11A, B Fournier's Disease. A 52-year-old man with perineo-scrotal swelling, erythema, and pain following treatment of a perineal abscess. Scrotal ultrasound shows a complex hydrocoele and locules of gas in the scrotal wall (arrow - A), more extensive gas locules seen elsewhere in the scrotum (B).

Cystic extra-testicular masses may be epididymal cysts, spermatoceles, cysts of the cord, or loculated hydroceles. Spermatoceles may have internal echoes not seen in an uncomplicated cyst and are always within the epididymal head but otherwise can be difficult to distinguish from simple epididymal cysts. As purely cystic masses are always benign and only treated if symptomatic, the distinction is unnecessary.

Cysts are smooth-walled. They may contain internal echoes if there has been infection or hemorrhage and with hemorrhage, a retractile clot may be seen. There will be no perfusion evident (Fig. 7.11C–E). A large cyst may mimic a hydrocoele, and careful interrogation of the extent of the fluid around the testes will be required to differentiate between the two.

Palpable solid extra-testicular masses most commonly arise from the epididymis, particularly in cases of epididymitis. Post-inflammatory change may be evident, resulting in a persistently enlarged and heterogenous epididymis that is not particularly tender. Chronic epididymitis is a cause of long-standing scrotal pain, and it can occur following an episode of acute epididymitis or be caused by granulomatous disease (tuberculosis), following a vasectomy, drug treatment (amiodarone), or systemic disease (e.g., Behçet's disease); in many cases no cause is identified. Ultrasound features are non-specific but include epididymal enlargement, heterogeneous echogenicity, and calcifications.[24]

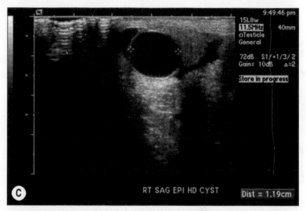

Fig. 7.11C Epididymal cysts demonstrate typical ultrasound features: anechoic, smooth-walled with post cystic enhancement clearly seen.

Sperm granulomas are well-defined, smooth, avascular round masses within the epididymis and commonly present 5–10 years post vasectomy but may also be seen in patients with no vasectomy history because of trauma or infection. No intervention is required unless the patient is symptomatic, particularly in lesions less than 2 cm. However, as there is a small theoretical risk of the lesions being a rare malignant lesion, a local policy of an interval scan or advice to the patient to return if any changes are felt would be prudent (Fig. 7.11F).

An adenomatoid tumor is the most common neoplasm of the epididymis but is still a rare tumor. The majority are benign and present as painless, slowly growing

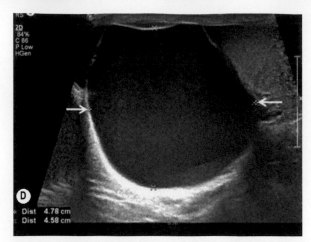

Fig. 7.11D Large epididymal cysts can mimic hydroceles. Careful assessment of the cyst wall is required.

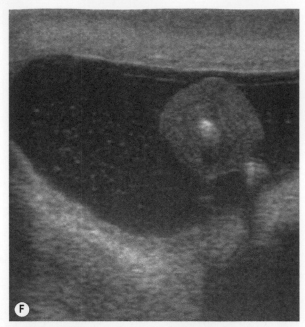

Fig. 7.11F Sperm granulomas are well-defined, smooth, avascular round masses within the epididymis.

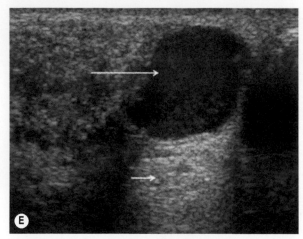

Fig. 7.11E A spermatocele (long arrow) will have typical smooth walls with post cystic enhancement (short arrow) of a simple cyst, but low-level, finely distributed echoes are seen within.

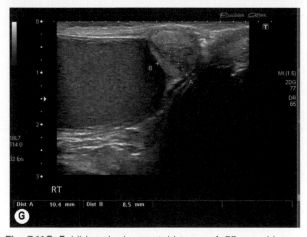

Fig. 7.11G Epididymal adenomatoid tumor. A 55-year-old man presenting with a one-year history of a slowly enlarging painless scrotal mass. Ultrasound shows an echogenic mass arising from the epididymal tail (between measurement calipers). The mass was surgically excised, and histology confirmed a benign adenomatoid tumor.

masses often in the epididymal tail. Although a solid, well-defined mass of variable echogenicity is most commonly seen, there are no characteristic ultrasound features (Fig. 7.11G).

Lipomas of the spermatic cord are the most common benign extra-testicular, extra-epididymal tumor and have sonographic appearances similar to lipomas elsewhere in the body; where there is uncertainty, MRI is diagnostic. Heterogenous, irregular, vascular solid masses of over 1 cm should be considered as suspicious for malignancy, particularly if the lesion is a new clinical finding or where the patient gives a history of localized pain or enlargement. Surgical excision will often be undertaken in this group.

Heterogenous irregular solid masses of less than 1 cm are more difficult to characterize but are still of concern, particularly when internal vascularity is detected. Management by a urologist will usually be indicated, and interval ultrasound is often the most appropriate management when surgical excision is not undertaken (Fig. 7.11H–K).

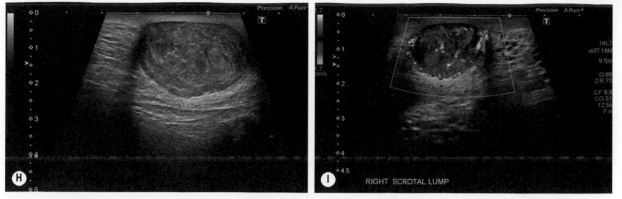

Fig. 7.11H, I Malignant extra-testicular mass. A 64-year-old man presenting with a painless but enlarging scrotal mass. Ultrasound shows a mass of mixed soft tissue echogenicity arising from the spermatic cord (H) showing high internal flow on Doppler examination (I). The mass was excised, and histology showed a malignant leiomyosarcoma.

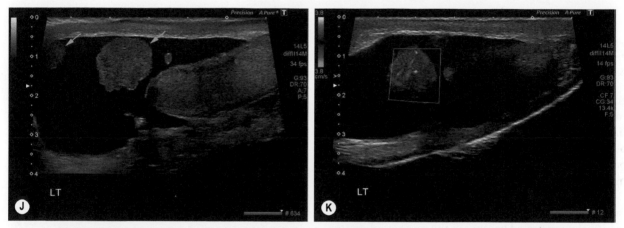

Fig. 7.11J, K Malignant extra-testicular mass. 83-year-old man with a palpable scrotal mass. Grayscale images show two extra-testicular masses separate from the testis, epididymis, and cord (arrows) with a moderate hydrocoele (J) which shows internal vascularity on Doppler examination (K). Surgical excision was undertaken, and histology showed malignant mesothelioma.

Epidermoid cysts can be present within the epididymis but more commonly in the testes. Appearances are similar regardless of location. (For detail, see: Benign Intratesticular Masses section.)

Scrotal Pearls

Mobile calcified masses within the scrotum are common. They are thought to be detached calcification of the appendix testis or appendix epididymis that may arise following appendiceal torsion. They are insignificant but may present as a mobile solid mass. They are termed scrotal pearls or scrotoliths (Fig. 7.12).

Hydroceles

A hydrocele is an abnormal amount of fluid between the tunica layers. However, what amounts to normal fluid is subjective. As a rule of thumb, if fluid can be seen to surround the entirety of the testis, then a hydrocoele is present (Fig. 7.13A).

Simple hydroceles are echo-free and may be idiopathic, secondary to inflammation, trauma, or rarely, testicular cancer. A congenital hydrocoele may occur in children because of a patent processus vaginalis where the scrotum is in direct communication with the peritoneal cavity. Complicated hydroceles contain internal

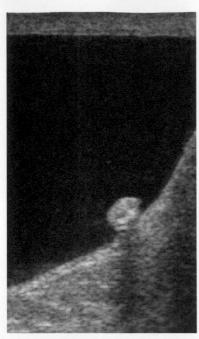

Fig. 7.12 Mobile calcified masses within the scrotum are common and insignificant. They are termed scrotal pearls.

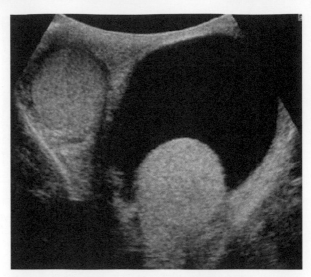

Fig. 7.13A Simple hydrocoele surrounds the testes. Large hydroceles can make imaging of the underlying testis with a standard linear high-frequency transducer challenging. Changing to a lower-frequency curvilinear, as in this case, can improve visualization.

echoes and are secondary to infection or trauma. Internal echoes in a hydrocoele post-trauma should alert the practitioner to hemorrhage, and careful assessment of the testicular capsule is required to evaluate for the presence of rupture. In scrotal infection, a complicated hydrocoele may indicate the presence of a pyocele.

In certain parts of the world, bilharzia is a common cause of hydrocele, and a coarse internal echo pattern may be demonstrated because of the presence of masses of eggs from this parasite. Calcification of the spermatic cord and tunica may be evident in chronic cases.

Loculated hydroceles can be seen post-infection or post-surgical intervention (either hernia repair or scrotal surgery). Intervention is usually not required (Fig. 7.13B).

Intratesticular Masses

Most patients with testicular tumors will present with painless testicular swelling. Mild scrotal ache or discomfort is less common. Most palpable testicular masses in younger men are malignant germ cell tumors (GCTs). Less commonly, testicular tumors may be impalpable and may be an incidental finding on scrotal ultrasound studies performed for other indications such as scrotal ache/pain, hydrocele, or infertility. Incidental

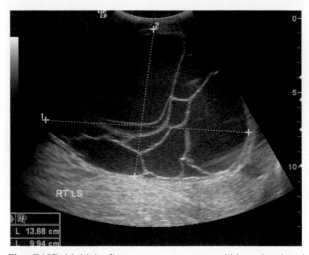

Fig. 7.13B Multiple fine septa are seen within a loculated hydrocele and are often present following infection or as a post-surgical complication.

non-palpable testicular masses will be identified in approximately 1%–7% of scrotal ultrasound studies and are particularly prevalent in men being scanned for infertility. Unlike palpable masses, most non-palpable testicular masses are benign with a direct correlation between lesion size and malignancy; management should avoid radical orchidectomy whenever possible.

Microlithiasis

Testicular microlithiasis (TML) is most often an incidental finding in an asymptomatic patient. Microlithiasis is defined as more than five echogenic non-shadowing foci measuring 1–3 mm per viewable image sector and is found in between 0.6%–9% of scrotal ultrasound examinations.[25] TML is frequently seen in patients with testicular GCTs; however, it is unclear whether there is a causal association between them. Current guidelines do not recommend routine ultrasound surveillance for men with TML unless they have a second risk factor for GCT (previous GCT, history of cryptorchidism or orchidopexy, testicular atrophy, or family history of GCT in a first-degree relative). All men with TML should be advised to perform regular self-examination and obtain an urgent ultrasound if any changes are detected. In a patient with a solid testicular mass, the finding of background testicular TML is a feature that increases the concern for a GCT (particularly seminoma) (Fig. 7.14A, Fig. 7.14B).[26,27,28]

Testicular macrocalcifications (>3 mm, often with acoustic shadowing) have traditionally been considered a benign finding. However, more recently, a link with GCT has also been suggested. There are no agreed-upon guidelines for management, but a similar strategy for the follow-up to TML should be considered (Fig. 7.14C).[25]

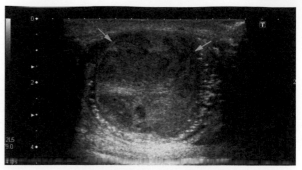

Fig. 7.14B Testicular seminoma in a patient with TML. A 25-year-old man presenting with scrotal ache and swelling. There is a large solid echo-poor mass in the testis (arrows); background TML can be seen in the adjacent testicular parenchyma.

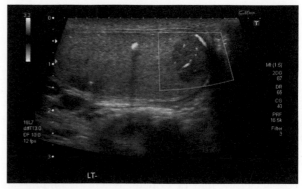

Fig. 7.14C Testicular seminoma in a patient with a testicular macrocalcification. A shadowing calcification is present in the middle third of the testis. In the lower pole, there is an echo-poor mass with internal blood flow. Radical orchidectomy was undertaken; histology showed testicular seminoma.

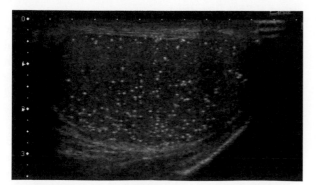

Fig. 7.14A Testicular microlithiasis (TML). The testis contains multiple small, non-shadowing, echogenic foci characteristic of TML.

Service providers are strongly advised to develop management guidelines that include necessary follow-up, onward referral, or alternative imaging in conjunction with their urological surgical colleagues and radiologists.

Benign Intratesticular Masses

The majority of palpable intratesticular masses are malignant, and it can be almost impossible to differentiate benign solid masses from malignant ones based on ultrasound appearances. However, in some benign conditions, such as diffuse orchitis, no normal testicular tissue is seen, whereas with malignancy tumors, a proportion of normal tissue will usually remain.

Intratesticular Cysts

Cysts that are entirely sonographically simple, can be assumed to be benign, and when asymptomatic, do not require follow-up or treatment. Cysts within the testis tend to be situated near the hilum or tunica. Dilatation of the ducts within the rete testes can mimic cysts. This is reported as ductal (cystic) ectasia of the rete testis and is a common benign finding in older men or following vasectomy (Fig. 7.15).

Any complex features within a testicular cyst are suspicious and may indicate a cystic or necrotic tumor (particularly non-seminoma GCT or teratoma in children), although benign causes such as infection or trauma are also possible. Further evaluation with a detailed clinical history, tumor marker measurement, and, where available, multi-parametric ultrasound is required.

Epidermoid Cysts

Epidermoid cysts represent 1% of testicular tumors, and rarely they may also occur in the epididymis. They are filled with keratin, so they appear solid but will usually demonstrate post cystic enhancement. They may have a characteristic pattern of concentric hyper- and hypoechogenic rings caused by layers of keratin.[29] Doppler imaging may demonstrate vascularity of the wall, but the central component will be avascular, and there will be no internal perfusion shown with CEUS. An anechoic capsule may be evident. Where the findings are typical, testis-preserving surgery is often possible for smaller lesions. Occasionally they may have a calcified or an atypical heterogenous appearance resulting in difficulties in confirming the diagnosis on ultrasound imaging alone. MRI may help, but excision will usually be required (Fig. 7.16A, Fig. 7.16B).

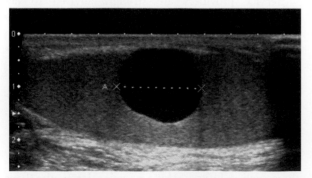

Fig. 7.15 Intratesticular cysts demonstrate typical ultrasound features: anechoic, smooth-walled with post cystic enhancement clearly seen.

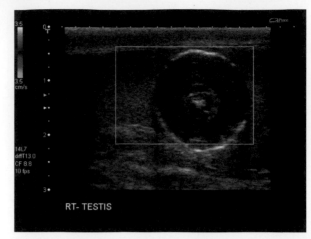

Fig. 7.16A Testicular epidermoid cyst. Characteristic appearances of a multilayered (onion-skin) avascular testicular mass.

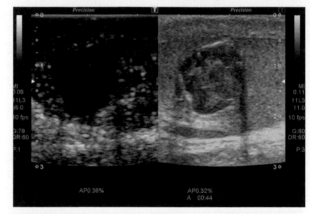

Fig. 7.16B Testicular epidermoid cyst – CEUS. Contrast ultrasound confirms that the mass is avascular, increasing diagnostic confidence.

Adrenal Rest Tumors

Adrenal rest tumors are the proliferation of ectopic adrenal tissue seen in patients with congenital adrenal hyperplasia, an inherited condition where there is an enzyme defect in adrenal hormone production. In some male patients, this leads to the development of adrenal tissue in the testis, particularly where there is difficultly in maintaining hormone replacement therapy.

These benign tumors are usually bilateral and may have a variety of sonographic appearances but most commonly are situated near the testicular hilum. They may mimic other benign and malignant conditions, and to prevent unnecessary orchidectomy, consideration

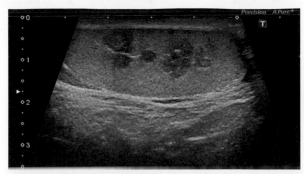

Fig. 7.17 Adrenal rest tumors. A 29-year-old man with known congenital adrenal hyperplasia. Ultrasound shows multiple echo-poor testicular masses adjacent to the mediastinum testis. In this clinical context, these are likely to represent adrenal rest tumors.

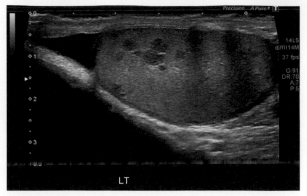

Fig. 7.18 Testicular sarcoidosis. Incidental discovery of multiple small non-palpable and bilateral testicular echo-poor nodules in a 43-year-old man with known pulmonary sarcoidosis. Following treatment, the testicular masses completely resolved on interval imaging.

of patient history is required. These tumors often regress with adequate hormone replacement treatment (Fig. 7.17).

Sarcoid

Sarcoidosis is a systemic disease of unknown cause characterized by non-caseating granuloma formation. Although the lungs are most commonly affected, there is frequently extrapulmonary disease, and the genitourinary tract may be involved. Scrotal sarcoid most commonly affects the epididymis, and testicular involvement is rare. On ultrasound, testicular sarcoid lesions are usually small echo-poor nodules; differentiation from malignancy based on ultrasound appearances alone can be difficult or impossible. In a patient with a known sarcoid history, the diagnosis may be suggested, particularly where the testicular lesions are multiple and if there is epididymal involvement (Fig. 7.18).[30]

Focal Orchitis

Focal orchitis may mimic a tumor. However, focal orchitis rarely presents without associated epididymitis or acute pain. If orchitis is the likely diagnosis, it is good practice to recommend a repeat scan in the non-acute phase to confirm resolution or identify a persistent and significant mass.

In conjunction with a raised white cell count and infective history or acute pain, a complex cystic mass within the testis may represent a testicular abscess. However, ultrasound findings may mimic a necrotic tumor, and clinical correlation will be required. Rescan in the post-acute phase may be required if orchidectomy is not performed.

Small Intratesticular Masses

Small (<5 mm) solid masses are now more regularly seen because of improvements in imaging technology, and the majority will be benign, often representing sex-cord stromal tumors. These small lesions can be very difficult to characterize by ultrasound. However, multi-parametric ultrasound (mp-US) using CEUS and elastography can help to differentiate benign from malignant lesions. Radical orchidectomy should be avoided whenever possible in tumor marker–negative patients.[31] Urological referral is required, and surveillance ultrasound or testis-preserving surgery is possible in most cases (Fig. 7.19).

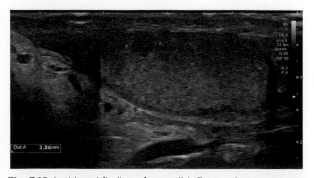

Fig. 7.19 Incidental finding of a small (<5 mm – between measurement calipers) echo-poor testicular mass in a 53-year-old man presenting with scrotal discomfort. The mass was non-palpable on clinical examination. Many such masses will be benign sex-cord stromal tumors, and radical orchidectomy should be avoided wherever possible.

Other Tumor-Mimicking Abnormalities

Post-trauma and post-inflammatory changes can mimic tumor, these changes can be permanent, and rescans may not help, although stability on surveillance is reassuring. Careful history taking and tumor marker assessment is essential.

Hematoma post testicular laceration/rupture can be complex, particularly as it retracts. Orchitis can result in post-infective calcification and areas of infarction, giving a heterogeneous texture to the testis (Fig. 7.20A, B).

Atrophy, either post-trauma or post-surgery, may produce similar appearances. Previous orchiopexy can result in testicular atrophy. Unfortunately, atrophied testes are at a higher risk of developing GCTs, and a small GCT may be difficult to identify within a heterogeneous atrophic testis. Patients reporting a change in symptoms or on self-examination require a follow-up scan (Fig. 7.20C).

Malignant Intratesticular Masses

Testicular malignancies occur in roughly six per 100,000 males. When testicular neoplasms peak in 15- to 34-year-olds, they are the most common tumors in men. History is important as there is a 3–5-fold increased risk of malignancy associated with cryptorchidism. Family history is another important fact; brothers of men with GCTs have an 8–10-fold increased risk. Previous cancer in one testicle is also a significant risk factor for later development of cancer in the contralateral testis. Careful follow-up is required.

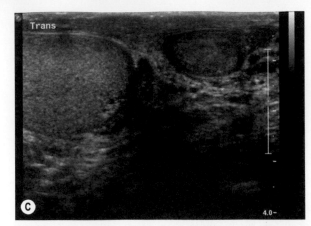

Fig. 7.20C Small abnormalities can be difficult to identify within atrophied testis, as seen here.

In the absence of relevant medical history (such as trauma, acute pain, fever, known or suspected relevant systemic disease), most palpable solid intratesticular masses are malignant. Most malignant tumors are unilateral (except lymphoma, which tends to be bilateral), although primary GCT is occasionally multifocal or bilateral.

Malignant intratesticular masses are usually solid, vascular, hypoechoic, and focal, although their appearance is variable, and it is usually impossible to differentiate the nature of the tumor on ultrasound imaging alone. Unlike diffuse diseases such as orchitis, malignant lesions commonly will have a rim of normal testicular tissue.

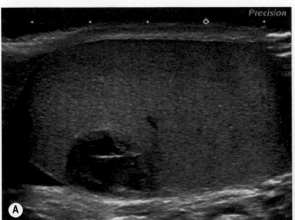

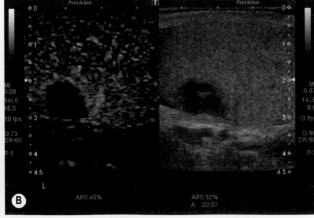

Fig. 7.20A, B Hematoma post testicular laceration/rupture can be complex, raising the suspicion of a sinister lesion. (A) CEUS can be utilized to characterize and reassure (B).

The role of ultrasound imaging is to confirm that a palpable abnormality is intratesticular, define its ultrasound characteristics and vascularity, differentiate between normal and abnormal testicular tissue, identify background testicular abnormality (such as TML), and confirm normality of the contralateral testis. Differentiation between benign and malignant masses is useful wherever possible in combination with clinical history and tumor marker measurement; multi parametric ultrasound is sometimes helpful in this context for indeterminate masses on a standard ultrasound. Some solid lesions, while malignant, may be because of underlying leukemia, lymphoma, or more rarely, metastases from non-hematological malignancy.

Serum tumor markers (human chorionic gonadotropin (β HCG), lactate dehydrogenase (LDH), and alfa-fetoprotein (AFP)) should be measured in all patients with suspicious testicular messes. Between 50%–60% of GCTs will produce markers that are of critical importance in diagnosis, staging, and monitoring response to treatment. Current tumor markers are, however, imperfect, lacking sensitivity and specificity; new markers are being developed that may have better accuracy, but these are not yet in routine clinical use.[32]

Primary Malignant Lesions

Most types of primary testicular cancer develop in the sperm-producing cells known as germ cells and are referred to as GCT. GCTs in men can arise in several parts of the body:

- The testicles, which is the most common location
- The back of the abdomen near the spine, called the retroperitoneum
- The central portion of the chest between the lungs, called the mediastinum
- The lower spine
- Very rarely in the pineal gland of the brain

There are two main categories of testicular GCTs.

Seminoma: A tumor is only called a seminoma if it is 100% seminoma. This means that the cancer does not include any of the types of tumors listed below.

Non-seminoma (NSGCT): A non-seminoma contains at least one of the following types of tumors:

- Choriocarcinoma
- Embryonal carcinoma
- Yolk sac tumor
- Teratoma

Each of these subtypes can occur alone or in any combination. Most NSGCTs are a mix of at least two different subtypes. NSGCTs may also be partly seminoma at any percentage level less than 100%. For example, a tumor that is 99% seminoma and 1% yolk sac tumor is still diagnosed and treated as a non-seminoma.

NSGCT tends to occur in younger patients than seminoma and tends to grow and spread more quickly than seminoma. Treatment of GCT is now highly effective for almost all patients, with a five-year survival of approximately 99% for patients with localized disease at presentation and high survival rates even for most patients presenting with non-visceral metastases because of modern cisplatin-based chemotherapy. However, delayed diagnosis is an adverse prognostic factor in patients presenting with high-stage NSGCT.

Ultrasound cannot reliably differentiate between seminoma and NSGCT, although a heterogeneous appearance with calcifications and cystic/necrotic areas makes NSGCT more likely, reflecting a mix of tumor types. Background TML in a patient with a homogeneous and sometimes lobulated echo-poor mass is likely to indicate a seminoma (Fig. 7.21A–D).

Other, less common types of testicular tumors include:

- Sex-cord stromal tumors (Leydig and Sertoli cell). Although representing only 5% of testicular tumors, they represent a high proportion of non-palpable incidentally discovered testicular masses. They cannot be reliably differentiated from GCTs on their ultrasound appearances. Most sex-cord stromal tumors are benign, but 10% are malignant.
- Adenocarcinoma of the rete testis is a rare, aggressive tumor with a poor prognosis, usually seen in older men. Symptoms are non-specific, and diagnosis is often delayed. Sparse ultrasound descriptions indicate that the tumor is usually echo-poor, ill-defined, and may have cystic components; it is most frequently situated at the testicular hilum or in the region of the epididymis.[33]
- Testicular lymphoma.

Testicular lymphoma is the most common tumor in older men and the most common bilateral testicular neoplasm. It may be part of more widespread non-Hodgkin's lymphoma, but primary extra-nodal testicular lymphoma may also occur. It usually presents

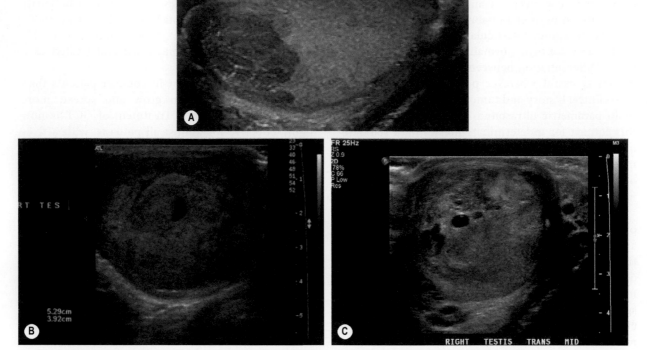

Fig. 7.21A–C Histology-proven pathology of seminoma, non-seminoma, teratoma, respectively, in these three cases. Ultrasound imaging demonstrates lobulated abnormal masses, but differentiation between tumor types is unreliable.

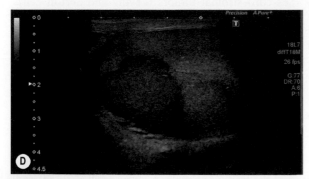

Fig. 7.21D Testicular seminoma. A 46-year-old man presenting with a palpable scrotal mass. Ultrasound shows a large uniformly echo-poor lobulated testicular mass. Histology showed pure seminoma GCT.

as a painless scrotal mass, often with a hydrocele. Testicular lymphoma may have a variety of appearances on ultrasound but is invariably echo-poor. Lesions may be solitary, multiple, or diffusely infiltrative and are usually hyper-vascular. Normal testicular vessels passing through the lymphoma deposits are a typical feature, reflecting the infiltrative nature of the tumor (Fig. 7.22A, B).[34]

Secondary Testicular Tumors

In addition to lymphoma, the testicles are a common site for involvement in the acute phase of leukemia and a common site for relapse. Multiple small, well-circumscribed masses are often present, all less than 1 cm in diameter. These nodules tend to follow the lines of the testicular septa. Alternatively, there is an infiltrative mass occupying a large part of the testes, and occasionally the whole testis is involved. This results in enlarged, hypoechoic testes compared to the unaffected contralateral side. Testicular leukemia is invariably hypervascular. Careful history taking is required to differentiate between a relapsed acute phase leukemia and orchitis (Fig. 7.23A, B).

Testicular metastases arising from other sites are uncommon and usually seen in patients with advanced

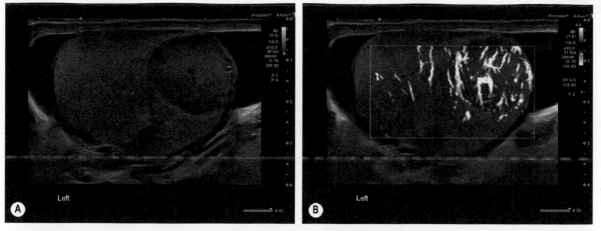

Fig. 7.22 Testicular lymphoma. A 78-year-old man with a painless scrotal mass. The grayscale image shows multifocal echo-poor testicular nodules and a small hydrocele (A). Color Doppler shows that the largest mass is highly vascular (B). The final histology was B-cell non-Hodgkin lymphoma. In patients over 60 years of age, lymphoma is the most common testicular malignancy.

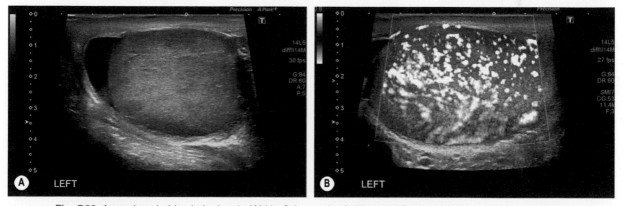

Fig. 7.23 Acute lymphoblastic leukemia (ALL) of the testis. A 50-year-old man with known ALL presenting with firm testicular swelling. Grayscale imaging shows that the testis is enlarged and mildly heterogenous (A) but without a discrete focal mass, indicating the infiltrative nature of leukemia. The mass is highly vascular on microvascular Doppler evaluation (B).

disease. Primary tumors of the prostate, lung, kidney, GI tract, and melanoma are the most common causes.[35]

THE PENIS

Anatomy

The penis is composed of the root, body, and glans. The root is situated within the perineum. The body of the penis contains three cylinders of tissue, the ventral corpus spongiosum, and paired dorsal corpora cavernosa. The corpus spongiosum contains the urethra and is expanded distally to form the glans penis. The corpora cavernosa are paired columns of spongy tissue that are responsible for erectile function. The penile corpora are easily identified and evaluated by ultrasound (Fig. 7.24).

The arterial blood supply of the penis arises from the pudendal artery (a branch of the internal iliac artery), which becomes the penile artery at the root of the penis. It divides into four branches to supply the penis, of which the cavernosal arteries are the most important. Venous drainage occurs via superficial and deep pathways into the saphenous and internal iliac venous systems.

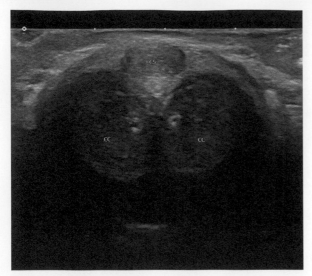

Fig. 7.24 Normal transverse image of the penis scanned from the ventral aspect. The paired corpora cavanosa (CC) and corpus spongiosum are clearly visualized.

Although ultrasound imaging of the penis is not a common examination, it is the imaging technique of choice for many conditions, including erectile dysfunction, trauma, Peyronie's disease, and priapism. An understanding of the anatomy and vascular supply is required to assist with image interpretation (Diagram 7.2).

Referrals for an ultrasound of the penis are rare. The main referral criteria are palpable penile masses, trauma, and hemodynamic studies in patients with erectile dysfunction. Ultrasound can be valuable in selected patients with priapism (prolonged painful erections) to differentiate ischemic from non-ischemic causes, although diagnosis is usually made through clinical history, examination, and analysis of cavernosal blood samples. Hemodynamic evaluations (often with pharmacological stimulation of erection) are usually undertaken in specialist centers and are not discussed further.

Palpable Penile Mass

Peyronie's Disease

The most common palpable mass is related to Peyronie's disease, which is found in at least 1% of men.[36] This occurs because of a build-up of fibrous plaques, usually within the tunica albuginea and most commonly on the dorsum of the penis. The fibrous plaques can cause bending of the penis on erection which may be painful and lead to sexual dysfunction. The fibrous plaques may resolve spontaneously, stabilize, or progress; some will calcify. Ultrasound may add additional information to clinical examination, with Peyronie's plaques usually appearing as areas of focal echogenic thickening of the tunica, which may progress to areas of focal calcification. Following pharmacological stimulation of erection, Doppler ultrasound can also assess erectile dysfunction sometimes associated with this condition. Treatment options include surgery to correct penile deformity, intralesional drug injections, and lithotripsy (Fig. 7.25A, B).

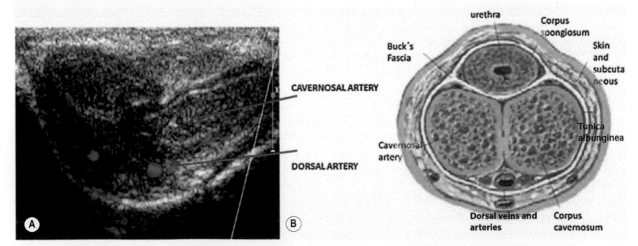

Diagram 7.2 (A) Ultrasonic image of the penis (transverse view) with a probe placed ventrally, depicting two cavernosa with cavernosal arteries and deep dorsal arteries. The corpus spongiosum can be appreciated. (B) Pictorial diagram of the ultrasonic image. (Source: JICC, ISSN: 1561–8811).

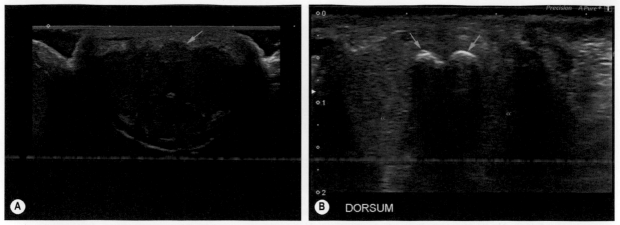

Fig. 7.25 (A) Non-calcified Peyronie's disease plaque. Scan performed from the dorsal surface of the penis shows an echogenic tunical mass between the corpora cavanosa (arrow). (B) Calcified Peyronie's plaque. Scan performed from the dorsal surface of the penis. There is shadowing high echogenicity (arrows) between the corpora cavenosa (CC) on the dorsal aspect of the penis.

Benign Penile Mass

Cysts can occur in the Cowper's or Littre's gland. The role of ultrasound is to differentiate between solid and cyst mass and provide reassurance where cysts are identified.

Cutaneous and subcutaneous lesions can occur but should be differentiated by physical examination. Ultrasound is not usually required.

Masses may also occur because of the malfunction of penile erection devices. While the prosthesis is well seen with ultrasound, it does not have a role in patient management and is rarely required. MRI may be useful in cases of suspected prosthetic failure.

> **TIP BOX**
>
> The penis can be scanned if a misplaced catheter is suspected. The tip or balloon of the catheter will be clearly seen within the urethra if not present within the bladder.

Malignant Penile Mass

Penile cancer is a rare disease in the western world; it is marginally more common in developing countries. Nearly all penile cancers are skin cancers, and squamous cell carcinoma (SCC) is the most common type.

Penile SCC most commonly presents between the ages of 50 and 70 years. The majority of lesions are found on the glans. Clinical presentation is variable. It may present as a small area of induration and erythema or a large ulcerating and infiltrative lesion. Assessment of lymphatic spread with palpation of inguinal lymph nodes is an essential component of the initial physical exam. Diagnosis is almost exclusively made by clinical examination and biopsy.[37] Imaging is rarely helpful for diagnosis, but MRI for local staging and computed tomography for distant staging are frequently required. Where there is a suspicion of inguinal lymph node metastases, ultrasound can be used to evaluate nodal morphology and guide fine-needle aspiration biopsy (Fig. 7.26A, B).

Other malignant penile masses are very rare but may be visualized by ultrasound. These include penile sarcomas, lymphoma, metastases, and urethral tumors. Ultrasound cannot provide a definite diagnosis but can be used to determine whether the mass is superficial or deep and determine its relationship to the penile corpora. A mass lying below the deep (Buck's) fascia is of most concern for a non-epithelial neoplasm (Fig. 7.27A, B).

THE PROSTATE

Anatomy

The prostate gland develops after puberty as a result of a testosterone surge. It is approximately the size of a walnut. The cranial aspect, the base, lies just under the bladder and is clearly defined by the bladder base. The apex of the prostate lies posterior to the symphysis pubis adjacent to the muscles of the pelvic floor. The apex

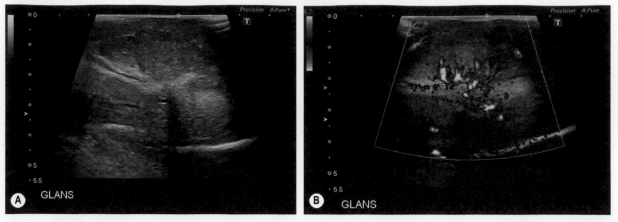

Fig. 7.26 Penile squamous cell carcinoma (SCC). A 92-year-old man with a visible mass on the glans penis. There is a poorly defined echo-poor mass infiltrating the glans penis (A), which is vascular on Power Doppler assessment (B). Surgical penectomy was performed with a final diagnosis of stage pT2 penile SCC. Ultrasound is not usually required for the diagnosis of penile cancer.

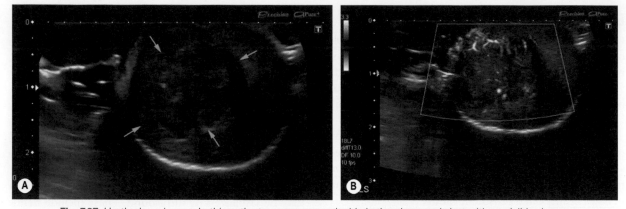

Fig. 7.27 Urethral carcinoma. In this patient, a mass was palpable in the glans penis but with no visible change on the skin surface. Grayscale ultrasound showed an echo-poor mass in the glans penis (arrows, A) that showed internal vascularity on Doppler examination (B). Urethroscopy and biopsy showed carcinoma arising from the urethra.

merges into the corpora spongiosum without a well-defined sonographic landmark.

There is no true capsule of the prostate but more of a fibromuscular stroma that disappears toward the apex of the gland. This fibromuscular stroma appears as a well-defined echogenic border on ultrasound imaging (Fig. 7.28A, B).[38]

The urethra provides an important landmark but does not run through the middle of the gland. It follows a curved course toward the anterior aspect of the gland. The seminal vesicles and vasa deferentia are paired structures on either side of the midline just above the prostate.

Zonal anatomy of the prostate was described by McNeal in 1981.[39] The prostate was divided into:

- Periurethral glands
- Transition zone
- Central zone
- Peripheral zone

Differentiation of the zones can be difficult on ultrasound imaging.[38] The advent of PI-RADS version 2.1 reporting of prostate MRI has subdivided the prostate into the transitional, central, and peripheral zones for the purposes of image reporting.[40] It is noted that central zones tumors, while recognized well on MRI, are rare (Figs. 7.29, 7.30).

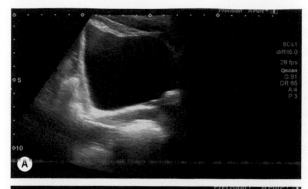

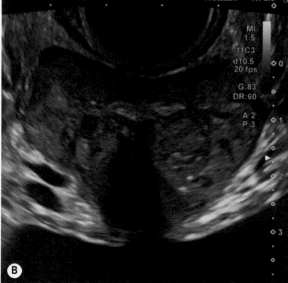

Fig. 7.28 (A) The detail of the prostate is poorly visualized on transabdominal imaging even with a full bladder as an acoustic window. (B) Transrectal imaging of the prostate yields far greater detail.

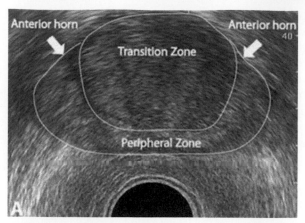

Fig. 7.29 The zones of the prostate can be identified with transrectal ultrasound, although the borders differentiating the zones can be indistinct.

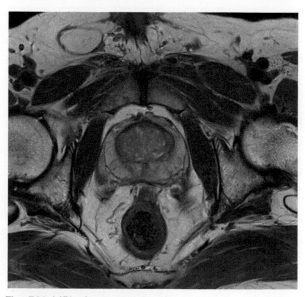

Fig. 7.30 MRI of prostate identifies the zones with greater differentiation.

The transitional zone is made up of two lobes of tissue sitting adjacent to the urethra bilaterally. The transitional zone has little in the way of glandular tissue. This zone enlarges commonly with age and is responsible for urethral constriction in cases of BPH.

The peripheral zone is largely at the base of the gland and forms the bulk of the glandular tissue. Prostate cancer arises in the peripheral zone in approximately 75%–80% of cases. However, prostate cancers arising from the transitional zone are larger at the time of diagnosis because of their central location and the decreased likelihood of detection on a digital rectal exam or systematic prostate needle biopsy schemes. Despite transitional zone cancer being larger on diagnosis, it is associated with favorable pathologic features and better recurrence-free survival than cancer arising with the peripheral zone.

Measurements

Measurements of the prostate are taken in the midline sagittal plane and the axial plane. The prostate has a volume of around 20 mL but with a normal range of 13–37 mL. The mean dimensions of a young adult prostate are 3 cm in length, 2.5 cm in depth, and 4 cm in length.

A precise prostate volume is required when planning radiotherapy, assessing suitability for radical prostate surgery, and calculating the prostatic specific antigen (PSA) density in men suspected of having prostate cancer. There is variability between the prostate volume measured by ultrasound and the volume measured by MR.[41] Care needs to be taken to ensure clinicians are aware of the technique used to calculate the prostate volume if treatment is being planned. The most accurate ultrasound method for measuring the prostate is use of a transrectal approach. However, in cases of suspected prostate enlargement causing bladder outflow issues, a transabdominal measurement is accurate enough for assessment purposes (Fig. 7.31).

> ### TIP BOX
>
> Prostate volume can be estimated by using the ellipsoid formula: length × width × height × 0.52.

Benign Prostate Disease
Benign Prostatic Hypertrophy (BPH)

BPH is an enlargement of the transition zone of the prostate resulting in a nodular enlargement of the inner gland. BPH is one of the most common diseases in aging men and the most common cause of lower urinary tract symptoms (LUTS).[42] BPH is an almost universal finding on imaging studies in older men; in many, it is asymptomatic but, in a substantial proportion, causes LUTS.

The resulting hypertrophy may result in the prostate bulging into the base of the bladder. This is commonly referred to as median lobe enlargement, although there is no true median lobe of the prostate. Insignificant calcification and cystic change may be present, but this is no indicator of the presence of malignant disease.

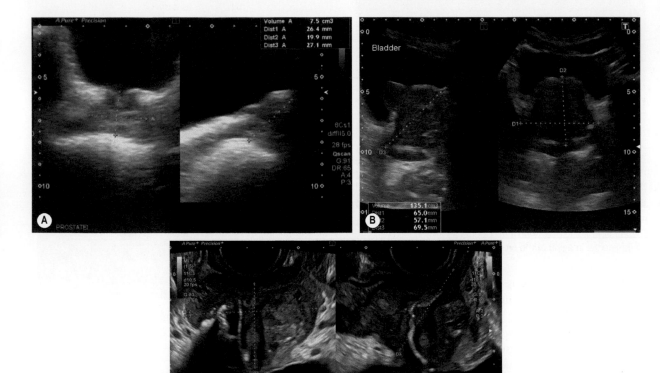

Fig. 7.31 Transabdominal volume measurements of the prostate are inaccurate because of the difficulty in distinguishing the true borders of the gland. TA volume measurements may suffice for assessment of BPH but should not be used when planning treatment or calculating PSAD. (A, B) TR volume measurements are more accurate than TA (C), but there is variability when compared to MRI.

The size of the prostate is a poor predictor of symptoms; however, BPH is commonly associated with bladder outflow obstruction. A transabdominal scan of the urinary tract in patients with LUTS is valuable. An assessment of the post-micturition residual bladder volume is essential. In younger patients, the bladder should empty almost completely post micturition; a residual volume of 50–100 mL is more commonly seen in older men. Anything above this level indicates potentially significant urinary retention (Fig 7.32, Fig 7.33)

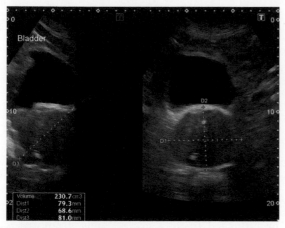

Fig. 7.32 Benign prostatic hyperplasia (BPH) is a common finding when undertaking investigations in the older population for LUTS. A volume of over 35 mL is reported as demonstrating hypertrophy, but the significance of this is based on clinical symptoms.

Cysts

Cysts of the prostate and seminal vesicles are recognized by their characteristic appearance. While cysts are benign, the location may be significant, and some cysts are associated with infertility.

Müllerian duct cysts are the most common congenital cyst of the prostate. They are a remnant of the Müllerian tubercle and arise in the midline, near the base of the prostate. They are usually asymptomatic but may be associated with infertility because of obstruction of the ejaculatory ducts (Fig. 7.34A, B).

Cysts of the seminal vesicles (arising from the Wolffian duct) are rare but are associated with renal agenesis on the ipsilateral side. A differential is the more common seminal duct ectasia, but the two can be difficult to differentiate. Upper renal tract examination is indicated in any case of seminal vesicle cyst.

Infection and Prostatitis

Prostatitis is the most common cause of a painful prostate. Chronic bacterial prostatitis is a common indolent cause of recurrent urinary tract infections.

There are two ultrasound features that are useful and provide a role for ultrasound in the management of prostatitis. The presence of calcification, while an insignificant finding in BPH, is relevant. The calcification can provide a nidus for infection and may complicate the treatment if this is not known. The second

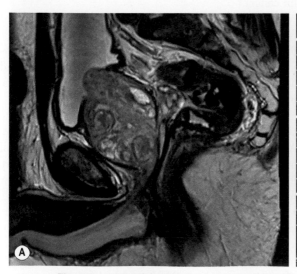
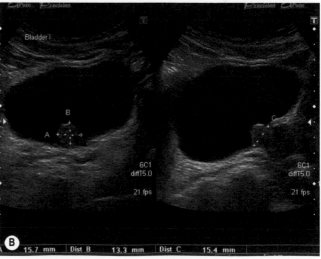

Fig. 7.33 Median lobe enlargement is well identified on MRI (A) but commonly seen on TA US and is not to be confused with bladder wall lesions (B).

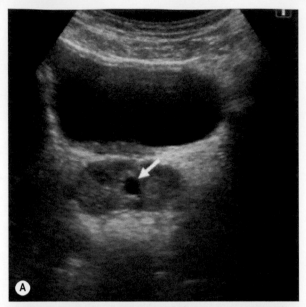

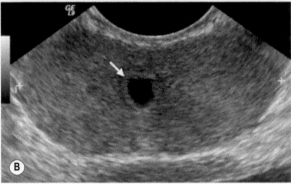

Fig. 7.34 A cyst within the prostate demonstrates typical ultrasound features and is seen well using both a TA (A) or TR approach (B).

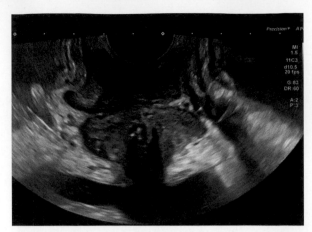

Fig. 7.35 Calcification can be seen within a gland when prostatitis is suspected. Care is needed when undertaking a TR examination because of the significant pain the patient may experience during the procedure.

relevant finding is that of fluid within the prostate. While this is likely to be a cyst, in the presence of prostatitis, the presence of an abscess, particularly if the fluid contains internal echoes, should be considered (Fig. 7.35).

Otherwise, sonography does not have a role in the management or imaging of prostatitis.

Infertility

The role of ultrasound of the prostate in the investigation of infertility is primarily for demonstrating normal anatomy and excluding the presence of congenital cysts, or BPH described above.[43,44]

The scan should document the presence of two seminal vesicles, two vasa deferentia, and where possible, two ejaculatory ducts.

Prostate Cancer

The estimated lifetime risk of being diagnosed with prostate cancer is 1 in 6 (18%) for males born after 1960 in the United Kingdom. Prostate cancer risk factors have not been conclusively identified, despite substantial research. However, older age remains the main risk factor for cancer.

Early prostate cancer is invariably asymptomatic and is usually identified in patients who have an elevated PSA level and/or an abnormal digital rectal examination. Advanced prostate cancer presents with local and distant symptoms including, but not exclusively, LUTS, pain, bone pain, and anemia.

PSA levels tend to increase with age, even in the absence of prostate cancer, which is not specific. Approximately 25% of men with PSA of 4–10 ng/mL will have prostate cancer. Calculating the PSA density, where PSA levels are divided by prostate volume, is a better predictor of the possibility of cancer being present.

Despite advances in imaging technologies, particularly multi-parametric MRI (mp MRI) and the advent of a standardized MRI reporting system, PI-RADS v2.1[40] imaging does not have a role in the routine diagnosis of prostate cancer. mpMRI can identify high-risk areas of abnormality within the prostate. Ultrasound imaging is essential to systematically guide biopsies. More recent developments in fusion technology have further improved the role of mpMRI and ultrasound in guiding targeted biopsies.[45] However, the diagnosis and grading of prostate cancer remain a histopathological process.

Ultrasound current has no role in the follow-up or assessment of prostate cancer disease progression. Its main role is to guide biopsies.

Ultrasound-guided biopsy of the prostate may be obtained from a transrectal (TR) or transperineal (TP) approach. An endocavity probe is used to image the prostate, accurately measure its volume, assess for any incidental findings, identify the anatomy, and guide needle placement for local anesthesia and biopsy (Figs. 7.36, 7.37).

Fusion-guided imaging allows the mpMRI to be fused with the live ultrasound image. This can be achieved for both TRUS and TP biopsy approaches. The use of fusion imaging can assist with accurate targeting of biopsy to areas of abnormality identified on the pre-biopsy mpMRI. The heterogeneous appearance of the prostate on B-mode imaging can lead to difficultly identifying focal areas of abnormality on US alone. While large series data is not available, small studies have indicated that a fusion approach to prostate biopsy provides a higher yield of significant cancer while reducing oversampling of insignificant disease.[46,47]

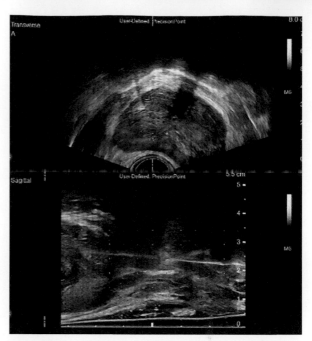

Fig. 7.37 TP US–guided biopsy under local anesthesia is emerging as the procedure of choice to minimize infection risk inherent with TRUS Bx.

REFERENCES

1. Tapping C, Cast J. Scrotal ultrasound: a pictorial review. *Ultrasound*. 2008;16:226–233.
2. Chetcuti K, Lam K, Belfield J. Testicular, epididymal and adnexal ultrasound: a pictorial review. Part 2: epididymal and adnexal ultrasound. *Ultrasound*. 2013;21:187–195.
3. Kim W, Rosen M, Langer J, Banner M, Siegelman E, Ramchandani P. US–MR imaging correlation in pathologic conditions of the scrotum. *RadioGraphics*. 2007;27:1239–1253.
4. Cochlin D, Dubbins P, Goldberg B, Halpern E. *Urogenital ultrasound*. Abingdon: Taylor & Francis; 2006.
5. Fu Z, Zhang J, Lu Y, et al. Clinical applications of superb microvascular imaging in the superficial tissues and organs: a systematic review. *Acad Radiol*. 2021 May;28(5):694–703.
6. Sidhu P, Cantisani V, Dietrich C, et al. The EFSUMB guidelines and recommendations for the clinical practice of contrast-enhanced ultrasound (CEUS) in non-hepatic applications: update 2017 (Long Version). *Ultraschall Med- Eur J Ultrasound*. 2018;39:e2–e44.
7. Ross J, Wilson K. *Anatomy and physiology in health and illness*. Edinburgh: Churchill Livingstone; 1993.
8. Tamir E. *The human body made simple*. Edinburgh: Churchill Livingstone; 2002.

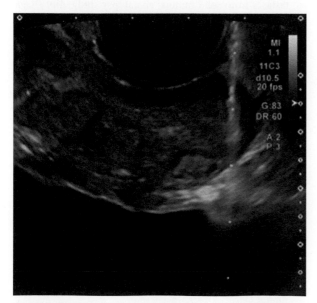

Fig. 7.36 TRUS-guided biopsy assists with needle placement.

9. MacLennan G, Hinman F. *Hinman's atlas of urosurgical anatomy*. Philadelphia: Elsevier/Saunders; 2012.

10. Caesar R, Kaplan G. Incidence of the bell-clapper deformity in an autopsy series. *Urol*. 1994;44:114–116.

11. Hsieh M, Huang S, Huang H, Chen Y, Hsu Y. The reliability of ultrasonographic measurements for testicular volume assessment: comparison of three common formulas with true testicular volume. *Asian J Androl*. 2009;11:261–265.

12. Jarvis LJ, Dubbins PA. Changes in the epididymis after vasectomy: sonographic findings. *Am J Roentgenol*. 1989;152:531–534.

13. Puttemans T, Delvigne A, Murillo D. Normal and variant appearances of the adult epididymis and vas deferens on high-resolution sonography. *J Clin Ultrasound*. 2006;34:385–392.

14. Kumar V, Abbas A, Aster J, Robbins S. *Robbins basic pathology*. 10th edn. Philadelphia: Elsevier; 2018.

15. Freeman S, Bertolotto M, Richenberg J, et al. Ultrasound evaluation of varicocoeles: guidelines and recommendations of the European Society of Urogenital Radiology Scrotal and Penile Imaging Working Group (ESUR-SPIWG) for detection, classification, and grading. *Eur Radiol*. 2019;30:11–25.

16. Pettersson A, Richiardi L, Nordenskjold A, Kaijser M, Akre O. Age at surgery for undescended testis and risk of testicular cancer. *New Engl J Med*. 2007;356:1835–1841.

17. Healthcare Safety Investigation Branch. *Final report-healthcare safety investigation branch*; Hsib.org.uk. 2020. Available at: https://www.hsib.org.uk/investigations-cases/primary-management-acute-onset-testicular-pain/final-report-page/.

18. Barbosa J, de Freitas P, Carvalho S, et al. Validation of the TWIST score for testicular torsion in adults. *Int Urol Nephrol*. 2021 Jan;53(1):7–11.

19. Kalfa N, Veyrac C, Lopez M, et al. Multicenter assessment of ultrasound of the spermatic cord in children with acute scrotum. *J Urol*. 2007;177:297–301.

20. Bandarkar A, Blask A. Testicular torsion with preserved flow: key sonographic features and value-added approach to diagnosis. *Pediatr Radiol*. 2018;48:735–744.

21. Chernyadyev S, Ufimtseva M, Vishnevskaya I, et al. Fournier's gangrene: literature review and clinical cases. *Urol Int*. 2018;101:91–97.

22. Thwaini A. Fournier's gangrene and its emergency management. *Postgrad Med J*. 2006;82:516–519.

23. Woodward P, Schwab C, Sesterhenn I. From the archives of the AFIP. *RadioGraphics*. 2003;23:215–240.

24. Nickel J. Chronic epididymitis: a practical approach to understanding and managing a difficult urologic enigma. *Rev Urol*. 2003;5:209.

25. Miller F, Rosario S, Clarke J, Sriprasad S, Muir G, Sidhu P. Testicular calcification and microlithiasis: association with primary intra-testicular malignancy in 3,477 patients. *Eur Radiol*. 2006;17:363–369.

26. Stephenson A, Eggener S, Bass E, et al. Diagnosis and treatment of early stage testicular cancer: AUA guideline. *J Urol*. 2019;202:272–281.

27. Richenberg J, Belfield J, Ramchandani P, et al. Testicular microlithiasis imaging and follow-up: guidelines of the ESUR scrotal imaging subcommittee. *Eur Radiol*. 2014;25:323–330.

28. Pedersen M, Bartlett E, Brown C, Rafaelsen S, Sellars M, Sidhu P. Is testicular macrocalcification a risk for malignancy? tumor development on ultrasonographic follow-up of preexisting intratesticular macrocalcification. *J Ultrasound Med*. 2018;37:2949–2953.

29. Atchley J, Dewbry K. Ultrasound appearances of testicular epidermoid cysts. *Clin Radiol*. 2000;55:493–502.

30. Stewart VR, Sidhu PS. The testis: the unusual, the rare and the bizarre. *Clin Radiol*. 2007;62:289–302.

31. Auer T, De Zordo T, Dejaco C, et al. Value of multiparametric US in the assessment of intratesticular lesions. *Radiol*. 2017;285:640–649.

32. Montgomery J, Weizer A, Filson C, Milose J, Hafez Khaled. Role of biochemical markers in testicular cancer: diagnosis, staging, and surveillance. Open Access. *J Urol*. 2011;1.

33. Tian Y, Yao W, Wang J, Wazir R, Wang K. Primary adenocarcinoma of the rete testis: a case report and review of the literature. *Oncol Lett*. 2013;7:455–457.

34. Bertolotto M, Derchi L, Secil M, et al. Grayscale and color doppler features of testicular lymphoma. *J Ultrasound Med*. 2015;34:1139–1145.

35. García-González R, Pinto J, Val-Bernal J. Testicular metastases from solid tumors: an autopsy study. *Ann Diagn Pathol*. 2000;4:59–64.

36. Smith B. Peyronie's disease. *Am J Clin Pathol*. 1966;45:670–678.

37. Marchionne E, Perez C, Hui A, Khachemoune A. Penile squamous cell carcinoma: a review of the literature and case report treated with mohs micrographic surgery. *An Bras Dermatol*. 2017;92:95–99.

38. Halpern E, Cochlin D, Goldberg B. *Imaging of the prostate*. London: Martin Dunitz; 2002.

39. McNeal J. The zonal anatomy of the prostate. *Prostate*. 1981;2:35–49.

40. Padhani A, Weinreb J, Rosenkrantz A, Villeirs G, Turkbey B, Barentsz J. Prostate imaging-reporting and data system steering committee: PI-RADS v2 status update and future directions. *Eur Urol*. 2019;75:385–396.

41. Murciano-Goroff Y, Wolfsberger L, Parekh A, et al. Variability in MRI vs. ultrasound measures of prostate volume and its impact on treatment recommendations for favorable-risk prostate cancer patients: a case series. *Radiat Oncol*. 2014;9.

42. Lim K. Epidemiology of clinical benign prostatic hyperplasia. *Asian J Urol*. 2017;4:148–151.

43. Ammar T, Sidhu P, Wilkins C. Male infertility: the role of imaging in diagnosis and management. *Br J Radiol.* 2012;85:S59–S68.

44. Mittal P, Little B, Harri P, et al. Role of imaging in the evaluation of male infertility. *RadioGraphics.* 2017;37:837–854.

45. Ahmed H, El-Shater Bosaily A, Brown L, et al. Diagnostic accuracy of multi-parametric MRI and TRUS biopsy in prostate cancer (PROMIS): a paired validating confirmatory study. *Lancet.* 2017;389:815–822.

46. Kasivisvanathan V, Rannikko A, Borghi M, et al. MRI-targeted or standard biopsy for prostate-cancer diagnosis. *New Engl J Med.* 2018;378:1767–1777.

47. Parker T, Morado P, Parker PC, Smith SL. *Fusion guided trans rectal ultrasound prostate biopsy. Does targeted biopsy following multi parametric magnetic resonance imaging (mpMRI) result in a more accurate detection of significant prostate cancer? British Medical Ultrasound Society, ASM, Harrogate*; 2019. Available at: https://www.bmus.org/ultrasound-2019.

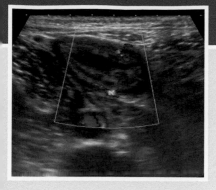

8

Ultrasound of the Retroperitoneum and Gastrointestinal Tract

Ruth Reeve and Catherine Kirkpatrick

CHAPTER OUTLINE

Normal Anatomy, 265
The Abdominal Aorta, 266
  Normal Anatomy, 266
  Technique, 266
  Abdominal Aortic Aneurysm (AAA), 268
    AAA Complications, 268
The Inferior Vena Cava, 271
  Normal Anatomy, 271
  Technique, 271
  Pathology of the IVC, 271
The Adrenal Glands, 274
  Normal Anatomy, 274
  Adenoma, 274
  Metastases, 274
  Other Adrenal Lesions, 274
Gastrointestinal (GI) Tract, 275
  Normal Anatomy, 276
  Technique, 276
  Esophagus and Stomach, 277

Pathology, 278
  Inflammatory Bowel Conditions, 278
    Appendicitis, 278
    Inflammatory Bowel Disease (IBD), 279
    Crohn's Disease, 279
    Colitis, 281
    Diverticulitis, 281
  Malignant Tumors, 281
  Obstruction, 282
  Other Retroperitoneal Abnormalities, 282
Abdominal Wall Hernia, 283
  Normal Anatomy, 283
  Technique, 283
    Epigastric Hernia, 286
    Umbilical and Paraumbilical, 286
    Spigelian Hernia, 286
    Incisional Hernia, 286
References, 286

NORMAL ANATOMY

The peritoneum is the large sheet of the serous membrane lining the abdominal cavity and surrounding organs. The peritoneum has several "extensions," which bind the organs together: the mesentery, which loosely anchors the small bowel, ensuring it does not twist; the transverse mesocolon, which attaches the transverse colon to the posterior abdominal wall; and the greater and lesser omentum. These projections coat the viscera and form pouches or sacs within the peritoneal cavity where dependent fluid can collect.

The retroperitoneal space contains the kidneys, ureters, adrenal glands, pancreas, and duodenal loop, great vessels, and the ascending and descending portions of the large bowel, including the caecum (Fig. 8.1).

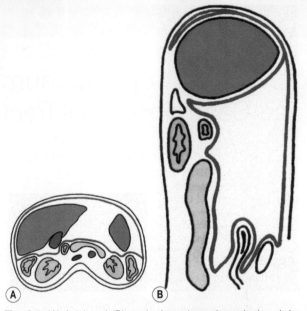

Fig. 8.1 (A) Axial and (B) sagittal sections through the abdomen showing the relationship of the abdominal viscera to the peritoneum (red).

THE ABDOMINAL AORTA

Normal Anatomy

The abdominal aorta is the continuation of the thoracic aorta, supplying arterial blood to all of the abdominal organs, the underside of the diaphragm, and abdominal wall, until its bifurcation in the pelvis. There are three main anterior branches of the abdominal aorta, including the celiac artery, superior mesenteric artery, and inferior mesentery artery, alongside other visceral branches, including the renal, suprarenal, and gonadal arteries. The aorta is positioned within the retroperitoneum, normally to the left of the IVC, often measuring ≤3 cm.[1]

Technique

The proximal abdominal aorta should be visualized in the midline, inferior to the xiphisternum. The celiac axis and superior mesenteric artery (SMA) are demonstrated in LS, arising from its anterior aspect (Fig. 8.2); the celiac axis branches – the main hepatic and splenic arteries – are better appreciated in TS. Just below this

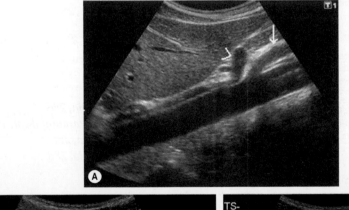

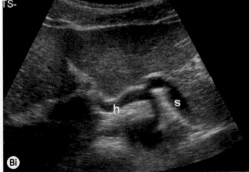

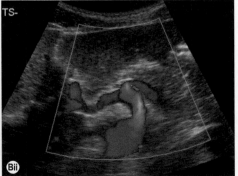

Fig. 8.2 (A) LS through the abdominal aorta demonstrating the celiac axis (arrowhead) and the superior mesenteric artery (SMA; arrow). The splenic vein is seen anterior to the SMA. (Bi) TS through the proximal abdominal aorta. The celiac axis divides into the hepatic (h) and splenic (s) arteries. (Bii) Color Doppler demonstrates the direction of flow with respect to the transducer.

Continued

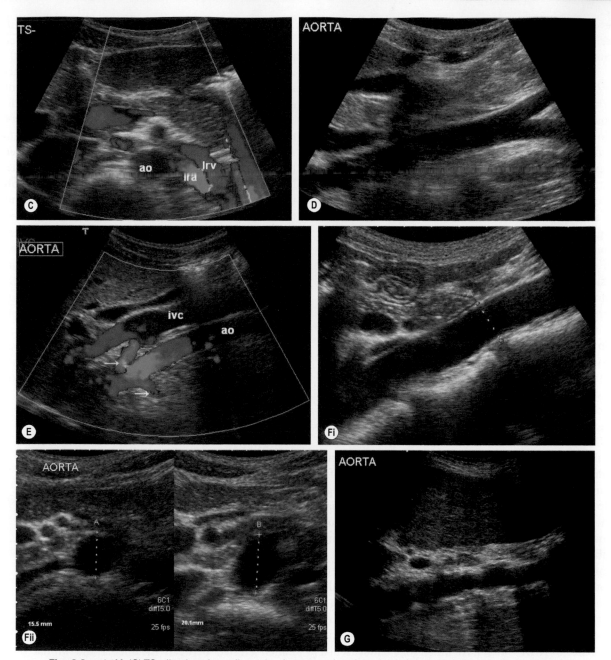

Fig. 8.2, cont'd (C) TS, distal to the celiac axis, demonstrating the origin of the renal arteries. The left renal vein (lrv, red) passes anterior to the left renal artery (lra, blue) and aorta (ao) to drain into the IVC. (D) A coronal plane from the patient's right side demonstrates the aortic bifurcation. (E) Coronal section, from the patient's right side, demonstrating the inferior vena cava and aorta at the level of the renal arteries (arrows). (Fi) Sagittal LS through the aorta demonstrating the correct measurement technique – calipers perpendicular to the walls. (Fii) Incorrect technique in TS: in the left image, the probe is angled caudally and is probably perpendicular to the vessel, but the right image has the probe perpendicular to the abdominal wall (similar to computed tomography), overestimating the aortic diameter by almost 20%. (G) The aorta of an elderly patient containing calcification in the walls, causing acoustic shadowing. (From Nagelhout JJ, Elisha S. Nurse Anesthesia. 6th ed. St. Louis, MO: Elsevier; 2018.)

level, the origin of the SMA is seen with the renal arteries inferior to this. The distal abdominal aorta runs more anteriorly toward the bifurcation.

Abdominal Aortic Aneurysm (AAA)

With age, the aorta often becomes ectatic and tortuous often with calcification of the walls (Fig. 8.2G). However, an AAA is a common and potentially deadly condition. AAA is defined as an aorta with a diameter over 1.5 times the normal diameter, >3 cm in total.[2,3] Risk factors for AAA include male sex, age over 65 years, smoking, and family history. The risk of aneurysm rupture increases with diameter, increasing dramatically when it reaches 6 cm.[4] Therefore, men are offered surgery once the AAA reaches 5.5 cm in diameter, women at 5 cm. Screening of the high-risk population with ultrasound is increasingly being adopted, as seen within the United Kingdom's AAA screening service.[4,5,6]

Currently, only men are offered screening in the United Kingdom. Studies have looked at whether women should also be included, but because of the significant reduction in women smoking since the 1970s and the lower predisposition risk, it is not considered economically viable. However, recent guidelines produced by National Institute for Clinical Excellence (NICE)[5] now recommend that women aged 70 or over being investigated for possible AAA should be considered for an ultrasound scan if they have any of a number of risk factors, including high cholesterol, high blood pressure, or are smokers or used to smoke. Small aneurysms may be monitored with ultrasound to allow timely treatment (open or endovascular repair) with a subsequent fall in mortality.[4,6] Postoperative complications of AAA repair include leaks, infections, or pseudoaneurysm, where such complications are usually monitored with computed tomography (CT) or magnetic resonance imaging (MRI).[7,8] Contrast-enhanced ultrasound (CEUS) has been incorporated into surveillance of AAA which have undergone endovascular repair (EVAR) as there is a risk that a leak can form, which results in leaking back into the aneurysm sac. Most AAA are associated with atherosclerosis, weakening the elasticity of the wall, causing the vessel to dilate and potentially rupture. Aneurysms may be fusiform or saccular in nature (Fig. 8.3). Blood flow within it is turbulent, and the slow-flowing blood at the edges of the vessel tends to thrombose.

The true maximum diameter of the aneurysm should be ascertained, where the calipers must be placed perpendicular to the walls for an accurate diameter at the widest part of the aneurysm. Measurements performed in the transverse plane tend to overestimate the diameter, as the aorta often runs obliquely (Fig. 8.2F). Therefore, a careful scanning technique is advised. It is recommended that the inner-to-inner diameter of the AAA be measured in both LS and TS.[9] Many centers have used outer to outer wall measurements, and there has often been discrepancy against measurements obtained as part of the screening program. NICE guidance (2020)[5] is that all measurements should be consistent and inner-to-inner wall measurements used. The ability of ultrasound to assess the aorta and locate the correct plane for measurement, regardless of vessel tortuosity, is an advantage over CT, which may overestimate the size of the aneurysm in an axial plane. Fortunately, most aneurysms are infrarenal, as surgery is always complicated by renal artery involvement. It may be difficult to determine the relationship of the aneurysm to the renal artery origins on ultrasound, and CT is helpful in such cases. Occasionally the aneurysm involves the bifurcation and common iliac arteries, and it is important to examine this when assessing the aorta.[10]

TIP BOX

When imaging the abdominal aorta, sonographers should be alert to the possibility of a thoracic aortic aneurysm extending into the abdominal aorta and creating a thoracoabdominal aortic aneurysm especially if the abdominal aneurysm is suprarenal.

AAA Complications

Dissection of the aneurysm, in which the intima becomes detached, is uncommon in the abdomen. Ultrasound may visualize the intimal flap, and the false lumen created between the media and intima often contains slower, more turbulent, or even reversed flow. Layers of thrombus may mimic a dissection, and color flow Doppler is particularly useful in such cases.

Leakage of an aneurysm may cause a retroperitoneal hematoma, but CT is usually more reliable in detecting leaks than ultrasound. CEUS has had success in identifying leaks following AAA repair and has been reported to be more sensitive than CT in this group

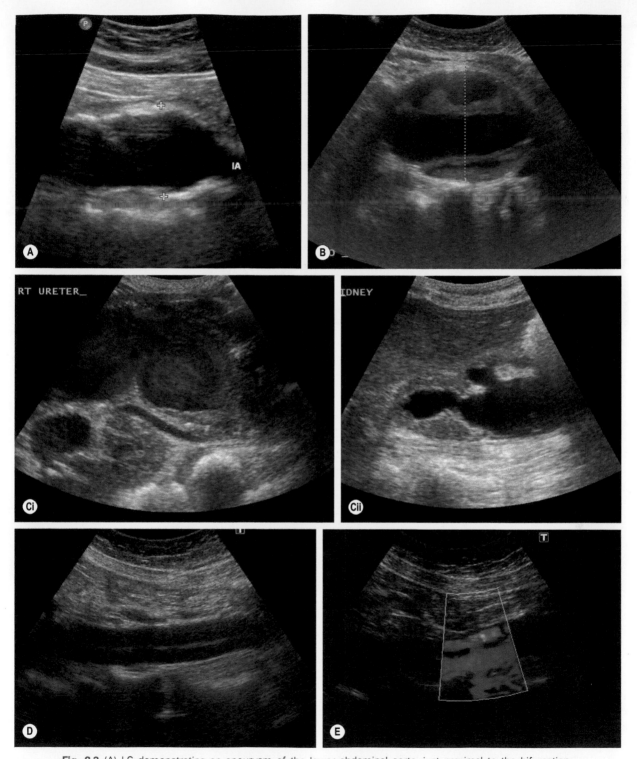

Fig. 8.3 (A) LS demonstrating an aneurysm of the lower abdominal aorta, just proximal to the bifurcation. *IA*, iliac artery. (B) LS through the aorta demonstrating an aneurysm containing thrombus. Measurement should be perpendicular to the axis of the aorta and include the adventitia ("outer to outer"). (Ci) A large abdominal aortic aneurysm full of thrombus is compressing the right ureter (calipers), causing right hydronephrosis (Cii). (D) LS of a dissecting aortic aneurysm. The detached intimal flap is clearly seen within the aortic lumen. (E) Color Doppler demonstrates flow on both sides of the intima.

Continued

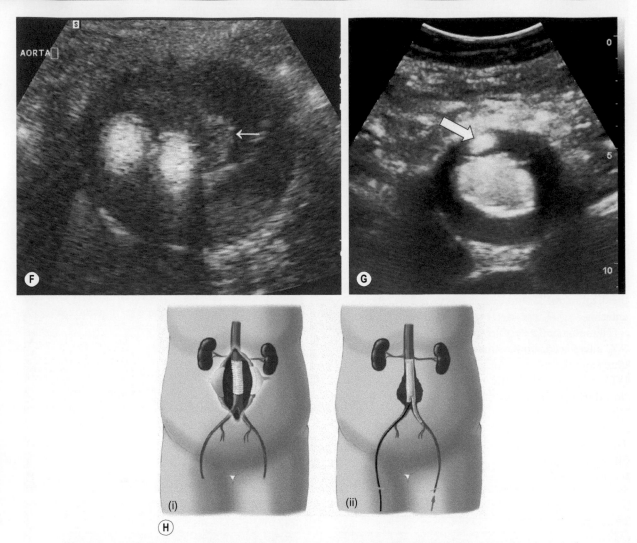

Fig. 8.3, cont'd (F) Contrast-enhanced ultrasound of the aorta post Y graft demonstrates enhancement of the lumens of the iliac arteries with slight leakage (arrow) in the region of the bifurcation. (G) Intraoperative contrast-enhanced ultrasound (CEUS) after endovascular aneurysm repair (EVAR): transverse view of type II endoleak (EL) from inferior mesenteric artery (arrow). (H) Comparison of (i) open surgical repair and (ii) EVAR. (Source: From Nagelhout JJ, Elisha S. Nurse Anesthesia. 6th ed. St. Louis, MO: Elsevier; 2018.; YMVA, ISSN: 0741-5214, 2018.)

(Fig. 8.3F, G).[11,12,13] This has the added advantage of reducing radiation dose because of CT, especially in patients who are regularly monitored with imaging.

Involvement of the renal arteries may cause renal artery thrombosis and subsequently small kidney(s). Therefore, it is important to check the kidneys at the time of scanning to ensure they are of normal size and appearance.

TIP BOX

In cases where bowel gas obscures the sagittal assessment of structures, a coronal approach can overcome this problem. Scanning from the patient's left side, the aorta can be demonstrated using the left kidney as an acoustic window, and from the right, the right lobe of the liver affords good access. A coronal view is also useful in displaying the origin of the renal arteries.

THE INFERIOR VENA CAVA

Normal Anatomy

The normal IVC has thinner walls and a more flattened profile than the aorta, and its lumen alters with changing abdominal pressure; for example, during respiration, the lumen decreases on inspiration or with the Valsalva maneuver (Fig. 8.4).

Technique

Ultrasound is highly successful in demonstrating the proximal IVC by using the liver as an acoustic window, especially if the patient is right side raised. The distal IVC may be obscured by overlying bowel gas and, unlike the aorta, is susceptible to compression, making visualization difficult in some cases. In comparison with the aorta in LS, the course of the IVC is anterior as it passes through the diaphragm. The main renal veins may be seen in TS, entering the IVC just below the level of the pancreas.

Hemodynamically, the blood flow spectrum from the IVC alters according to the distance of the sample volume from the right atrium. The blood flow through the IVC and proximal hepatic veins is pulsatile, with reverse flow during right atrial systole.

Pathology of the IVC

The most common anomaly of the IVC is that of duplication. However, this is infrequently noticed in ultrasound and is best demonstrated with CT or MRI. Transposition of the IVC may be seen in situs inversus.

Thrombus in the IVC may be because of benign causes or the result of a tumor. It is not usually possible to tell the difference on gray-scale appearances alone, but vascularity may be demonstrated on power or color Doppler and CEUS within tumor thrombus. A Wilm's tumor is a common renal tumor in pediatrics and has been reported to invade the IVC in 4%–8% of cases.[14] Tumor thrombus invades the renal vein and enters the IVC in around 10% of renal carcinoma cases. Tumor thrombus from hepatic or adrenal masses can also invade the IVC (Fig. 8.5).

Coagulation disorders, which cause Budd–Chiari syndrome (see Chapter 2), predominantly affect the hepatic veins but may also involve the IVC (Fig. 8.6). Patients may require the insertion of an IVC filter, which is performed under fluoroscopy guidance but may be monitored for patency using ultrasound with Doppler. Dilatation of the IVC is a finding commonly associated with congestive heart failure and is frequently accompanied by hepatic vein dilatation.

Compression of the IVC by large masses is not uncommon. This may be because of retroperitoneal masses, such as lymphadenopathy, or liver masses, such as a tumor or caudate lobe hypertrophy. Color or power Doppler is particularly useful in confirming the patency of the vessel and differentiating extrinsic compression from invasion. Insertion of metallic stents may be performed under angiographic control to maintain the vessel patency, particularly if the compression is because of inoperable hepatic metastasis (Fig. 8.6C).

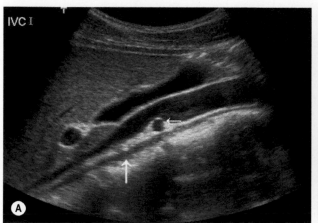

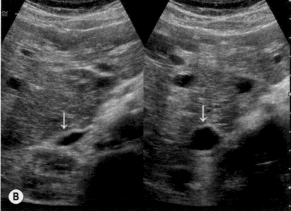

Fig. 8.4 (A) LS through the inferior vena cava (IVC). The right renal artery (small arrow) is seen passing posterior to the IVC. The diaphragmatic crus lies posterior to this (large arrow). (B) TS through the IVC demonstrating the difference in profile during the Valsalva maneuver (left) than normal expiration (right). (Liver cysts are present.)

Continued

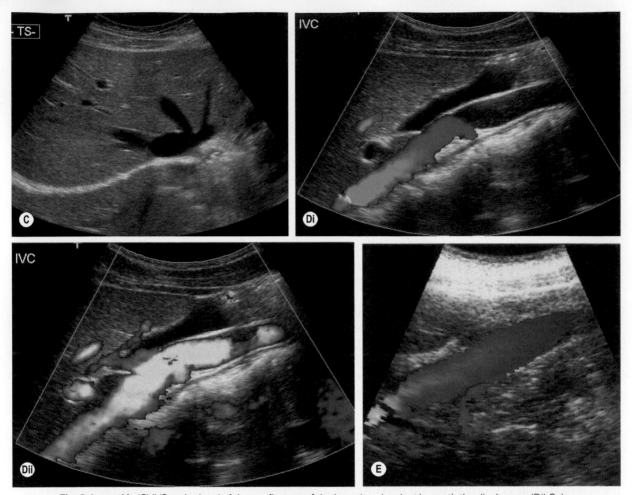

Fig. 8.4, cont'd (C) IVC at the level of the confluence of the hepatic veins, just beneath the diaphragm. (Di) Color Doppler fails to demonstrate flow when the IVC is perpendicular to the beam. (Dii) Power Doppler overcomes this, as it is less angle-dependent. (E) The right renal vein (in red) is seen draining into the IVC on color Doppler.

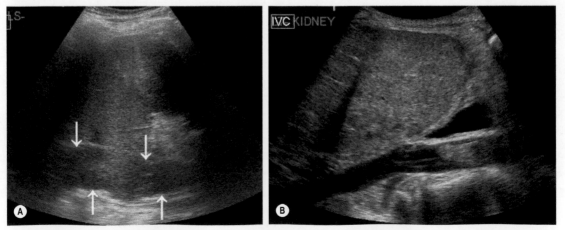

Fig. 8.5 (A) Tumor thrombus from a left renal carcinoma completely occludes the inferior vena cava (IVC; arrows). (B) Advanced renal carcinoma. The IVC contains a tumor thrombus.

Continued

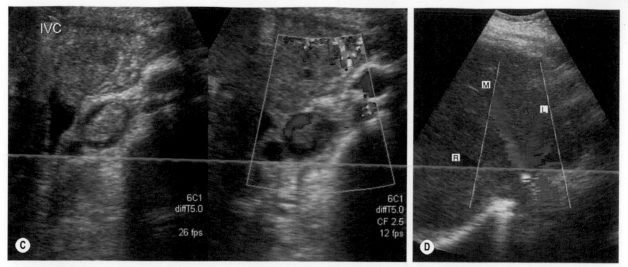

Fig. 8.5, cont'd (C) TS through the IVC containing non-occlusive thrombus. Flow is demonstrated around the thrombus on the right-hand image. (D) Tumor thrombus from a renal carcinoma has spread up the IVC and invaded the right hepatic vein, causing a partial Budd–Chiari effect. M, L, R: middle, left, and right hepatic veins.

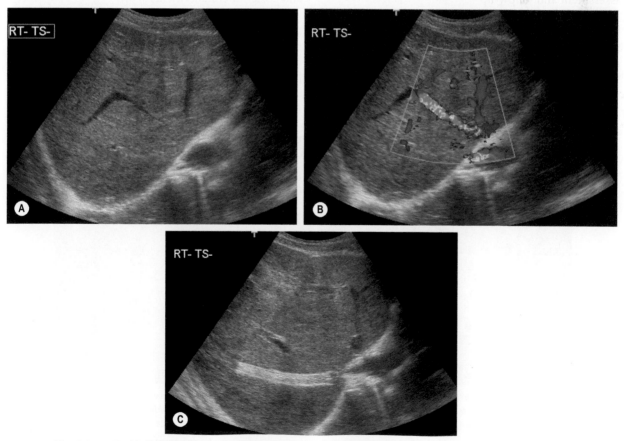

Fig. 8.6 (A) Budd–Chiari syndrome, with an occluded right hepatic vein. (B) Confirmed with color Doppler. (C) A stent has been inserted under angiographic guidance to restore flow in the vein.

Tumors of the IVC are rare. Leiomyosarcoma is a primary IVC tumor, appearing as a hyperechoic mass in the lumen of the vein.[15] This may cause partial or complete obstruction of the IVC, resulting in Budd–Chiari syndrome. The hepatic veins and proximal IVC may be considerably dilated in partial occlusion.

THE ADRENAL GLANDS

Normal Anatomy

Each adrenal gland is constructed with a central fold or ridge, which points anteromedially, from which extend two thin "wings" of tissue – a medial and a lateral wing (Fig. 8.7), giving rise to an "arrowhead" or "pyramid" shape effect. Although ultrasound is not routinely used to assess the adrenal glands, an abnormality identified at the upper pole of the kidneys should include adrenal mass as part of the differential diagnosis. CT is the imaging modality of choice for assessment and follow-up.

Adenoma

Small (less than 3 cm) solid adrenal nodules are a common, incidental finding in non-symptomatic patients. Where characteristics are of small, well-defined, and hypoechoic structure on ultrasound in a patient with no clinical history, it is usually safe to assume that this represents a small adrenal nodule.

Metastases

Adrenal metastases have similar appearances to adenomas. The adrenal glands are a common site for metastases, particularly from lung, breast, and bowel cancer, and melanoma, and may be accompanied by liver metastases (Fig. 8.8A). The adrenal glands are also commonly involved in non-Hodgkin's lymphoma.

Other Adrenal Lesions

Simple cysts are uncommon in the adrenal gland but are easily differentiated from solid lesions with ultrasound. Some cysts may be the sequelae of previous hemorrhage, but most are simple epithelial cysts. The usual acoustic characteristics of a cyst (anechoic, thin, regular capsule, and posterior enhancement) apply.

Primary adrenal carcinomas are rare in adults. They are commonly endocrinologically inactive in adults and therefore tend to present late when they are quite large, where they may invade the IVC and metastasize to the liver.

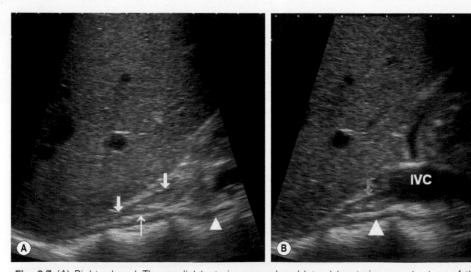

Fig. 8.7 (A) Right adrenal. The medial (anterior arrows) and lateral (posterior arrow) wings of the gland lie just anterior to the diaphragmatic crus (arrowhead). (B) The medial ridge of the right adrenal (arrow) is seen anterior to the diaphragmatic crus (arrowhead). The hyperechoic medulla is surrounded by the hypoechoic adrenal cortex.

Continued

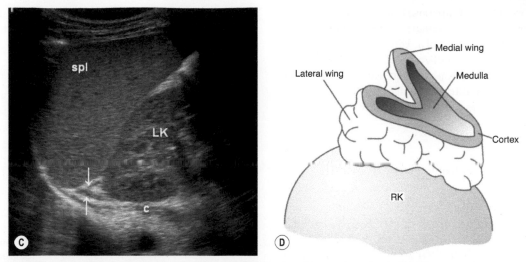

Fig. 8.7, cont'd (C) The two hypoechoic wings of the left adrenal (arrows) can be seen in the space between the spleen, left kidney, and the crus, c. (D) Diagram of the right adrenal gland showing the structure and anatomical relationship to the right kidney.

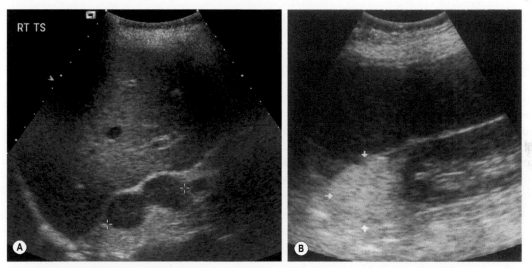

Fig. 8.8 (A) Right adrenal metastasis from primary lung carcinoma. (B) Left adrenal myelolipoma – an incidental finding confirmed on computed tomography that remained stable over three years. Its high-fat content makes it hyperechoic.

GASTROINTESTINAL (GI) TRACT

Historically contrast radiographic investigations, including CT, MRI, and fluoroscopy, were frequently the first-line of investigation for suspected GI tract disease, in conjunction with an endoscopic examination. Over the past few years, technological advancement and the increasing experience of ultrasound practitioners have meant that ultrasound is now an important tool for visualizing bowel conditions, giving practitioners the ability to diagnose a range of different pathologies within the GI tract.

The advantages of examining the GI tract with ultrasound are the non-invasive method of assessing the luminal and mural appearances of physiological conditions and the extra-intestinal features such as mesentery and lymphadenopathy. Ultrasound practitioners undertaking abdominal ultrasound should have an understanding of the ultrasound appearances of the GI tract to reduce the rate of misdiagnosis for normal GI anatomy and increase the sensitivity for detecting GI tract diseases.

Normal Anatomy

Comprising the esophagus, stomach, small and large bowel, rectum, and anus, the GI tract has a tortuous course over the length of approximately 3–5 m. The small bowel is comprised of the duodenum, jejunum, and ileum. The terminal ileum connects to the colon by the ileocecal valve (Fig. 8.9A).

The colon is a combination of the cecum, ascending colon, transverse colon, sigmoid colon, rectum, and anal canal. The colon frames the abdominal cavity beginning in the right iliac fossa to the right upper quadrant. The ascending and descending colon are usually fixed to the retroperitoneum, whereas the transverse and sigmoid colon may have a different course because of the different lengths in the mesocolon.

Normal stomach, duodenum, jejunum, and ileum appear as fluid and gas-filled lumens, demonstrating varying degrees of valvulae conniventes. Normal colon is often seen as a gas-filled lumen, with a haustral pattern noted in sagittal scanning. The wall of the GI tract consists of five layers (Fig. 8.9B), which can be examined on ultrasound. Normal wall thickness of the GI tract is <2–3 mm when distended,[16] other than that seen in the duodenal bulb and rectum where this may be more (Fig. 8.9C).

Technique

The scanning technique is variable but should be performed in a systematic way. Bowel assessment usually involves utilizing a low-frequency abdominal probe to provide an overview of the position and pathologic conditions before switching to a higher frequency probe for a more detailed assessment. Assessment is best made initially scanning in the transverse/axial section of the lumen, following the tract back and forth until an adequate assessment is made along the entire course of the bowel. This technique advocated by many bowel imaging experts is known as "mowing the lawn" (Fig. 8.9D).

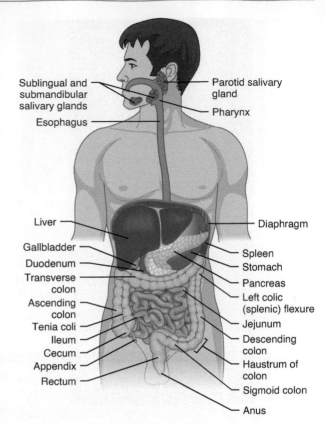

Fig. 8.9A Diagram of the digestive system showing different parts of the bowel. (Source: Goodman and Fuller's Pathology: Implications for the Physical Therapist , Fifth Edition, 2021.)

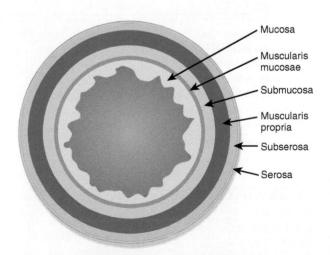

Fig. 8.9B Diagram showing the layers of the bowel wall. (Source: Problem Solving in Abdominal Imaging, First Edition, 2009.)

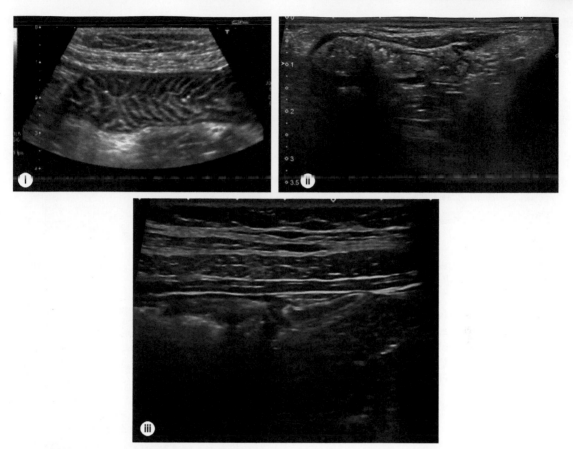

Fig. 8.9C (i) Normal appearances of the jejunum. (ii) Normal appearances of the colon. (iii) Normal appearances of the ileocecal junction.

> **TIP**
>
> The flexures are often located high in the abdomen and may need sub and intercostal imaging.
>
> Using external references to identify fixed anatomy can help assess the bowel; for example, the right iliac region over the iliopsoas muscle will help locate the ileocolic region. Similarly, the descending-sigmoid junction can be identified over the left iliac crest.

Esophagus and Stomach

The esophagus is not usually accessible to percutaneous ultrasound. However, the upper esophagus can be identified in the neck, usually adjacent to the left lobe of the thyroid. The lower end can be demonstrated as it passes through the diaphragm in the midline, just anterior to the aorta (Fig. 8.9E). Its normal appearances should

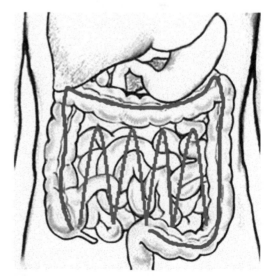

Fig. 8.9D Diagram showing the bowel scanning technique in ultrasound.

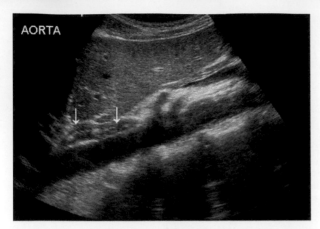

Fig. 8.9E Normal esophagus (arrow) between the aorta and the left lobe of the liver. Thin, hypoechoic walls with a hyperechoic lumen because of the presence of air.

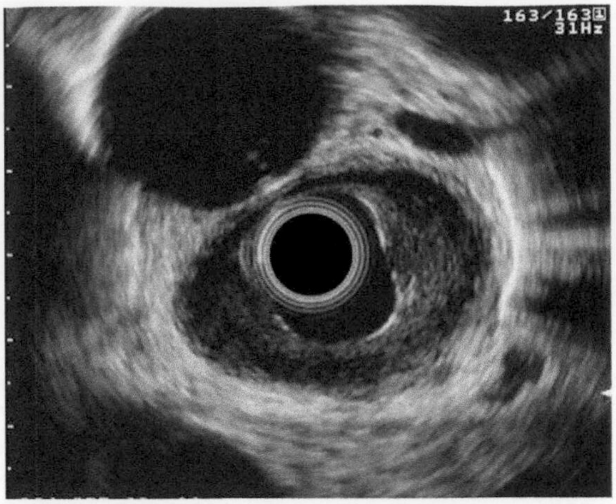

Fig. 8.9F Endoscopic ultrasound demonstrates the thickened wall of esophageal carcinoma prior to stent insertion.

not be confused with a mass. Occasionally, ultrasound demonstrates the thickened wall associated with an esophageal carcinoma involving the lower esophagus. Endoscopic ultrasound (EUS) is excellent for imaging the esophagus as it can also be used for biopsy and stent placement (Fig. 8.9F).

PATHOLOGY

Inflammatory Bowel Conditions

Appendicitis

Acute appendicitis is a common diagnosis on admission to the casualty department with right lower abdominal pain. However, around 15%–25% of patients who undergo laparotomy turn out to have normal appendices (Fig. 8.10). The use of ultrasound in the investigation of acute abdominal pain is well-established and increases the reliability of the diagnosis of acute appendicitis when performed by an experienced operator.[17]

The ultrasound features of acute appendicitis may include a thickened, non-compressible appendix with a mural thickness ≥6 mm in diameter (if not distended). The mesentery is expanded and hyperechoic. Other secondary signs include lymphadenopathy and free fluid or collections (Fig. 8.11A). Both the appendicular wall and the mesentery demonstrate increased signal using Doppler. These features have a high sensitivity and specificity for acute appendicitis (74% and 94%, respectively).[17]

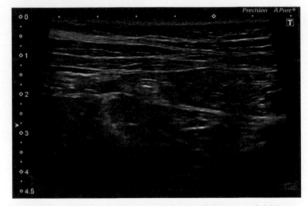

Fig. 8.10 Normal appendix. Normal stratification and thickness of the wall of the appendix. Gas-filled lumen.

Appendicitis is most often caused by a luminal obstruction, such as an appendicolith or tumor. Occasionally, a hyper-reflective appendicolith may be seen in the blind end of the inflamed appendix, casting an acoustic shadow (Fig. 8.11C). However, care must be taken to fully assess the appendix in cases of acute appendicitis to ensure that there is no malignant cause, as this will affect patient management. Furthermore, complications should be assessed and reported to referring clinicians. Common complications of acute appendicitis include perforation, resulting in ultrasound appearances of a simple or complex peri-appendiceal fluid collection (Fig. 8.11B).

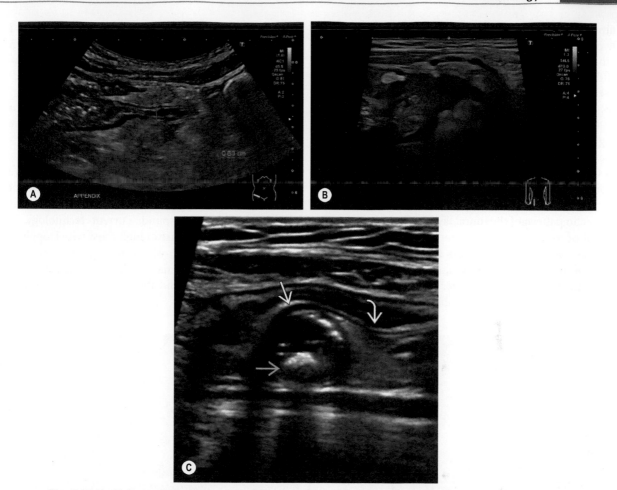

Fig. 8.11 (A, B) Acute appendicitis with a thickened, tender edematous wall, complex peri-appendiceal fluid, and hyperechoic peri-appendiceal fat. (C) Short axis ultrasound of an inflamed distended appendix containing appendicoliths. The adjacent fat is inflamed. (Source: Diagnostic Ultrasound for Sonographers, 2019.)

TIP
The appendix can be located using graduated compression over the cecal edge, inferior to the terminal ileum. However, the appendix can be located in a number of different positions. If unable to visualize the appendix in the more typical position over the iliopsoas region, turning the patient onto their left side can reveal a retrocecal appendix. Also, it can be longer than commonly expected – up to 27 cm, and therefore subhepatic appendicitis can also be appreciated.

Often an abnormal appendix is highlighted by the abnormal appearance of the appendicular mesentery. However, care should be taken not to misinterpret mesenteric changes from Crohn's disease as appendicitis.

Inflammatory Bowel Disease (IBD)

Radiological investigations have a useful role to play in the management of patients with IBD. The advantages of using ultrasound over other techniques such as MR and CT enterography are the ability to dynamically assess the bowel without ionising radiation or contrast mediums, resulting in ultrasound becoming useful in monitoring disease and identifying extra-luminal complications.[18]

Crohn's Disease

Crohn's disease is a common cause of inflammation affecting the small bowel and particularly the terminal ileum. It often presents with pain, changes in bowel habits (diarrhea), and weight loss. The terminal ileum/ileocecal junction is involved in the majority of cases. Initial ultrasound assessment may suggest the initial diagnosis. It can be used to evaluate the bowel wall and identify other complications of Crohn's disease with sensitivity and specificity comparable to CT.[19] Ultrasound is also used to screen patients at risk and monitor patients for recurrence of disease following surgery.[20]

Ultrasound features of Crohn's disease vary depending on the stage of disease and complications/treatments. Wall thickening is the more important feature of Crohn's disease on ultrasound (>3–4 mm measured from the interface between the serosa to the proper muscle to the interface between the mucosa and lumen). The echo pattern of the mural layers will depend on the extent of the disease. In cases of clinical and biochemical disease activity, the layers become ill-defined. In cases of fibrosis and ulceration, the stratification of the layers may be indistinguishable.[21] The important ultrasound feature that is recognizable in Crohn's disease is the presence of mesenteric fat hypertrophy.[21] Fat wrapping or fat creep is seen as the mesenteric tissue around the diseased bowel (Fig. 8.12). This is pathognomonic of Crohn's disease. Prominent mesenteric lymph nodes may also be present.[21]

In addition, there may be evidence of "skip lesions," whereby there is a segment of diseased bowel followed by a normal segment followed by another stretch of thickened bowel.

In acute flare-ups of Crohn's disease, there is often increased Doppler signal in the outer layers. The use of color and Power Doppler is well documented in Crohn's assessment with ultrasound; current technology has seen the advent of the use of high sensitivity Doppler or microvascular imaging, which has seen an increase in the detection of inflammatory changes but also a redefinition of normality, and therefore caution is advised when using.

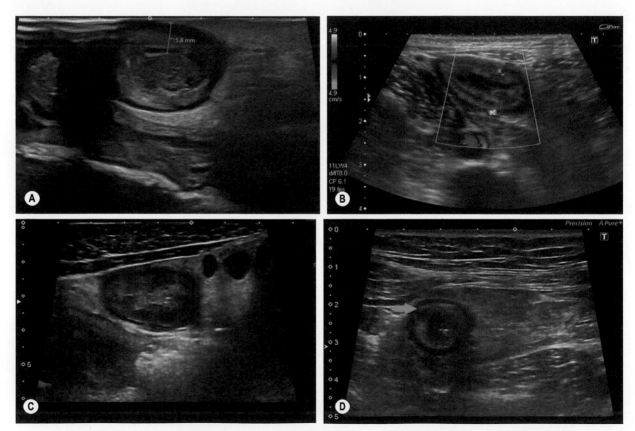

Fig. 8.12 (A) Wall thickening in Crohn's disease. (B) Hyperemia in thickened bowel wall associated with Crohn's disease. (C) Mesenteric lymphadenopathy with thickened bowel and creeping fat (images supplied with the kind permission of Dr. R. Beable). (D) Terminal ileal Crohn's disease. Transmural fibrotic disease on the mesenteric border (red arrow). Mesenteric hypertrophy with hypoechoic echogenicity. Hypoechoic region within the submucosa (green arrow) representing ulcerative disease.

Colitis

Ultrasound is effective at assessing for bowel wall thickening seen in colitides, although it has limited value in differentiating the differing causes. The main ultrasound feature of colitis is wall thickening.

Unlike Crohn's disease, ulcerative colitis (UC) only involves the mucosa and begins from the rectum, often progressing proximally to the rest of the colon. Colonoscopy is often the method of choice for diagnosing UC. However, ultrasound has a role in assessing the extent of disease and excluding other pathologic conditions. Ultrasound features of UC include thickening of the bowel wall involving the mucosa and submucosa without the involvement of the muscularis propria or the peri-colonic fat.[21] Other findings in UC include an irregular appearance of the mucosal surface because of deep ulcerations and loss of normal haustral pattern.[22]

Diverticulitis

Diverticulitis may also be recognized on ultrasound as outpouchings from the bowel wall (Fig. 8.13).[23] Acute diverticulitis usually appears as outpouchings from the bowel wall on ultrasound with extra-colonic inflammation. Ultrasound in experienced hands can rival CT in terms of sensitivity and specificity in the diagnosis of acute diverticulitis.[17] Perforation of a diverticulum may give rise to a diverticular abscess, where CT is still the method of choice for the complications of diverticulitis because of the frequent pelvic location of disease.

> **TIP**
>
> In cases where patients have pelvic segments of the bowel, transvaginal assessment where indicated can be useful in evaluating distal diverticular disease.

Malignant Tumors

Malignant tumors often appear as ill-defined soft tissue areas that have disturbed the normal stratification of the bowel wall layers. Tumors are often visualized because of the lack of normal distension of the lumen at the diseased segment because of the fibrotic nature of the tissue. Doppler flow can usually be visualized in malignant bowel masses, although it is also present in inflammatory masses (Fig. 8.14). The absence of a bowel mass on ultrasound does not exclude bowel carcinoma but can be reassuring to clinicians where more invasive testing is not appropriate. However, the finding of a colonic mass on ultrasound should result in a subsequent staging by CT.

The role of ultrasound in patients with known and suspected bowel carcinoma in experienced hands is useful to help confirm and stage disease, identifying invasion into adjacent structures such as the abdominal wall and adjacent loops of the bowel, where the dynamic nature of ultrasound allows assessment for movement with regards to adjacent structures. EUS is useful for staging rectal cancers and in the follow-up of rectal cancer and can detect early recurrence of disease.

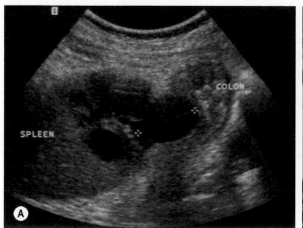
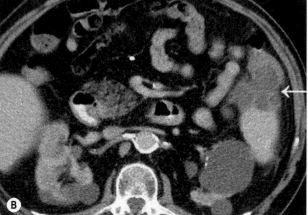

Fig. 8.13 (A) A diverticular abscess arising in the left colon has invaded the spleen. (B) Appearances are confirmed on computed tomography.

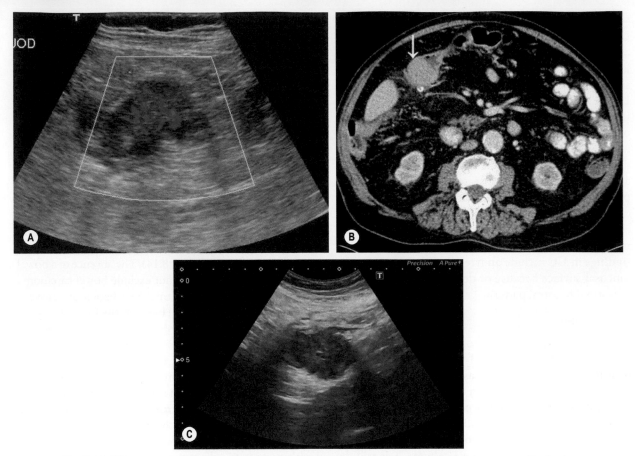

Fig. 8.14 (A) A suspected bowel carcinoma was found in a patient presenting with right upper quadrant pain. (B) Computed tomography confirms the carcinoma in the transverse colon (arrow). (C) Sigmoid tumor with extramural invasion. Loss of mural layers and empty lumen. Central cystic area suggesting necrotic change.

Obstruction

Ultrasound has been found to be helpful in the investigation of acute obstruction with a sensitivity of 89% in the diagnosis of small bowel obstruction[24] and 88% in establishing the level and cause of obstruction in the colon.[25] Although non-specific, it can help confirm obstruction by demonstrating dilated, fluid-filled bowel loops with ineffective peristalsis (Fig. 8.15). The benefit of ultrasound is that fluid-filled loops of the bowel are highly amenable to scanning, with an additional advantage of visualizing peristalsis, unlike a plain X-ray. It is possible to trace the dilated bowel to the site of obstruction, distal to which are normal loops of collapsed bowel.[26] Ultrasound is also useful in demonstrating herniation of bowel (Fig. 8.15B), especially in acute cases associated with obstruction.

Other Retroperitoneal Abnormalities

Ultrasound is useful for identifying retroperitoneal masses, but CT and MRI are more effective in establishing the extent and nature of many of these masses, particularly those partly obscured by gas-filled bowel.

The majority of malignant retroperitoneal tumors are renal or adrenal in origin. Other primary tumors, apart from lymphomas, are rare and include liposarcoma and leiomyosarcoma. These tend to be large when they present and have variable/complex ultrasound appearance. Encasement of major vessels by tumor is a further characteristic of the retroperitoneal origin of the mass,

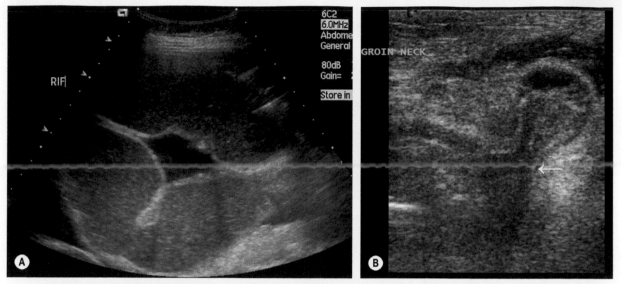

Fig. 8.15 (A) Dilated, fluid-filled loops of the bowel because of an obstructing cecal carcinoma. Ascites are also present. (B) A loop of bowel is demonstrated herniating through into the right groin. The neck of the hernia is indicated by the arrow.

together with anterior displacement of structures such as the pancreas, kidneys, aorta, and IVC.

Ultrasound can also identify peritoneal and omental deposits in patients with late-stage carcinoma. These are particularly amenable to diagnosis when surrounded by ascites (Fig. 8.16) and usually arise from gynecological or urological tumors. On ultrasound, other identifiable retroperitoneal masses include mesenteric panniculitis, hematoma, psoas abscesses, lymphadenopathy (Fig. 8.17), and pancreatic pseudocysts.

ABDOMINAL WALL HERNIA

Investigation for the diagnosis of a hernia and its differential diagnoses (which can also be appreciated within the same ultrasound examination) is a common request in the ultrasound department. A hernia is the abnormal protrusion of tissue, either an organ or fatty tissue, through a discontinuity in the musculature or fascia, which would usually contain it. They are usually classified by location and the type of tissue they contain. While most hernias are located in the groin (inguinal or femoral), this is frequently covered by musculoskeletal texts. There are several subcategories of anterior abdominal wall hernia which the generalist ultrasound practitioner may also frequently encounter. They may include epigastric,

umbilical, paraumbilical, Spigelian, and incisional.[28] The general principles of hernia scanning can apply to most hernia scanning. Hernia may be congenital (may not always present in pediatric patients) or acquired.

Normal Anatomy

Several layers make up the anterior abdominal wall, including fascia, muscle, fat, and peritoneum (Fig. 8.18A).[27]

Technique

It is essential that the ultrasound practitioner takes a clinical history from the patient prior to scanning, including pointing to the location of concern, as hernia often presents in a specific area with a history of lump which may or may not be reducible, pain, previous surgery, exacerbating movements, and duration of symptoms along with any other relevant history which may provide alternative differential diagnoses where required.

Light probe pressure should be employed in the first instance to avoid iatrogenic reduction of a hernia in the first instance. Dynamic scanning while increasing abdominal pressure is almost always essential. Various methods can be employed to do this, including the Valsalva maneuver,[28] straining, or changing the patient position to elicit the lump, e.g., standing. Eliciting a cough is often not useful because of the sudden

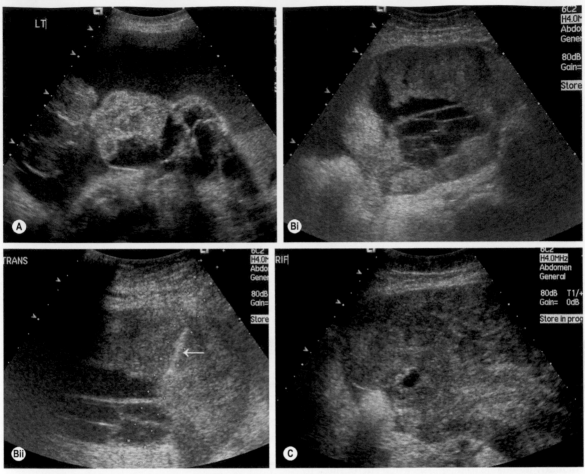

Fig. 8.16 (A) Late-stage ovarian carcinoma demonstrates abdominal ascites with hyperechoic omental deposits. (Bi) Carcinoma of the peritoneum. An ultrasound-guided biopsy was performed prior to treatment; (Bii) the needle is seen (arrow) entering the solid peripheral area of the mass for histological diagnosis. (C) A large solid peritoneal tumor.

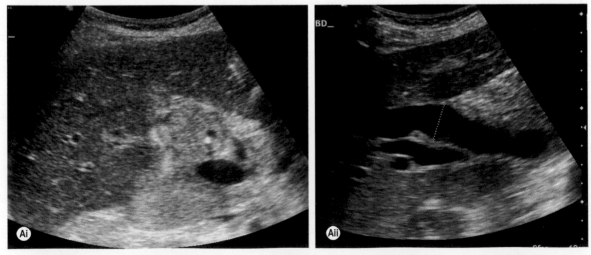

Fig. 8.17 (Ai) A hyperechoic mass of enlarged lymph node around the porta hepatis is causing obstructive jaundice, with dilatation of the common bile duct (CBD) (Aii).

Continued

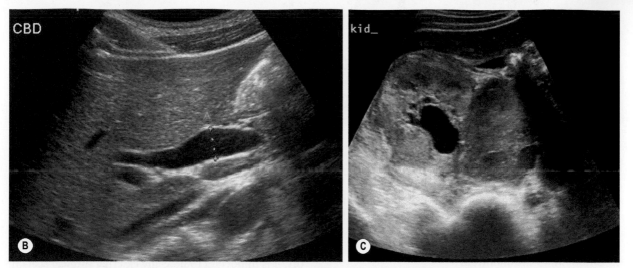

Fig. 8.17, cont'd (B) Lymphadenopathy may be the cause of obstructive jaundice. Small lymph nodes are present around the porta, dilating the CBD (calipers). (C) Large retroperitoneal lymph node mass causing a right renal obstruction.

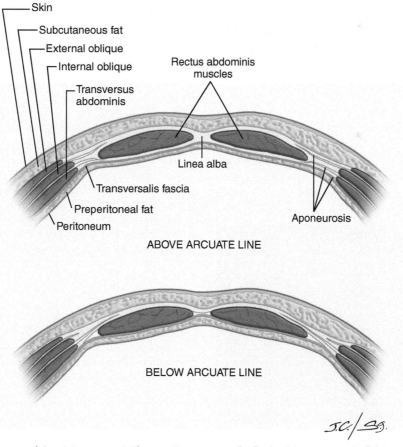

Fig. 8.18A Layers of the abdominal wall. (Source: Hysterectomy for Benign Disease: Female Pelvic Surgery Video Atlas Series, 2010.)

movement of the patient, which can lead to misinterpretation of findings in the inexperienced operator.

> **TIP**
>
> Cine-loop clips are a useful way of imaging and recording the hernia and its dynamics.

Epigastric Hernia

An epigastric hernia presents as a bulge between the xiphoid process and the umbilicus through the linea alba. It is usually only a fat-containing hernia unless it is a particularly large gap (Fig. 8.18B).

Umbilical and Paraumbilical

Umbilical hernias are usually clinically obvious in presentation, may be painful, and contain bowel and fat. They are more common in female patients and have an increased risk of strangulation. They can also result in complications such as bowel obstruction.

Paraumbilical hernia occur close to the umbilicus. As with umbilical hernias, they are often painful and can be noted to have external discoloration of the skin.

Spigelian Hernia

Spigelian hernias are not often clinically obvious. There can be pain provoked by Valsalva but no evidence of reducible mass. They occur in the "semi lunar line" (linea semilunaris) as a herniation of tissue between lateral rectus and oblique muscles. Spigelian hernia is a rare en-

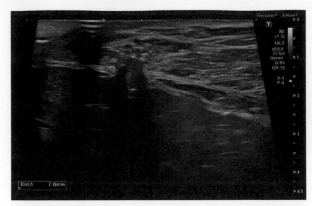

Fig. 8.18C Incisional hernia in an obese patient with a previous history of four laparotomies.

tity. It is important to note any external surgical scars in the region to ensure that the suspected Spigelian hernia is not an incisional hernia.

Incisional Hernia

Any patient who has undergone surgery is at risk of an incisional hernia. This risk is increased if the patient has a high body mass index or a postoperative infection. The hernia will be apparent on ultrasound close to the surgical scar (Fig. 8.18C).

> **TIP**
>
> Ultrasound practitioners should be aware that mimics of anterior abdominal hernia are not uncommon. For example, divarication of the rectus muscles (Diastasis Recti) is a common clinical presentation (especially in obese men and post-partum females) which may be misinterpreted as a ventral hernia on clinical presentation as it presents as a bulge or "ridge" in the midline when the patient moves from lying to "sit-up."

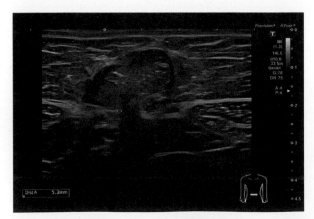

Fig. 8.18B Transverse section of a small fat-containing partially reducible epigastric hernia.

REFERENCES

1. Lema PC, Kim JH, St James E. Overview of common errors and pitfalls to avoid in the acquisition and interpretation of ultrasound imaging of the abdominal aorta. *J Vasc Diagn Interv.* 2017;5:41–46.
2. Thrush A, Hartshorne T. *Vascular ultrasound how, why and when.* 3rd edition. Churchill Livingstone; 2010.
3. Birkmeyer JD, Upchurch G. Evidence based screening and management of abdominal aortic aneurysms. *Ann Int Med.* 2007;146:749–750.

4. Akil Y, Khodabakhsh P, Naylor M, Sharpe R, Walker J, Hartshorne T. Small abdominal aortic aneurysms are not all the same. *Angiol.* 2020;71:205–207.

5. National Institute of Clinical Excellence. *Abdominal aortic aneurysm: diagnosis and management.* NICE (NG156). London: UK; 2020. Available at: https://www.nhs.uk/conditions/abdominal-aortic-aneurysm-screening.

6. Cosford PA, Leng GC. Screening for abdominal aortic aneurysm. *Cochrane Database Syst Rev.* 2007;18(CD002945).

7. Brown PM, Zelt DT, Sobolev B. The risk of rupture in untreated aneurysms: the impact of size, gender and expansion rate. 2003;37(2). https://doi.org/10.1067/mva.2003.119.

8. Waton S, Johal A, Heikkila K, Cromwell D, Boyle J, Loftus I. *National vascular registry: 2017 annual report.* London: The Royal College of Surgeons of England, November 2017. https://www.vsqip.org.uk/content/uploads/2018/05/2017-NVR-Annual-Report.pdf.

9. Public Health England. *NHS abdominal aortic aneurysm (AAA) screening programme essential elements in providing an AAA screening and surveillance programme,* version 5. London: UK; 2017.

10. Guidelines for professional ultrasound practice, version 3. British Medical Ultrasound Society and Society and College of Radiographers, London; 2019, p. 81.

11. Iezzi R, Basilico R, Giancristofaro D, et al. Contrast-enhanced ultrasound versus color duplex ultrasound imaging in the follow-up of patients after endovascular abdominal aortic aneurysm repair. *J Vasc Surg.* 2009;49:552–560.

12. Yang X, Chen YX, Zhang B, et al. Contrast-enhanced ultrasound in detecting endoleaks with failed computed tomography angiography diagnosis after endovascular abdominal aortic aneurysm repair. *Chin Med J (Engl).* 2015;128:2491–2497.

13. Clevert DA, Minaifar N, Weckbach S, et al. Color duplex ultrasound and contrast-enhanced ultrasound in comparison to MS-CT in the detection of endoleak following endovascular aneurysm repair. *Clin Hemorheol Microcirc.* 2008;39:121–132.

14. Smillie RP, Shetty M, Boyer AC, et al. Imaging evaluation of the inferior vena cava. *RadioGraphics.* 2015;35.

15. Moncayo KE, Vidal-Insua JJ, Troncoso A, et al. Inferior vena cava leiomyosarcoma: preoperative diagnosis and surgical management. *Surg Case Rep.* 2015;1:35.

16. EFSUMB. *EFSUMB recommendations and guidelines for gastrointestinal ultrasound.* EFSUMB: Thieme; 2017.

17. Zeidan BS, Wasser T, Nicholas GG. Ultrasonography in the diagnosis of acute appendicitis. *J R Coll Surg Edinb.* 1997;42:24–26.

18. Carucci LR, Levine MS. Radiographic imaging of inflammatory bowel disease. *Gastroenterol Clinics North Am.* 2002;31:93–117.

19. Horsthius K, Bipat S, Bennink RJ, Stoker J. Inflammatory bowel disease diagnosed with US, MR, scintigraphy and CT: meta-analysis of prospective studies. *Radiol.* 2008;247:64–79.

20. Andreoli A, Cerro P, Flasco G. Role of ultrasonography in the diagnosis of postsurgical recurrence of Crohn's disease. *Am J Gastroenterol.* 1998;93:1117–1121.

21. EFSUMB. *EFSUMB recommendations and guidelines for intestinal ultrasound (GIUS) in inflammatory bowel diseases.* EFSUMB: Thieme; 2018.

22. Bru C, Sans M, Defelitto MM, et al. Hydrocolonic sonography for evaluating inflammatory bowel disease. *Am J Roentgenol.* 2001;177:99–105.

23. O'Malley M, Wilson S. Ultrasound of gastrointestinal tract abnormalities with CT correlation. *Radiographics.* 2003;23:59–72.

24. Schmutz GR, Benko A, Fournier L. Small bowel obstruction: role and contribution of sonography. *Eur Radiol.* 1997;7:1054–1058.

25. Lim JH, Ko YT, Dee DH, et al. Determining the site and causes of colonic obstruction with sonography. *AJR Am J Roentgenol.* 1994;163:1113–1117.

26. Ogata M, Mateer JR, Condon RE. Prospective evaluation of abdominal sonography for the diagnosis of bowel obstruction. *Ann Surg.* 1996;223:237–241.

27. Sandring S. *Gray's anatomy. The anatomical basis of clinical practice.* 41st edition. London: Elsevier; 2016.

28. Jayaram PR, Pereria FDA, Barrett JA. Evaluation of dynamic ultrasound scanning in the diagnosis of equivocal ventral hernias with surgical comparison. *Br J Radiol.* 2018;91:20180056.

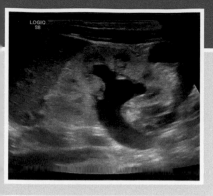

9

Ultrasound of the Pediatric Abdomen

Lorraine C. Walsh

CHAPTER OUTLINE

Introduction, 290
General Pediatric Ultrasound Hints and Tips, 290
  Equipment, 290
  Pediatric Abdomen and Pelvis Ultrasound
    Technique, 290
Liver and Hepatobiliary Pathologic
  Conditions, 290
  Normal Pediatric Ultrasound Appearances, 290
  "Starry Night" Liver/Hyperechoic Periportal
    Cuffing (ErPC), 291
  Biliary Atresia, 291
  Ultrasound Findings that Support the Diagnosis of
    Biliary Atresia, 291
  Choledochal Cysts, 293
  Cystic Fibrosis, 293
Focal Liver Lesions, 295
  Congenital Hepatic Hemangioma (CHH) and
    Infantile Hepatic Hemangioma (IHH), 295
    Ultrasound Appearances, 296
  Hepatoblastoma, 296
  Hepatocellular Carcinoma (HCC), 296
Spleen, 298
Pancreas, 299
Urinary Tract, 301
  Ultrasound Technique, 301
    Renal Size, 302
    Normal Kidney Appearances, 302
Congenital Anomalies, 303
  Renal Agenesis, 303
  Renal Fusion and Ectopia, 303
  The Duplex System, 304

    Complete Duplication, 304
    Partial Duplication, 305
  Urachal Remnant, 306
  Posterior Urethral Valves (PUV), 306
Renal Cystic Disease, 307
  Simple Renal Cysts, 307
  Genetic Renal Cystic Disease, 308
    Autosomal Recessive Polycystic Kidney Disease
    [ARPCKD] and Autosomal Dominant
    Polycystic Kidney Disease [ADPCKD], 308
    Multicystic Dysplastic Kidneys (MCDK), 308
Malignant Renal Tumors, 309
  Nephroblastoma (Wilms Tumor), 309
  Neuroblastoma, 310
    Role of US in the Assessment of Renal Tumors, 310
Renal Tract Dilatation, 311
  Postnatal Renal Dilatation, 311
  Obstructive Uropathy, 311
  Non-Obstructive Uropathy, 311
  Vesicoureteric Reflux, 311
Gastrointestinal Tract, 313
  Congenital Abnormalities, 313
    Intestinal Malrotation and Volvulus, 313
    US Signs of Malrotation +/- Volvulus, 314
Acquired Disorders, 314
  Infantile Hypertrophic Pyloric Stenosis (IHPS), 314
    Tips for Ultrasound Examination of the
    Pylorus, 315
  Intussusception, 316
References, 318

INTRODUCTION

Ultrasound (US) is the primary imaging modality in children, with the tissue composition and body habitus of most resulting in superior image quality compared to adults. However, children remain one of the most challenging groups of patients to image, requiring different techniques and skills. The presenting symptoms and pathological processes in children can differ from those in adults, and special considerations are required in relation to diagnosis and imaging techniques. This chapter addresses only the most common pediatric situations likely to present in a general department, and further specialist reading is recommended at the end of the chapter.

GENERAL PEDIATRIC ULTRASOUND HINTS AND TIPS

- Preparation is key; reducing the examination time minimizes anxiety. The sonographer must understand the clinical referral details and review prior imaging before the child enters the examination room.
- The use of toys and electronic devices to play cartoons or music can be invaluable distractions. Sterile dummies and oral sucrose solution can help calm a fractious hungry baby.
- Speak directly to the child and the guardian; never underestimate the positive impact of a smiling face on a young child.
- Adapt the examination where necessary; lie the child on top of their guardian or examine the kidneys in prone erect while the child is embraced in a "bear hug."
- A systematic scanning technique is essential, but the sonographer must be able to adapt the examination as required, keeping a mental "checklist" to ensure US imaging protocol requirements are met.

Equipment

- The sonographer must have a detailed knowledge of the ultrasound equipment, and a full range of presets are essential, including abdominal and renal, bowel, and superficial settings with different settings for neonates and older children.
- A range of high-frequency (5–15 MHz) dynamic transducers with small and conventional footprints are required. Always use the highest-frequency transducer available based on the child's body habitus. Linear high-frequency probes are required for the assessment of superficial structures.
- A rapid frame cine loop enables multiple still images to be obtained in fractious patients.

Pediatric Abdomen and Pelvis Ultrasound Technique

- Examine the whole abdomen, including the pelvis, unless a focused examination such as renal tract is indicated. In cases of nonspecific abdominal pain or appendicitis, assess the bowel architecture and mesentery with a high-frequency linear probe using a bowel preset.
- A subcostal/intercostal approach is often required with children to examine major organs. Asking the child to push their tummy out (Valsalva) can improve image quality.
- Vascular assessment using Doppler is essential for hepatobiliary and acute abdomen referrals.
- When examining the spleen, the longest axis or largest spleen if multiple, should be measured in the sagittal/coronal plane and assessed for enlargement for age using an appropriate size chart.
- Kidneys should be additionally examined in prone/prone erect with a high-frequency linear probe, with high-resolution images because of the superficial location and lack of overlying muscle bulk in pediatric patients.

LIVER AND HEPATOBILIARY PATHOLOGIC CONDITIONS

Normal Pediatric Ultrasound Appearances

The sonographer should have a knowledge of the normal fetal and neonatal circulatory system, and assessment of liver vasculature using pulsed-wave and color Doppler is essential.[1] The normal liver in children should be homogenous and slightly more echogenic than the right kidney and less than the pancreas and spleen. The interface between the hepatic parenchyma and the portal triads and vessel walls should be visible. The right lobe of the liver should not extend below the lower pole of the right kidney, and the liver should have a smooth contour. The normal gallbladder is thin-walled and distended after fasting (Table 9.1).

TABLE 9.1 Normal Pediatric GB and Biliary Measurements			
Age	Mean Gallbladder Length[2]	Gallbladder Wall Thickness[2]	CBD Diameter[2,3]
Birth to 12 months	2.5 cm (range 1.3–3.4 cm)	≤3 mm	1–2 mm
12 years to 16 years	6.1 cm (range 3.8–8 cm)	≤3 mm	Maximum of 4 mm

Sources: Refs. 2 and 3.

"Starry Night" Liver/Hyperechoic Periportal Cuffing (ErPC)

"Starry night" liver or hyperechoic/echo-rich periportal cuffing (ErPC) is caused by a diffuse hypo-echogenicity of the liver causing prominence of the small portal branches compared to the liver parenchyma (Fig. 9.1).[4]

A "starry night" liver is nonspecific and has been observed in healthy patients. However, it has been reported as having high sensitivity and specificity in pediatric patients presenting with abdominal inflammation, including gastroenteritis, acute/perforated appendicitis, mesenteric lymphadenitis, and acute hepatitis.[5,6] In our clinical trust, operators report a "starry night" appearance of the liver. However, all US findings must always be evaluated in the context of a full clinical history, laboratory parameters, and other US appearances.

Biliary Atresia

Physiological jaundice is common, affecting up to 60% of neonates, and normally resolves by day 14. Any continuing jaundice beyond this requires urgent investigation.[7] Extrahepatic biliary atresia and neonatal hepatitis are the cause of 60%–90% of conjugated hyperbilirubinemia, and infants typically present aged one to two months with jaundice, dark urine, and pale stools.[2] Biliary atresia (BA) is a serious liver disease and can be fatal if untreated. Therefore its early diagnosis is crucial. The cause of biliary atresia remains unclear but results in progressive inflammation, destruction, and fibrosis of the biliary tree resulting in biliary cirrhosis. The treatment for biliary atresia is a Kasai portoenterostomy, which is successful in up to 60% of neonates. If unsuccessful, a liver transplant during infancy is required.[7,8,9]

Ultrasound Findings that Support the Diagnosis of Biliary Atresia

There are two primary diagnostic features of biliary atresia:[8]

- Abnormal gallbladder – absent or small, irregular contour or wall
- Triangular cord sign – an area of increased echogenicity anterior to the bifurcation of the portal vein

Due to its narrow caliber, the absence of a common bile duct (CBD) is not diagnostic of biliary atresia.[8,10,11] It is essential for the neonate to be fasted for 3 h and the gallbladder and liver carefully examined using a high-frequency transducer (Fig. 9.2A, B).

Biliary atresia causes cirrhosis, leading to portal hypertension, hepatosplenomegaly, and a heterogenous hepatic parenchyma. The hepatic artery becomes hypertrophied, appearing dominant on color Doppler compared to the adjacent portal vein (Fig. 9.2C, D).

Approximately 10%–20% of infants with biliary atresia have splenic malformation syndrome, with associated congenital abnormalities, including situs inversus, polysplenia, preduodenal portal vein, and interruption of the inferior vena cava (IVC) with azygous continuation, all of which may be detected on US (Fig. 9.3).[7,9,10]

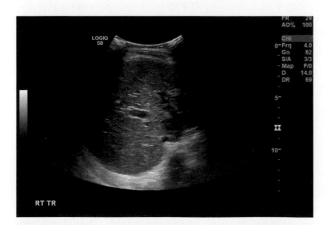

Fig. 9.1 Liver demonstrating prominence of small portal branches compared to the liver parenchyma, giving a "starry night."

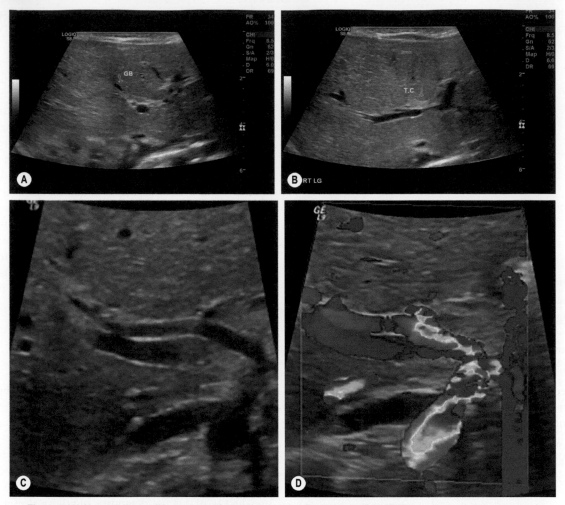

Fig. 9.2 (A) Abnormally small irregular walled gallbladder in biliary atresia (BA). (B) Triangular cord sign; increased echogenicity seen anterior to the bifurcation of the portal vein in a five-week-old infant with BA. (C) Hypertrophy of the hepatic artery in BA. (D) Color Doppler image of hypertrophy of the hepatic artery in BA.

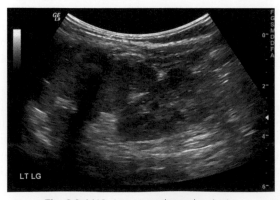

Fig. 9.3 LUQ demonstrating polysplenia.

Cystic biliary atresia is an abnormal cystic structure at the porta hepatis containing bile or mucous, with an obliterated biliary tree and accounts for 8% of cases of biliary atresia (Fig. 9.4A, B).[10] This can be misdiagnosed as a choledochal cyst or gallbladder. The presence of a triangular cord sign supports a diagnosis of cystic biliary atresia, while intrahepatic biliary duct dilatation is suggestive of a choledochal cyst. Further diagnostic examinations, including an intraoperative cholangiography, hepatobiliary scintigraphy, or magnetic resonance cholangiopancreatography (MRCP), may be required to make a definitive diagnosis.[10]

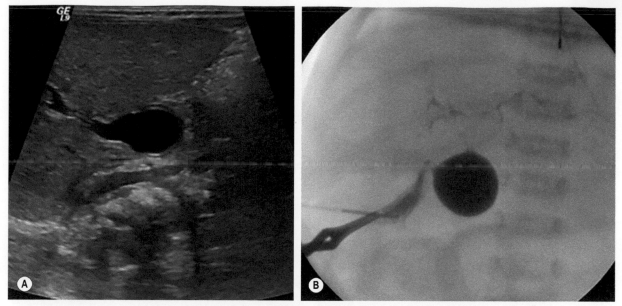

Fig. 9.4 (A) Cyst at porta hepatis. (B) Cholangiogram demonstrating cyst.

Choledochal Cysts

Choledochal cysts are a congenital dilatation of the biliary tree. The exact cause is unknown; however, many patients have an abnormal pancreaticobiliary junction allowing reflux of pancreatic enzymes into the biliary tree, causing dilatation. Choledochal cysts are classified by the seminal work of Todani.[12]

There are five types with two subgroups.

- **Type I** (80%–90% of cases). Consists of focal/diffuse dilatation of the CBD, may involve the common hepatic duct or cystic duct, and may cause intrahepatic ductal dilatation.
- **Type V** (Caroli disease). Consists of saccular/fusiform dilatation of the intrahepatic ducts. Associated with autosomal recessive polycystic kidney disease (ARPCKD), demonstrating the importance of a full abdominal assessment in pediatric patients.[3]

Choledochal cysts are well-defined cysts close to the porta hepatis, in continuity with the biliary tree, often containing biliary sludge and calculi (Fig. 9.5A). There is often associated dilatation of the proximal bile ducts supporting differentiation from cystic biliary atresia. An MRCP is often performed for larger and inconclusive lesions because of the associated complications, including cholangitis, pancreatitis, liver abscess, and cyst rupture.[2] A technetium-99

hepatobiliary iminodiacetic acid (HIDA) scan can also differentiate between the two conditions. Choledochal cysts will demonstrate contrast entering the duodenum on a HIDA scan compared to cystic biliary atresia, where there is an absence of contrast emptying into the duodenum (Fig. 9.5B, C).

Cystic Fibrosis

Cystic fibrosis (CF) is a common, autosomal recessive multisystem disease affecting the lungs, pancreas, intestine, liver, sweat glands, and in males, the Wolffian ducts.[13] Mucous accumulates in the bronchi leading to progressive destruction of the terminal bronchioles. Improved treatment and management of CF pulmonary disease have resulted in increased survival rates. However, there is a resultant increase in cystic fibrosis liver disease (CFLD).

CFLD results from mucosal hyperplasia in the gallbladder and bile ducts resulting in increased biliary sludge with gallstones, cholecystitis, and biliary strictures.[13] Secondary atrophy of the gallbladder results in a micro gallbladder in 4%–45% of cases (Fig. 9.6A).[14] Progressive fibrosis causes the liver to be hyperechoic with a coarse nodular echotexture and increased periportal echogenicity (Fig. 9.6B). Eventually, cirrhosis develops, causing portal hypertension, with associated

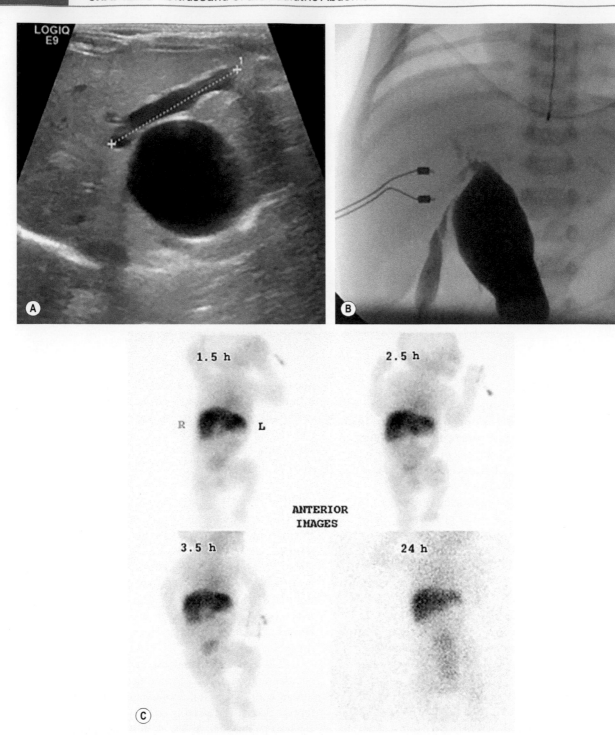

Fig. 9.5 (A) Choledocal cyst closely adjacent to gallbladder. (B) Fluoroscopy demonstrates a large cystic structure which is the choledochal cyst to the left of a normal gallbladder (smaller cystic structure). A non-dilated biliary system is demonstrated. (C) Tibida. The tibida scan demonstrates an initial filling defect in the inferior border of the liver relating to the choledochal cyst (1.5 h, 2.5 h, 3.5 h) but after 24 h, there is filling in the duodenum confirming choledochal cyst with no impediment to the flow of bile. This enables differentiation from cystic biliary atresia, where there would be an absence of biliary excretion into the duodenum.

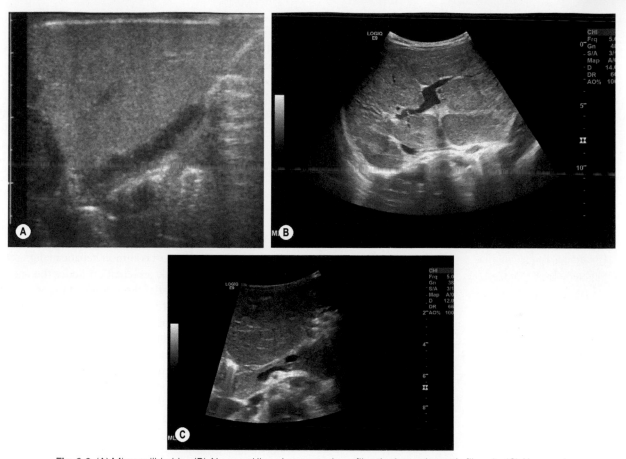

Fig. 9.6 (A) Microgallbladder. (B) Abnormal liver demonstrating a fibrotic change in cystic fibrosis. (C) Abnormal cystic pancreas in cystic fibrosis.

varices and splenomegaly, so assessment of the portal venous system with color and spectral Doppler is essential. CFLD is a significant cause of morbidity and mortality in children with CF, and US is the primary diagnostic examination to monitor disease progression.[13,15] Shear wave elastography offers the potential to diagnose, stage, and monitor liver fibrosis.

The pancreas is also affected by CF with a wide range of abnormal appearances on US, including complete atrophy of the pancreas, pancreatic cysts, and ductal dilatation. (Fig. 9.6C). The pancreas often demonstrates increased echogenicity, calcification, and heterogeneity with features of acute and chronic pancreatitis.[13,14]

FOCAL LIVER LESIONS

This section provides an overview of the most common pediatric liver lesions, with further reading recommended at the end of the chapter (Table 9.2).

Congenital Hepatic Hemangioma (CHH) and Infantile Hepatic Hemangioma (IHH)

Hemangiomas and vascular tumors are the most common benign tumors in infancy, affecting 4%–5% of infants. There are two forms, and the agreed standardized terms advised are CHH and IHH.[7,10]

- CHHs evolve *in utero,* so may be detected antenatally, and are fully developed at birth. They can present postnatally as an abdominal mass or heart failure in the newborn because of the shift from fetal blood flow via the umbilicus to postnatal flow (Fig. 9.7A, B).[7,10,16]
- IHHs typically appear within weeks of birth, undergo proliferation during the first few months, and gradually involute over the next few years. IHHs are often associated with cutaneous hemangiomas, so US is used to screen for associated internal hemangiomas. Most IHHs are clinically asymptomatic and diagnosed incidentally or during screening.[10]

TABLE 9.2 **Causes of Focal liver Lesions in Children**
Congenital Masses
Hepatic cyst
Choledochal cyst
Congenital hepatic hemangioma
Primary Liver Masses
Infantile hepatic hemangioma
Hepatic adenoma
Focal nodular hyperplasia
Mesenchymal hamartoma
Regenerative nodule
Hepatoblastoma
Hepatocellular carcinoma
Fibrolamellar hepatocellular carcinoma
Undifferentiated (embryonal) sarcoma
Angiosarcoma
Lymphoma
Rhabdomyosarcoma
Metastatic Disease
Liver metastases may occur from most pediatric malignancies, including neuroblastoma, rhabdomyosarcoma, Wilms tumor
Infection
Bacterial infection
Fungal infection
Parasitic infection
Conditions That Can Mimic Focal Hepatic Masses
Focal fatty proliferation
Hepatic infarction
Extrahepatic masses

The potential complications of IHH and CHH overlap, but it must be noted that CHHs are at peak size and vascularity at birth, while IHHs continue to proliferate until approximately six to 12 months of age. Serial US monitors hemangioma progression or regression.[10,7]

Ultrasound Appearances

- CHHs are often large, well-circumscribed lesions that appear heterogeneous because of hemorrhage, necrosis, fibrosis, and calcification during their involution. CHHs often contain large vascular channels, so color Doppler assessment is essential, but the presence of a discrete parenchymal mass enables differentiation

from an arterio-vascular malformation. It is important to exclude malignancy.[10]
- IHHs are rarely unifocal, presenting as multifocal lesions with normal intervening parenchyma or as a diffuse mass with innumerable lesions that replace the normal hepatic parenchyma. IHHs rarely contain calcification.

Most hepatic hemangiomas do not require treatment and involute spontaneously, but complications include hemorrhage, thrombocytopenia, hypofibrinogenemia, high-output cardiac failure, and thrombus formation. In these cases, computed tomography (CT) may be used to localize the vessels (Fig. 9.7C), and fluoroscopic guided embolization is required (Fig. 9.7D).[10]

Hepatoblastoma

Hepatoblastoma is the most common hepatic malignancy in childhood, with a peak presentation under the age of 18 months. Presentation after three years is rare, and there is a male predominance of 3:2. The most common presenting features are palpable abdominal mass with distension, anorexia, weight loss, vomiting, pain, and jaundice.[7,17] Complications include rupture, hemorrhage, and metastases, with the primary metastatic site being the lungs.[10] Hepatoblastoma are associated with genetic syndromes such as Beckwidth-Wiedmann, hemihypertrophy, low birth weight below 1500 g, and precocious puberty.[7,10,18]

Hepatoblastoma usually presents on US as a large solid solitary mass measuring 12 cm or more in 80% of cases, with the remaining 20% manifesting as multiple hepatic masses (Fig. 9.8A, B). The mass is often hyperechoic compared to normal liver parenchyma; however, it is often heterogeneous because of necrosis, calcification, and hemorrhage. There may be associated ascites, invasion/compression of the hepatic vasculature, and IVC, so a detailed assessment with color and spectral Doppler is essential.[10,18,19] Hepatoblastoma is associated with elevated alpha-fetoprotein blood levels, which enables differentiation from hepatic hemangiomas.[3,19] Management is dependent on the extent of the disease, and treatment includes neoadjuvant chemotherapy, tumor resection, or liver transplantation.[7,10]

Hepatocellular Carcinoma (HCC)

Hepatocellular carcinoma (HCC) is the most common malignant liver tumor in older children, often with a history of liver disease, including hepatitis B, with peak incidences of four to five years and 12–14 years.[7,18] The US appearance of HCC is variable. Smaller HCCs are usually hypoechoic to normal liver parenchyma but may appear hyperechoic.

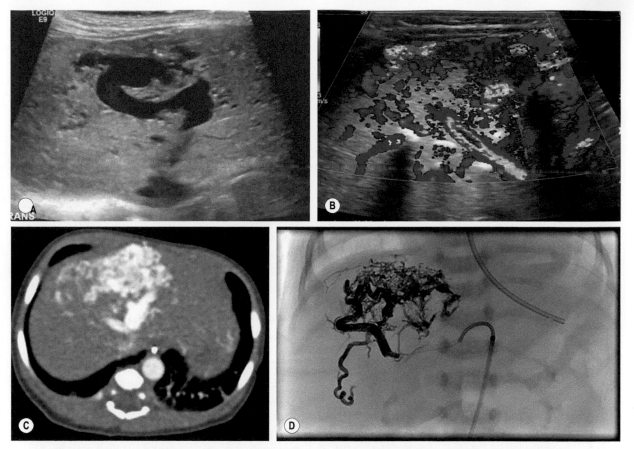

Fig. 9.7 (A) B mode ultrasound image of infantile hepatic hemangioma. (B) Color Doppler ultrasound of infantile hepatic hemangioma. (C) Computed tomography of infantile hepatic hemangioma. (D) Interventional radiography image demonstrating abnormal vasculature within infantile hepatic hemangioma.

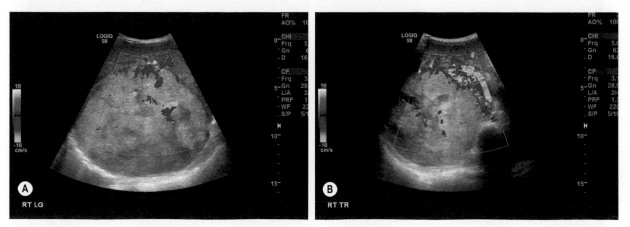

Fig. 9.8 (A) Large vascular heterogeneous mass in the right lobe of the liver. (B) Large heterogeneous mass in right lobe deviating the portal vein and hepatic artery.

Larger HCC lesions are commonly heterogeneous, while infiltrative HCCs may appear as a diffuse disruption of the normal liver echotexture. HCC is well vascularized with high-velocity arterial flow, so Doppler assessment of the mass and hepatic vasculature and IVC is essential.[18]

CASE STUDY (Fig. 9.9A–G)

The sonographer should always be aware of multiple pathologic conditions and the role of US compared to other imaging modalities. This case regards a teenage patient referred with pyrexia, rigors, and pain in the right upper quadrant (RUQ). Ultrasound revealed two large avascular complex masses in the right lobe of the liver (Fig. 9.9A–C). In addition, there was collapse and consolidation in the right lower lobe, which demonstrates hepatization on ultrasound (Fig. 9.9D). This is demonstrated on chest radiograph (Fig. 9.9F). A CT scan confirms the liver mass, and with clinical correlation, a diagnosis of a liver abscess was made (Fig. 9.9E). US was used to guide drainage of the liver abscess (Fig. 9.9G).

SPLEEN

The spleen should be routinely measured for every pediatric abdominal examination and the size assessed against age.[2,20] Polysplenia (Fig. 9.3) is associated with biliary atresia, while cardiac anomalies are associated with a right-sided or absent spleen. Portal hypertension can result in splenomegaly, splenic varices, and the development of a splenorenal shunt.[2,20]

The presence of an accessory spleen or splenunculi is significant in conditions that may require a splenectomy, including hereditary spherocytosis or sickle cell disease, because of potential hypertrophy of any residual splenic tissue post-surgery. Acute splenic sequestration is an emergent cause of splenomegaly in children with sickle cell disease and trauma. Children commonly present with tachycardia, hemodynamic instability, severe abdominal pain and distention, and massive splenomegaly. Children with long-standing sickle cell disease often present with a small, fibrotic, and calcified spleen because of auto-infarction.[2]

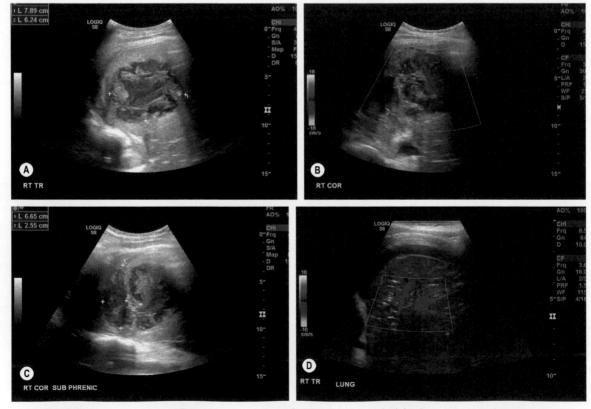

Fig. 9.9 (A) Heterogeneous liver abscess on B mode ultrasound in right lobe liver. (B) Liver abscess color Doppler. (C) Liver abscess sub-phrenic. (D) Right lower lobe lung consolidation with color Doppler.

Continued

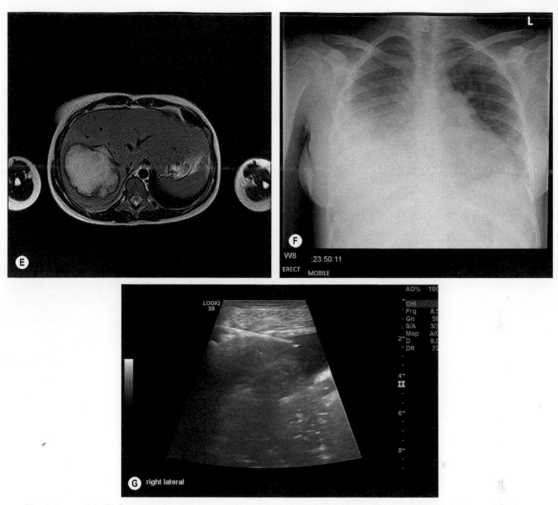

Fig. 9.9, cont'd (E) Computed tomography of an abscess. (F) Chest X-ray demonstrating right lower lobe lung consolidation. (G) Ultrasound-guided liver abscess drainage, with echogenic linear artifact caused by a needle.

PANCREAS

The pancreas is often well visualized in children, and the appearances of the pancreas vary with age. The pancreas is bulky and hypoechoic in neonates compared to adults; this should not be misinterpreted as pancreatitis (Fig. 9.10A, B). In older children, echogenicity is equal to or slightly greater than that of the liver, and the pancreas reaches adult size in the late teens.[2]

Normal pancreatic duct diameter should not be greater than:[19]

- 1.5 mm in children between one to six years of age
- 1.9 mm at ages seven to 12 years
- 2.2 mm at ages 13–18 years

Although pancreatic trauma is rare, it is a significant injury in children, who have a higher incidence than adults. The pancreas can be completely transected, initiating pancreatitis and peritonitis with pancreatic pseudocysts developing in 15%–20% of pediatric patients.[19]

Fig. 9.10C, D demonstrates pseudocyst following traumatic pancreatic rupture (Table 9.3).

CASE STUDY

Fig. 9.11A–D demonstrates chronic pancreatitis with a pancreatic pseudocyst, dilated pancreatic duct, and loculated pelvic collection.

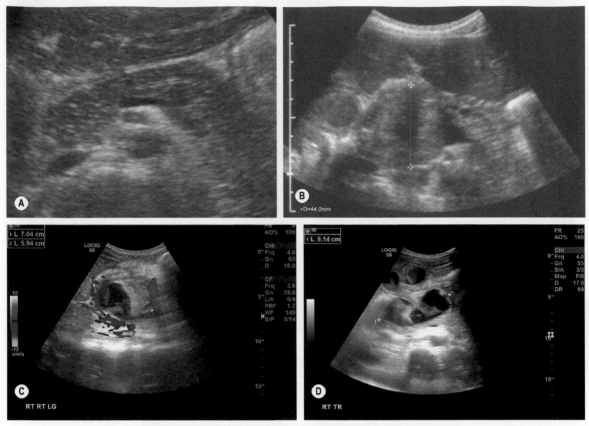

Fig. 9.10 (A) Normal pancreas in a five-year-old boy – relatively hypoechoic and bulky compared to the adult gland. (B) A complex mass in the head of the pancreas and a dilated pancreatic duct in a seven-year-old boy. Ultrasound-guided biopsy revealed a complex malignant vascular tumor, and he underwent a Whipple's procedure. (C) Longitudinal image of heterogeneous collection consistent with pancreatic rupture and surrounding vasculature. (D) Transverse ultrasound image of heterogenous collection consistent with pancreatic rupture.

TABLE 9.3   Pediatric Pancreatic Abnormalities

Increased Echogenicity

Cystic fibrosis	Fatty replacement of the pancreas, calcifications, ectatic pancreatic duct, coarse texture, cysts
Pancreatitis	Hereditary
	Trauma (physical abuse, road traffic accident)
	Congenital anomaly, e.g., choledochal cyst
	Drug toxicity
	Viral and parasitic infection
Hemochromatosis	Pancreatic fibrosis, iron deposition in liver and pancreas

Focal Lesions

Cysts	Isolated congenital cyst
	Autosomal dominant polycystic disease
	Von Hippel–Lindau disease
	Meckel–Gruber syndrome
Solid lesions	Primary pancreatic neoplasms are very rare in children

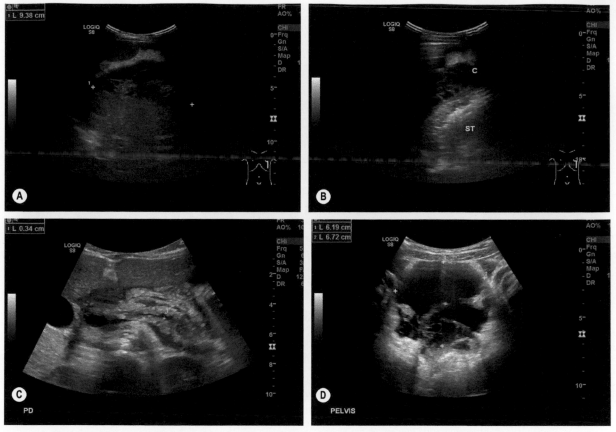

Fig. 9.11 (A) Large heterogeneous pancreatic pseudocyst because of chronic pancreatitis. (B) Pancreatic pseudocyst (C) in the pancreatic tail closely adjacent to the stomach (ST). (C) Echogenic pancreas with chronic pancreatitis and dilated pancreatic duct. (D) Pelvic collection with known chronic pancreatitis.

URINARY TRACT

Ultrasound Technique

- Examine the bladder first. This enables assessment before the child micturates or additional fluid intake if the bladder is inadequately filled.
- Pre- and post-micturition bladder volumes are required where possible.
- Color Doppler is essential to identify the ureteric orifices, ureteric jets, and differentiation of dilated ureters, ovaries, and iliac vessels.
- Assess the bladder contents for urinary debris or calculi, optimizing the TGC.
- Assess the bladder wall for wall thickness, irregularity, presence of bladder diverticula or ureterocele.
- Examine the kidneys in supine, coronal, and prone/prone erect positions, confirming the number, size, and location of both kidneys. Both kidneys should

be comparable in size, and a difference of more than 10% should prompt detailed investigation.

- Assess renal outline and contour, looking for evidence of fetal lobulation or scarring. The US appearances of scarring include a focal reduction in cortical thickness, irregular outline, interruption of or loss of the renal capsule echo, or a disruption in the renal architecture.
- Assess for renal pelvis dilatation (RPD). If present, determine the presence and extent of calyceal dilatation. For standardization, consistency, and reproducibility of measurements, the RPD is measured as follows: the child in a prone position, with the kidney in transverse, at the renal hilum with the calipers positioned at the edge of the renal parenchyma (Fig. 9.12A). A 10 mm cutoff is acceptable in cases of *isolated* RPD, with no ureteric or calyceal dilatation.
- Color Doppler can assist in identifying "crossing vessels" in cases of pelvic ureteric junction (PUJ) obstruction.

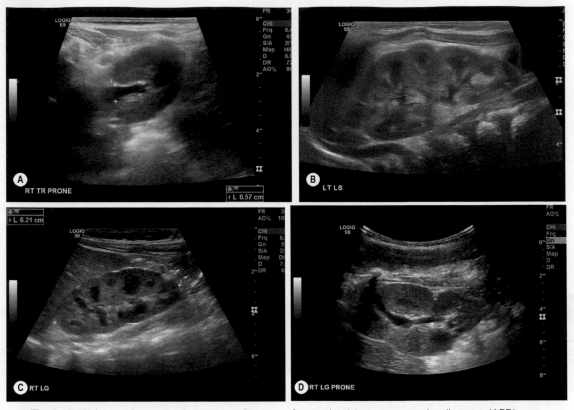

Fig. 9.12 (A) Image demonstrating correct placement for renal pelvis anteroposterior diameter (APD) measurement. (B) Neonatal kidney demonstrating increased echogenicity due to Tamms-Horsfall protein deposits. (C) Follow-up of the same patient demonstrating normal neonatal appearances, with the prominence of corticomedullary differentiation with fetal lobulation. (D) Focal loss of normal cortical thickness consistent with renal scarring. Compare with normal neonatal lobulations between the renal pyramids.

- Assess for normal corticomedullary differentiation; do not mistake renal pyramids for hydronephrosis.
- Look for evidence of urolithial thickening, which can be seen in infection or reflux.
- Exclude a horseshoe kidney by identifying the lower pole of the left kidney and the IVC in the coronal plane.

Ultrasound is often the first line investigation for renal assessment or may be used in conjunction with other imaging modalities (Table 9.4).

Renal Size

Record the maximum bipolar renal length ensuring accurate caliper placement, and do not assess renal size for age in the presence of hydronephrosis. Accurate evaluation of renal size is essential. The simplest method is by comparison of the maximum bipolar renal length to age-based reference charts, plotted manually. An example is the seminal works of Rosenbaum et al.[21] However, there are recognized limitations with this study, includ-

ing the date of publication, small sample size, and lack of information on the ethnicity of the sample population. There are web-based multivariable renal nomograms available for standardized renal centiles.[22]

Single kidney charts should be used for children with one functioning kidney; an example is Spira et al.[23]

Normal Kidney Appearances

There are several differences between the infant and the adult kidney. In neonates, the renal cortex is hyperechoic in contrast to the hypoechoic medullary pyramids, resulting in marked corticomedullary differentiation, which should not be mistaken for hydronephrosis. Several pathological conditions result in increased neonatal renal medullary echogenicity, but in our center's experience, this can be an isolated transient abnormality, thought to be because of deposits of Tamm-Horsfall protein and is associated with dehydration (Fig. 9.12B).[24] In the absence of renal biochemical abnormalities, we

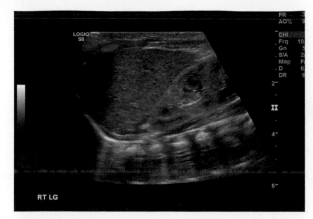

Fig. 9.13 Normal neonatal right adrenal gland.

perform a follow-up scan in four weeks to ensure the renal echogenicity returns to normal.

Fetal lobulations are smooth indentations of the renal outline lying between the renal pyramids (Fig. 9.12C) and should not be confused with renal scarring (Fig. 9.12D), which is irregular indentations usually overlying the renal pyramids. Over time the renal cortex becomes less hyperechoic, the corticomedullary differentiation lessens, and fat deposition in the renal sinus becomes more evident.

The adrenal glands are large and easily demonstrated on US in neonates. They are recognized as a typical wishbone or inverted V over the kidneys (Fig. 9.13). The adrenals gradually involute after birth, and by two to four months, have attained their normal "adult" configuration.

CONGENITAL ANOMALIES

Renal Agenesis

The kidneys form from the ureteric bud, which arises from the pelvic area during the fifth to sixth week of gestation. The bud undergoes numerous divisions, forming the ureters, renal pelvis, calyces, and renal tubules. Any interruption of this process may cause renal agenesis or ectopia.

Bilateral renal agenesis is lethal because of pulmonary hypoplasia and is usually diagnosed antenatally. Unilateral renal agenesis (URA) has an incidence of one in 2000 live births,[25] and one in three patients with URA have additional renal abnormalities. URA is associated with VATER syndrome (vertebral, anal, trachea, esophagus, and radius anomalies) and with ipsilateral gynecological anomalies in girls.

Renal Fusion and Ectopia

A horseshoe kidney is the most common form of renal fusion with an incident rate of one in 500 births, with a 2:1 male to female ratio. There is an association with chromosomal abnormalities, including Edwards Syndrome (67%), Turners Syndrome (14%–20%), and Downs Syndrome (1%).[26] The lower poles of the kidneys have a medial orientation and are fused with a central isthmus or "bridge" across the front of the spine, which can be difficult to detect lying behind gas-filled bowel. Sonographers should be suspicious for a horseshoe kidney when the lower poles of the kidneys cannot be clearly visualized, and both kidneys are small for age. Visualization of the left lower pole is often improved scanning coronally in the left mid-axillary line, turning the child if necessary.[27] Other forms of renal fusion include an "L" shape, where one kidney lies horizontally across the midline; crossed fused ectopia where both kidneys lie on the same side; "H" shaped fusion of the hilar regions; and complete fusion to form a "cake"-shaped solitary kidney (Fig. 9.14).

Dimercapto succinic acid (DMSA) will only detect functioning renal tissue. Therefore, an isthmus composed of a fibrous band of non-functioning tissue will not be identified. There may be a variable number of ureters with renal fusion, and as the ureters pass anterior to the conjoined lower poles, resultant compression with obstruction, hydronephrosis, and urinary tract infections (UTIs) is common. Additional complications include: vesicoureteral reflux (VUR), nephrocalcinosis, and an increased risk of malignancy, including Wilms tumor.[26]

The incidence of renal ectopia is 0.2%, and the ureteral bladder insertion may be on the same or opposite

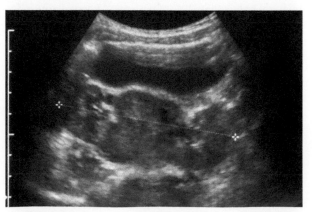

Fig. 9.14 Renal fusion forming a "cake"-shaped solitary kidney in the pelvis.

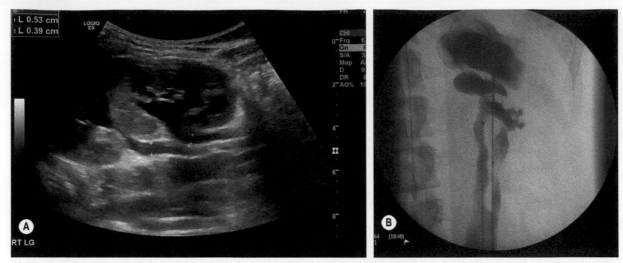

Fig. 9.15 (A) Ultrasound image demonstrating the presence of two ureters in a duplex right kidney. (B) Fluoroscopic examination demonstrating dilated upper and lower moieties and two ureters.

side of the ectopic kidney. Crossed fused ectopia occurs when there is a fusion of both kidneys. Most ectopic kidneys demonstrate malrotation, but the incidence of associated anomalies is low compared to horseshoe kidneys. The most common abnormality is VUR. Ectopic kidneys occur most frequently in the pelvis and, like a horseshoe kidney, are susceptible to blunt abdominal trauma.[26,27]

The Duplex System

Duplex kidneys are a common incidental finding in adults and usually of no clinical concern, but can be a significant finding in children. Almost 50% of pediatric patients investigated for UTI and found to have duplex kidneys had complications requiring treatment.[28] Duplex kidneys are twice as common in females than males and bilateral in less than 20% of patients.[28] Recognizing a duplex kidney is essential for the pediatric sonographer because of the associated complications, which can result in scarring and functional impairment of the kidney.

There is a wide variation with complete or partial renal duplication.

Complete Duplication

Results in two separate pelvicalyceal systems that arise from two ureteral buds from the mesonephric duct and are demonstrated on US as a kidney which is longer than normal with two renal sinuses separated by a parenchymal bridge. This results in two ureters, each independently draining sections of a kidney (Fig. 9.15A, B).

The opposing ends of the kidney are described as upper and lower moieties.[29] Ectopic insertion of the upper pole ureter can be a cause of urinary incontinence in girls.

The Weigert-Meyer rule[29] is applicable to a completely duplicated collecting system and states that:

- The ureter arising from the lower pole of the kidney inserts more superiorly and laterally into the bladder, resulting in a short intramural course that predisposes the ureter to reflux.
- The ureter arising from the upper pole moiety, which inserts more inferiorly and medially, frequently forms an obstructed uretercele (Fig. 9.16).

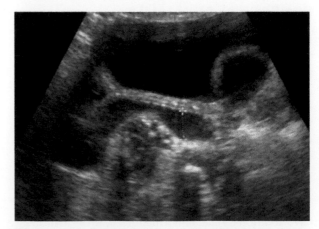

Fig. 9.16 Dilated ureter (calipers) of the upper moiety of a duplex kidney terminating in a ureterocele seen in the base of the bladder.

CASE STUDY

Duplex kidney with left upper moiety nephrectomy and incision of ureterocele now left lower moiety pelvic ureteric junction obstruction. With urolithial thickening and urinary debris. Normal right kidney. Renal scintigraphy using 99mTc-mercaptoacetyltriglycine (MAG3) demonstrates 39% left and 61% right renal function (Fig. 9.17A–C).

Partial Duplication

Arises when a single ureteric bud divides prematurely, prior to fusion with the mesenchyme. This leads to bifid moieties and ureters, which fuse to form a single ureteric insertion distally with a resultant range of incomplete duplications within a kidney and ureter.

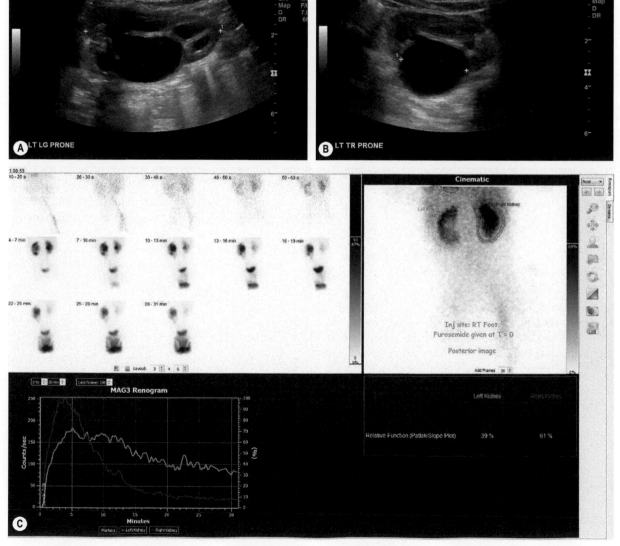

Fig. 9.17 (A) Ultrasound image demonstrating urolithial thickening. (B) Left renal pelvis APD measurement. (C) MAG3 image demonstrating delayed excretion in the left kidney compared to the right.

There is a range of complications associated with duplex kidneys which are specific to the moiety. Upper moiety complications include ectopic ureteric insertion, with or without a ureterocele and multicystic dysplastic moiety. Lower moiety complications include VUR, renal scarring, and PUJ obstruction. Further imaging may be required to characterize a detected abnormality, including contrast US, nuclear medicine studies, micturating cystourethrograms (MCUG), CT, and magnetic resonance (MRI).[28]

Urachal Remnant

The urachus is the embryological remnant of the allantois and extends from the umbilicus to the bladder dome. This normally closes before birth; incomplete regression of the urachus can result in a range of abnormalities, and a diagnosis should be considered if a diverticulum of the anterosuperior aspect of the bladder is present.[27]

Posterior Urethral Valves (PUV)

PUV affects males and is caused by an obstructing membrane that restricts the passage of urine through the urethra, causing lower urinary tract obstruction. It has an incidence of one in 5000 at birth and is associated with high fetal and neonatal mortality (30%) and significant lifelong morbidity.[30,31] The obstructed valves and associated reflux result in the following abnormalities on US:
- Abnormal distended, thickened trabeculated bladder wall (Fig. 9.18A).
- Ureteric dilatation – usually bilateral.
- Pelvicalyceal dilatation – usually bilateral (Fig. 9.18B, C).
- Echogenic dysplastic kidneys.
- Occasionally a dilated urethra can be visualized inferior to the bladder.

PUV is often accompanied by abnormal renal development, and 30%–42% of patients develop end-stage renal failure, with PUV the most common cause for

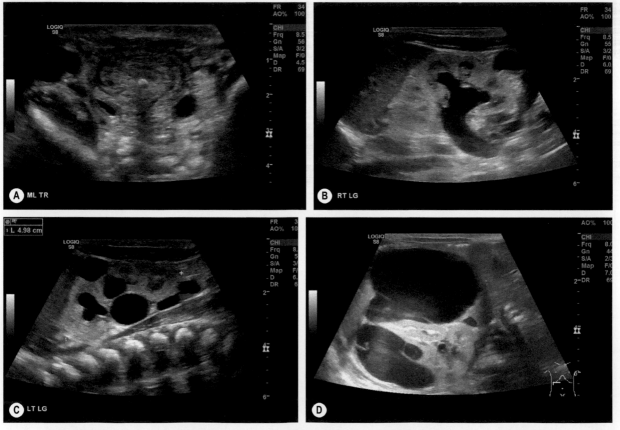

Fig. 9.18 (A) Abnormal thick-walled bladder and bilateral dilated ureters because of posterior urethral valves. (B,C) Bilateral abnormal kidneys because of posterior urethral valves. (D) Abnormal right kidney with urinoma extending around the kidney because of posterior urethral valves in a three-day-old baby.

TABLE 9.4	Imaging the Pediatric Renal Tract
Ultrasound	First-line investigation in all cases. Excellent structural detail
	Limited sensitivity for duplex kidneys, reflux, ureteral pathologic conditions, and small scars
	Monitoring of disease progression
	Monitoring of treatment
Contrast sonocystography	Alternative to X-ray or radionuclide cystography. Poor structural detail, unsuitable for the demonstration of urethral anomalies
Diuretic renogram (dynamic) – Tc^{99M} MAG3	Outlines the pelvicalyceal system. Diagnosis of obstruction and relative renal function by analysis of excretion curves
Radionuclide cystography (dynamic)	Diagnosis of reflux
Direct (via a catheter or suprapubic injection of isotope into the bladder) or indirect (following diuretic renogram)	
Cortical scintigraphy (static) – Tc^{99M} DMSA	Demonstrates uptake in the renal cortex
	Superior detection of renal scarring in vesicoureteric reflux and acute pyelonephritis
	Demonstration of congenital anomalies, e.g., ectopic or solitary kidney
	Analysis of differential renal function
Intravenous urography	Limited use in children
	Assessment of level of ureteric obstruction
	Assessment of congenital anomalies, e.g., ectopic ureters and duplex kidney
	Postoperative evaluation
Micturating cystourethrogram	Accurate diagnosis of reflux, polyps, diverticula, strictures, and urethral anomalies, but involving a significant radiation dose
Contrast-enhanced voiding urosonography	Enables assessment of the structure of the urethra and bladder, with the benefit of real-time assessment of voiding function without the need for radiation, making this a proposed alternative to micturating cystourethrograms
Plain X-ray	Some calculi – mainly those in the ureter
	Of limited value in a pediatric renal workup
	May show gross spinal anomalies
CT	Reserved mainly for confirmation and staging of malignant tumors because of significant radiation dose
	Renal trauma
	Increasingly used for ureteric calculus detection
MRI	Assessment of difficult congenital anomalies and focal masses. Staging of malignancy

renal transplantation.[30] US and MCUG are the primary diagnostic tests, but there is the potential for contrast-enhanced voiding urosonography (ceVUS) to replace the MCUG (Fig. 9.18D) (Table 9.4).[31,32]

RENAL CYSTIC DISEASE

Simple Renal Cysts

Simple renal cysts are a common finding in adults (see renal section) but are an abnormal finding in the pediatric population, prompting further investigation as they may be associated with genetic renal cystic disease. The cysts should be confirmed in two different planes using a high-frequency linear US transducer, and the following documented:

- Unilateral or bilateral.
- Size, number, and location of the cysts.
- US appearances. Are cysts simple; being anechoic, thin-walled, and avascular on Doppler insonation? Any internal echoes or calcification?

- Is the surrounding kidney parenchyma normal in appearance and echogenicity, with normal corticomedullary differentiation?
- Extend the examination to exclude cysts in the liver, spleen, and pancreas.

Genetic Renal Cystic Disease

Autosomal Recessive Polycystic Kidney Disease [ARPCKD] and Autosomal Dominant Polycystic Kidney Disease [ADPCKD]

Genetic disease is usually bilateral, with a wide spectrum of severity. It is important to differentiate between ARPCKD and ADPCKD.

ARPCKD is associated with hepatic fibrosis and portal hypertension and can be diagnosed antenatally. US appearances:

- Enlarged kidneys above 95th centile in size for age.
- Presence of multiple cysts of between 1–2 mm, which are poorly differentiated because of their small size.
- Echogenic renal parenchyma with loss of corticomedullary differentiation (Fig. 9.19A).

Serial US is used to monitor the following:

- Size of the kidneys.
- The number and size of any visible cysts.
- Examination of the liver for evidence of portal hypertension, including Doppler assessment of the portal vein and hepatic veins.

- Assessment of splenic size and assessment of the splenic vein, and evidence of splenic varices.

In comparison, **ADPCKD** has a wide spectrum of severity. In severe forms, cysts are present in childhood, but in many cases, cysts are not detected until screening in the second or third decade of life. There is also an associated risk of intracranial berry aneurysms (Fig. 9.19B).[27,33]

Multicystic Dysplastic Kidneys (MCDK)

MCDK is because of complete, early ureteric obstruction *in utero* before ten weeks and is frequently diagnosed antenatally. The resulting kidney is non-functioning and contains multiple non-communicating cysts of varying sizes, separated by hyperechoic "dysplastic" renal parenchyma (Fig. 9.20A).[33]

MCDK is usually unilateral and is considered a benign condition, although there is a slight risk of malignancy and hypertension in later life. A DMSA scan differentiates a non-functioning MCDK from a grossly hydronephrotic kidney, and this distinction cannot always be reliably made on US. The contralateral kidney should be closely examined in MCDK because of a 33% risk of associated renal abnormalities, including ureterocele, VUR, or PUJ obstruction. Serial US are performed to ensure the involution of the affected kidney, as there is a slight increased risk of Wilms tumor and to monitor the growth of the contralateral kidney (Fig. 9.20B, C).[27,33,34]

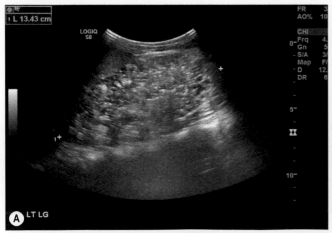 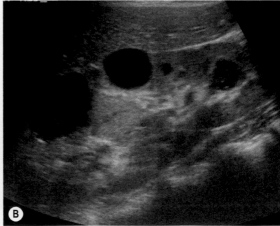

Fig. 9.19 (A) Large hyperechoic kidney due to autosomal recessive polycystic kidney disease. (B) Frank cysts seen in the kidneys of a 10-year-old girl with autosomal dominant polycystic kidney disease.

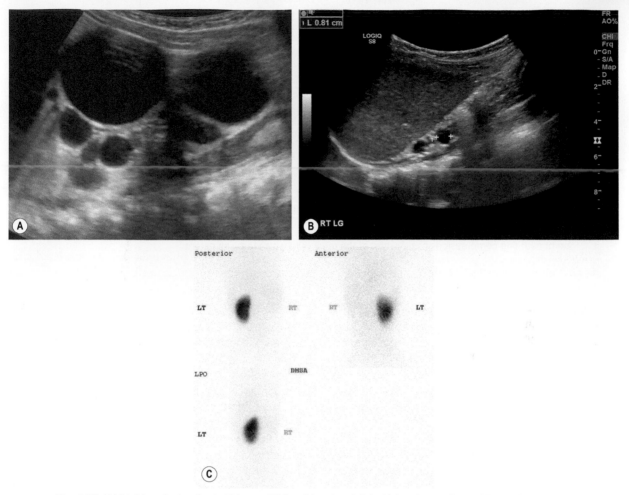

Fig. 9.20 (A) Multicystic dysplastic kidneys. (B) Small involuted right kidney in a patient with multicystic dysplastic kidney. (C) Dimercapto succinic acid scan, right multicystic dysplastic kidney with no functioning renal tissue, and left hydronephrotic kidney with scarring.

MALIGNANT RENAL TUMORS

Two common tumors present in childhood: nephroblastoma, commonly known as a Wilms tumor, and neuroblastoma. The natural histories and clinical courses of these two tumors are very different, and US is often the primary investigation for children with an abdominal mass, a common presenting feature in both tumors.

Nephroblastoma (Wilms Tumor)

A Wilms tumor is an embryonic type of renal cancer and the most common malignant mass in children, accounting for 90% of all pediatric malignant renal masses, with 80% of children presenting before the age of five years.[27,35,36] Patients usually present with a large, painless abdominal mass and are frequently otherwise well. Wilms tumors are usually unilateral, but in 10% of cases, there is bilateral or multifocal disease that may present at an earlier age. The ultrasound appearances of a Wilms tumor are of a large, well-defined heterogeneous mass, which often replaces the whole of the affected kidney. The mass is typically heterogeneous in echotexture containing cysts and large hypoechoic areas because of central necrosis and hyperechoic areas (Fig. 9.21A–B).[35]

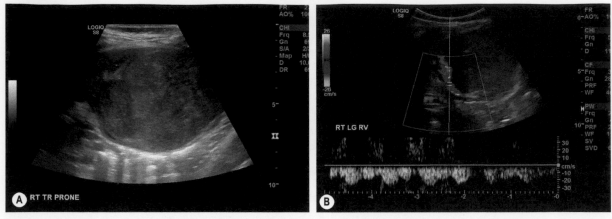

Fig. 9.21 (A) Large heterogeneous mass in the right kidney – Wilms tumor. (B) Right kidney with Wilms tumor demonstrating compression and deviation of the renal vein, which remains patent.

In contrast to neuroblastoma, Wilms tumors often cause displacement, rather than encasement, of major blood vessels, with vascular invasion in approximately 5%–10% of cases, so the renal vein and IVC should be assessed with Doppler. IVC tumor thrombus extension occurs in 4% of cases, which may extend into the heart. Wilms tumors commonly metastasize to the lungs, so a chest radiograph is normally required.[35]

Wilms tumors are usually sporadic occurrences, but there are predisposing conditions that have a higher risk of developing a tumor, including hemihypertrophy, sporadic aniridia, and the following syndromes: Beckwith–Wiedemann; Denys-Drash; and Wilms tumor, aniridia, genitourinary, and range of development delays (WAGR); these children will require regular US screening.[27]

Neuroblastoma

Neuroblastoma are located within the adrenal gland but can also be found in the retroperitoneum, posterior mediastinum, neck, or pelvis. Neuroblastoma occur in early childhood, with up to 90% diagnosed by six years of age, with a slightly higher incidence in Caucasians. They are often metastatic at diagnosis and frequently present in an unwell child. The heterogeneity of the tumor, and its biological characteristics, mean the prognosis is highly variable at different ages. Some tumors are very aggressive, while others, typically in infancy, may spontaneously regress.[35]

Neuroblastomas are usually large on presentation, displacing the kidney downwards and laterally invading the adjacent kidney, making it difficult to distinguish from a Wilms tumor. They are predominantly solid on ultrasound, heterogeneous in echotexture, frequently contain calcification, and rarely appear cystic. Neuroblastoma tumor margins are ill-defined and, unlike a Wilms tumor, tend to encase rather than invade vascular structures (Fig. 9.22A, B). Lymphadenopathy is common with nodes surrounding and elevating the aorta and IVC (Fig. 9.23).[35]

Contrast MRI of the abdomen and pelvis is recommended for disease staging with preoperative CT prior to surgery. MRI Apparent Diffusion Coefficient (ADC) mapping has the potential to provide additional information for optimal treatment management. Nuclear medicine examinations, including bone scintigraphy and metaiodobenzylguanidine (MIBG) scans are also useful in demonstrating metastases.[36]

Role of US in the Assessment of Renal Tumors

- Confirm the presence and size of a primary abdominal mass, providing an estimate if very large.
- Determine, if possible, if the mass is extra- or intrarenal in location.
- Describe the ultrasound appearances of the mass.
- Confirm the presence of a normal, non-obstructed contralateral kidney and assessment of the urinary bladder.

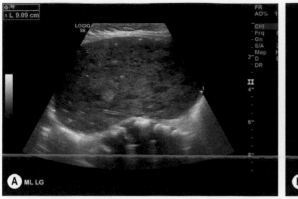
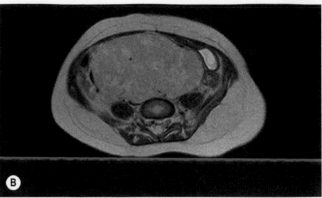

Fig. 9.22 (A) Ultrasound of a large midline abdominal mass with neuroblastoma. (B) Magnetic resonance imaging of same patient – neuroblastoma.

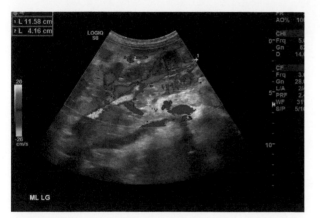

Fig. 9.23 Midline longitudinal image of midline lymphadeonapthy.

- Determine, if possible, the patency of the affected main renal artery and vein.
- Assess the IVC for the presence of tumor thrombus.
- Check the abdomen and pelvis for liver metastatic disease, lymphadenopathy, and the presence of ascites.

RENAL TRACT DILATATION

Postnatal Renal Dilatation

Antenatal hydronephrosis is a common US finding which can lead to renal complications, so early diagnosis is essential. However, many cases detected antenatally will spontaneously resolve with observation, so there is a risk of unnecessary investigations and medical follow-up. The challenge is to predict the children diagnosed antenatally who would benefit from further diagnostic

imaging, including US and corrective surgery, before they develop potentially irreversible renal damage.[37,38]

Postnatal US can assist in identifying the cause of renal dilatation, which can be from obstructive or non-obstructive causes.[38]

Obstructive Uropathy

- VUJ (Vesicoureteric Junction)
- PUJ (Pelvi-ureteric Junction Obstruction)
- PUV (Posterior Urethral Valve Obstruction)
- Obstructed upper moiety of a duplex kidney +/− ureterocele

Non-Obstructive Uropathy

- Urinary reflux

Ideally, the ultrasound examination should be performed two to three days after birth, unless there is severe dilatation, as dehydration can cause an obstructed/dilated kidney to appear normal. A follow-up US at six weeks is generally recommended even if the initial US is normal. A dilated renal tract is predisposed to infection because of ascending infection in reflux or hematogenous infection in an obstructed system, where a pyonephrosis requiring percutaneous nephrostomy may develop. Therefore, consider changing to prophylactic antibiotics in neonates with significant renal tract dilatation (Fig. 9.24A–B).[39]

Vesicoureteric Reflux

Vesicoureteric reflux (VUR) is defined as the retrograde flow of urine from the bladder up the ureter and into the renal pelvis. It can be unilateral or bilateral and graded

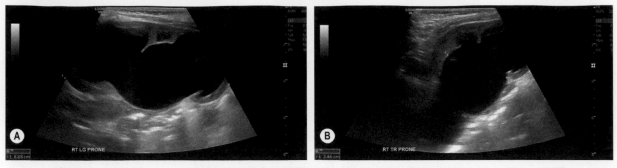

Fig. 9.24 (A) PUJ obstruction in the right kidney. LS demonstrating urinary debris. (B) PUJ obstruction with TS renal pelvis APD measurement and urinary debris.

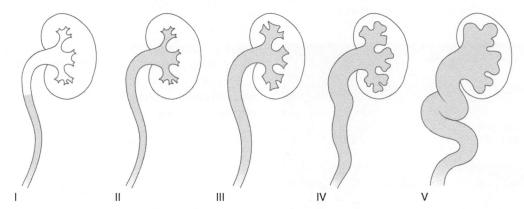

Diagram 9.1 Vesicoureteric Reflux Grading System. (Source: From Lebowitz RL, Olbing H, Parkkulainen KV, et al. International reflux study in children: international system of radiographic grading of vesicoureteral reflux: International Reflux Study in Children. *Pediatr Radiol.* 1985;15:105.)

in severity from I to V using the International Reflux Study in Children.

Grade I indicates reflux of urine into part of the ureter. Grade V indicates gross dilatation and tortuosity of the ureter and renal pelvis, with blunting of the calyces (Diagram 9.1).

VUR is common in the first year of life and often resolves spontaneously, suggesting VUR is a physiological phenomenon in many children. However, VUR is associated with UTIs, with a reported incidence rate of 8%–40% of children investigated for a first UTI, and 59% of children with confirmed VUR on MCUG had at least one scarred kidney.[40] VUR has a genetic basis affecting identical twins in almost 100% of cases and has a 27% prevalence in siblings.[30,41]

The use of prophylactic antibiotics in cases of VUR may reduce the incidence of UTI and associated reflux neuropathy but has side effects and may increase

microbial resistance. A normal US does not exclude high-grade VUR; an MCUG or contrast-enhanced voiding sonography is required for a definitive diagnosis, and the most reliable method of scar detection is a DMSA scan, all of which are invasive tests. The challenge remains in trying to identify children with high-grade VUR with the risk of UTIs and associated reflux nephropathy without subjecting children to unnecessary diagnostic examinations and prophylactic treatment.[30,40]

High-grade VUR is associated with further urological malformations, including a developmental anomaly at the vesicoureteric junction, a neurogenic bladder, partial outlet obstruction, or calculi, so a detailed US examination is vital.[41] Fig. 9.25A–C demonstrate multiple renal calculi and significant urinary bladder debris. Postoperative kidney with a stent *in situ* demonstrates abnormal renal parenchyma (Box 9.1).

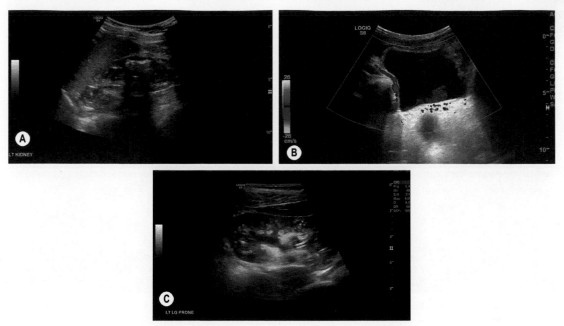

Fig. 9.25 (A) Multiple echogenic renal calculi with posterior acoustic shadowing. (B) Bladder containing urinary debris. (C) Postoperative image of kidney post calculi removal demonstrating stent in the renal pelvis and abnormal renal parenchyma.

BOX 9.1 Conditions Associated with Urinary Tract infection

- Vesicoureteric reflux
- Obstruction
  - Pelviureteric junction
  - Vesicoureteric junction
  - PUV
  - Duplex kidney with obstructed moiety/ectopic ureter
  - Ureterocele
- Other structural anomalies
  - Duplex and/or ectopic renal anatomy
  - Multicystic dysplastic kidneys
  - Prune belly syndrome
- Calculi
- Neurogenic bladder

BOX 9.2 Pediatric Abdominal Malignancies

- Neuroblastoma
- Wilms tumor
- Hepatoblastoma
- Hepatocellular carcinoma
- Rhabdomyosarcoma
- Leukemia
- Lymphoma

BOX 9.3 Abdominal Fluid-filled Masses in Pediatrics – Differential Diagnoses

- Choledochal cyst
- Mesenteric cyst
- Duplication cyst
- Hepatic cyst
- Pancreatic pseudocyst
- Epidermoid cyst of the spleen
- Lymphangioma
- Ovarian cyst
- Encysted fluid associated with ventriculoperitoneal shunt tubing
- Renal cyst or renal dilatation
- Cystic renal tumor

GASTROINTESTINAL TRACT

Congenital Abnormalities

Intestinal Malrotation and Volvulus

Intestinal malrotation occurs when the midgut fails to undergo the normal rotation around the axis of the superior mesenteric artery (SMA) during fetal development. Obstructing Ladd's bands are associated with malrotation and the cecum abnormally sited in the RUQ.

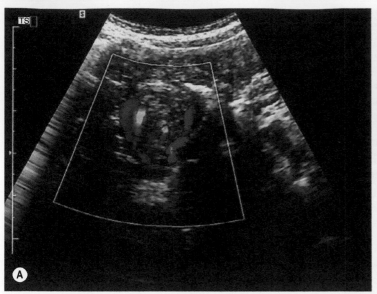
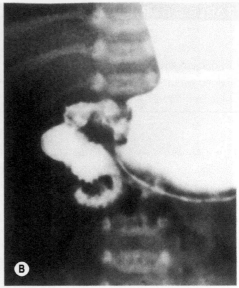

Fig. 9.26 Volvulus. (A) Mesentery and superior mesenteric vein are twisted around the superior mesenteric artery, which is seen in the cross-section at the center of the film. (B) Barium meal shows corkscrewing of the duodenum away from the midline, consistent with malrotation and volvulus. (By kind permission of Dr. Delia Martinez, Leeds.)

Early diagnosis is important, as malrotation can rapidly develop into volvulus, a life-threatening emergency because of obstruction caused by twisting (volving) of the small bowel resulting in bowel obstruction, vascular ischemia, and necrosis of most of the small bowel.[42] Clinical presentation symptoms of midgut volvulus are acute abdominal pain and bile-stained vomiting with a flat nondistended abdomen. Most neonates usually present within seven days of birth and up to 80% within the first month of life.[42,43]

US Signs of Malrotation +/− Volvulus

Some authors advocate instilling 50 mL of distilled water via a nasogastric tube to dispel air within the bowel and evaluate for dilatation and bowel wall edema.[42,43]

- In cases of malrotation, the normal relationship of the superior mesenteric vein (SMV) to the SMA is reversed, with the SMV lying anteriorly and/or to the left of the SMA.
- "Whirlpool sign" with the SMV winding around the SMA – there may be a small bowel mass in this area.
- Dilatation of distal SMV compared to proximal.
- A dilated, fluid-filled duodenum with distal tapering (may be difficult to visualize because of gas).
- The duodenal jejunal flexure may be lower and in a more medial position than is normal.

- Duodenal wall thickness greater than 2 mm (when duodenum fluid-filled).
- Presence of ascites.

Diagnosis on US can be limited because of gaseous bowel, so fluoroscopic contrast examinations of the gastrointestinal (GI) tract or CT and MRI are required to confirm malrotation +/− volvulus (Fig. 9.26A–B).[44,45]

ACQUIRED DISORDERS

Infantile Hypertrophic Pyloric Stenosis (IHPS)

IHPS has a peak occurrence of six weeks of age with a male-to-female prevalence of 4:1.[46] IHPS occurs when the pyloric muscle becomes hypertrophied and elongated, restricting the passage of gastric contents, causing obstruction and prolonged projectile vomiting. US has been so successful in demonstrating IHPS that clinical skills have declined, so US is now routinely used to make a definitive diagnosis of IHPS with a reported sensitivity of 98% and specificity of 100%.[46]

IHPS diagnostic features:

- Thickened and elongated pyloric muscle
- Increased but ineffective peristalsis
- Failure of the pylorus to relax and open (Table 9.5)

Measurements of canal length and muscle thickness can support the ultrasonographic diagnosis of

TABLE 9.5	**Pyloric Muscle Dimensions**	
	Normal Pylorus	Hypertrophic Pyloric Stenosis
Pyloric length	<15 mm	≥16 mm
Pyloric width	<11 mm	≥11 mm
Muscle thickness	<2.5 mm	≥3 mm

IHPS. However, measurements can be low in cases of dehydration and prematurity. The US examination should be repeated post-hydration in cases with borderline measurements or persistent non-bilious vomiting to exclude evolving pyloric stenosis.[46,47]

Tips for Ultrasound Examination of the Pylorus

It must be stressed that the examination of the pylorus is a dynamic examination performed in real-time. The infant should be fasted for 3 h prior to examination for improved visualization of the pylorus, and a sterile dummy and sucrose solution can soothe a hungry fractious baby, improving image quality.

- The baby lies in the right posterior oblique position, encouraging gastric emptying and displacing air, and examination performed using a high-frequency linear probe.

- Scan the epigastrium in the transverse plane; the pylorus is usually medial to the GB.
- Rotate the transducer into the sagittal oblique plane to achieve a long axis of the pylorus and assess. Rotate the probe through 90 degrees to view the pylorus in transverse – target sign.
- A dynamic assessment of the pylorus should be undertaken after 15 mL of dioralyte/sterile water, administered orally/via a nasogastric tube to aid visualization of the gastric antrum to observe pyloric function. The pylorus is observed in real time.
- Pyloric stenosis can be excluded if the pylorus is of normal caliber and seen to relax with gastric contents moving freely into the duodenum.
- It can take 15–20 min for the delayed opening of the pyloric muscle, so focus on the pylorus initially. If the pylorus is not seen to open, examine the remaining abdomen, returning to the pylorus at regular intervals.
- If the examination is negative for pyloric stenosis, other causes for vomiting should be assessed, so a full abdominal examination should be performed with an assessment of the SMV/SMA axis for malrotation.
- If pyloric stenosis is confirmed, then a focused assessment of both kidneys should be made for any associated hydronephrosis or renal abnormalities (Fig. 9.27A–E).

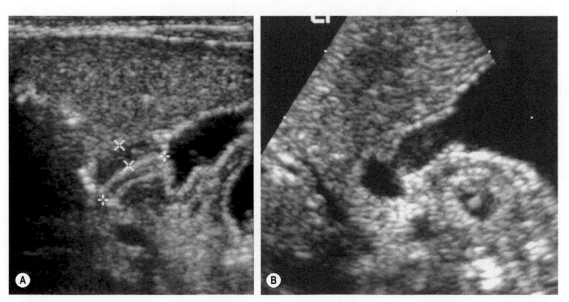

Fig. 9.27 Hypertrophic pyloric stenosis. (A) Normal pylorus demonstrating measurement of the length of the pyloric canal and thickness of the muscle. (B) A few minutes later, the pylorus relaxed and opened widely, excluding the diagnosis of hypertrophic pyloric stenosis.

Continued

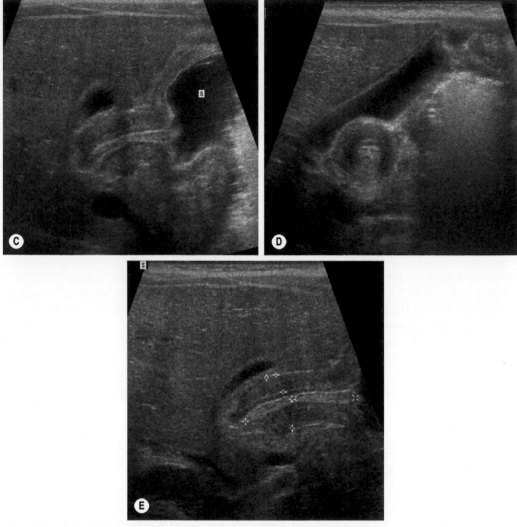

Fig. 9.27, cont'd (C) Thickened and elongated pylorus of hypertrophic pyloric stenosis seen in longitudinal section. S represents a fluid-filled stomach. (D) TS view of the thickened pylorus. (E) Demonstrates the measurements of pyloric length, muscle thickness, and pyloric width.

Intussusception

Intussusception is a common cause of acute abdominal pain in young children between three months and three years of age, with a peak incidence at five to six months and a male-to-female prevalence of 2:1.[48] The classic triad of symptoms associated is drawing up legs and crying because of colicky abdominal pain, bloody "redcurrant jelly–like" stool, and a palpable abdominal mass. However, less than 50% of affected infants present with all three symptoms, and there is significant overlap with other acute abdominal conditions.[48,49]

Intussusception occurs when a segment of the bowel (the intussusceptum) telescopes into an adjacent segment (the intussuscipiens). Secondary intussusception occurs in the presence of a pathological "lead point," and this occurs in 57% of intussusceptions in children over four years of age.[48] Early diagnosis of intussusception is essential as it can progress to to ischemia, bowel necrosis, perforation, and peritonitis.[49] Over 80% of idiopathic intussusceptions occur in the ileocecal region. US is the primary investigation for intussusception, with high sensitivity (>90%) and specificity (>90%) when performed by a trained operator,[48,49] replacing

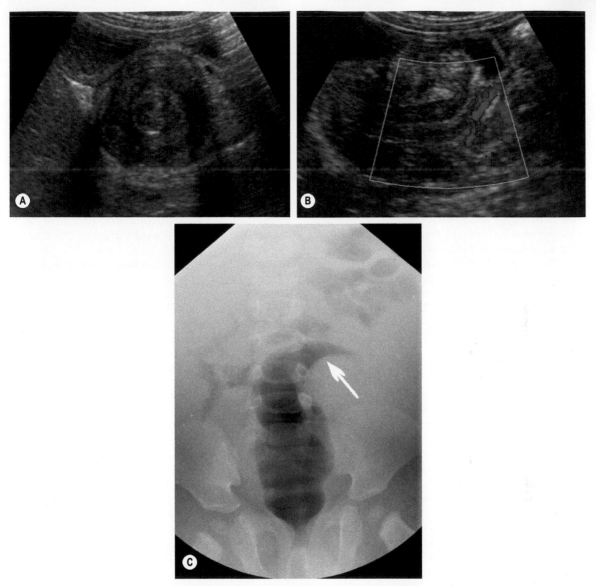

Fig. 9.28 Intussusception. (A) The characteristic "doughnut" appearance of bowel within bowel because of an intussusception. (B) Color Doppler demonstrates blood flow within the intussuscepted bowel, and dilated fluid-filled loops of obstructed bowel are seen proximal to it. (C) Air enema; the intussusception is seen indenting into the lumen of the air-filled sigmoid colon during a successful air enema reduction (arrow).

the fluoroscopic contrast enema. An abdominal radiograph is not sensitive for diagnosing intussusception but may be used to assess features of intestinal obstruction or perforation. CT/MRI are used in cases of a suspected pathological lead point or in atypical or recurrent cases.[48]

The ultrasound appearances of bowel within bowel are characteristic. In cross-section, the bowel assumes a "doughnut" or target sign, with concentric rings of

the bowel wall and the "pseudo kidney sign" when it is seen on the longitudinal section (Fig. 9.28 A–C). Dilated loops of fluid-filled, obstructed bowel may be demonstrated proximal to the intussusception.

In approximately 20% of cases, spontaneous reduction of intussusception occurs without treatment.[48] In the United Kingdom, 95% of intussusception reductions are performed with a non-operative air enema reduction under fluoroscopy control.[48]

REFERENCES

1. Chavhan GB, Parra DA, Mann A, Navarro OM. Normal Doppler spectral waveforms of major pediatric vessels: specific patterns. *Radiographics*. 2008;28(3):691–706.

2. Back SJ, Maya CL, Khwaja A. Ultrasound of congenital and inherited disorders of the pediatric hepatobiliary system, pancreas and spleen. *Pediatric Radiol*. 2017;47:1069–1078.

3. Shamir SB, Kurian J, Kogan-Liberman D, Taragin BH. Hepatic imaging in neonates and young infants: state of the art. *Radiol*. 2017;285:763–777.

4. Tulin-Silver S, Babb J, Pinkney L, et al. The challenging ultrasound diagnosis of perforated appendicitis in children: constellations of sonographic findings improve specificity. *Pediatric Radiol*. 2015;45:820–830.

5. Di MS, Severino R, Gioioso M, et al. Paediatric liver ultrasound: a pictorial essay. *J Ultrasound*. 2019.

6. Fidan N, Yetis EU, Murat M, Yucesoy C, Turgal E, Metin M. Is the presence of echo-rich periportal cuffing in the liver indicator for abdominal inflammation in pediatric patients? *Med Ultrason*. 2019;21:225–231.

7. Kelly D, Sharif K, Hartley J, eds. *Atlas of pediatric hepatology* (Chapter 4: The child with abdominal distension by Khalid Shah). Springer; 2018.

8. Zhou L, Shan Q, Tian W, Wang Z, Liang J, Xie X. Ultrasound for the diagnosis of biliary atresia: a meta-analysis. *Am J Roentgenol*. 2016;206:W73–W82.

9. Götze T, Blessing H, Grillhösl C, Gerner P, Hoerning A. Neonatal cholestasis–differential diagnoses, current diagnostic procedures, and treatment. *Front Pediatr*. 2015;3:43.

10. Shamir SB, Kurian J, Kogan-Liberman D, Taragin BH. Hepatic imaging in neonates and young infants: state of the art. *Radiol*. 2017;285:763–777.

11. Mittal V, Saxena AK, Sodhi KS, et al. Role of abdominal sonography in the preoperative diagnosis of extrahepatic biliary atresia in infants younger than 90 days. *Am J Roentgenol*. 2011;196:W438–W445.

12. Todani T, Watanabe Y, Narusue M, Tabuchi K, Okajima K. Congenital bile duct cysts: classification, operative procedures, and review of thirty-seven cases including cancer arising from choledochal cyst. *Am J Surg*. 1977;134:263–269.

13. Gillespie CD, O'Reilly MK, Allen GN, McDermott S, Chan VO, Ridge CA. Imaging the abdominal manifestations of cystic fibrosis. *Int J Hepatol*. 2017;5128760.

14. Lavelle LP, McEvoy SH, Ni Mhurchu E, et al. Cystic fibrosis below the diaphragm: abdominal findings in adult patients. *Radiographics*. 2015;35:680–695.

15. van Mourik ID. Liver disease in cystic fibrosis. *Paediatr Child Health*. 2017;27(12):552–555.

16. Iacobas I, Phung TL, Adams DM, et al. Guidance document for hepatic hemangioma (infantile and congenital) evaluation and monitoring. *J Pediatr*. 2018;203:294–300.e2.

17. Thyagarajan MS, Sharif K. Space occupying lesions in the liver. *Indian J Pediatr*. 2016;83:1291–1302.

18. Chung EM, Lattin Jr GE, Cube R, et al. From the archives of the AFIP: pediatric liver masses: radiologic-pathologic correlation part 2. Malignant tumors. *Radiographics*. 2011;31:483–507.

19. Di Serafino M, Severino R, Gioioso M, et al. Paediatric liver ultrasound: a pictorial essay. *J Ultrasound*. 2020;23:87–103.

20. De Bruyn R, Darge K. *Pediatric Ultrasound, How, Why and When*. 3rd edn. Elsevier; 2016.

21. Rosenbaum DM, Korngold E, Teele RL. Sonographic assessment of renal length in normal children. *Am J Roentgenol*. 1984;142:467–469.

22. Chen JJ, Mao W, Rongviriyapanich C, Luisiri A, Steinhardt GF. A multivariable assessment of renal size and growth of scarred kidneys in children. *J Urol*. 2005;174:2358–2362.

23. Spira EM, Jacobi C, Frankenschmidt A, Pohl M, von Schnakenburg C. Sonographic long-term study: paediatric growth charts for single kidneys. *Arch Disease Childhood*. 2009;94:693–698.

24. Hemachandar R, Boopathy V. Transient renal medullary hyperechogenicity in a term neonate. *BMJ Case Rep*. 2015. bcr2015211285.

25. Westland R, Schreuder MF, Ket JC, van Wijk JA. Unilateral renal agenesis: a systematic review on associated anomalies and renal injury. *Nephrol Dialysis Transplant*. 2013;28:1844–1855.

26. Kirkpatrick JJ, Leslie SW. *Horseshoe kidney*. Treasure Island (FL): StatPearls Publishing; 2020. Available at: https://www.ncbi.nlm.nih.gov/books/NBK431105/.

27. Paliwalla M, Park K. A practical guide to urinary tract ultrasound in a child: pearls and pitfalls. *Ultrasound*. 2014;22:213–222.

28. Doery AJ, Ang E, Ditchfield MR. Duplex kidney: not just a drooping lily. *J Med Imaging Radiation Oncol*. 2015;59:149–153.

29. Chao TT, Dashe JS. Duplicated collecting system. In: *Obstetric imaging: fetal diagnosis and care*. Elsevier; 2018:50–53.

30. Diamond DA, Chan IH, Holland AJ, et al. Advances in paediatric urology. *Lancet*. 2017;390:1061–1071.

31. Deshpande AV. Current strategies to predict and manage sequelae of posterior urethral valves in children. *Pediatr Nephrol*. 2018;33:1651–1661.

32. Duran C, Beltrán VP, González A, Gómez C, Riego JD. Contrast-enhanced voiding urosonography for vesicoureteral reflux diagnosis in children. *Radiographics*. 2017;37:1854–1869.

33. Chang A, Sivananthan D, Nataraja R, Johnstone L, Webb N, Lopez PJ. Evidence-based treatment of multicystic dysplastic kidney: a systematic review. *J Pediatric Urol*. 2018.

34. Bergmann C. ARPKD and early manifestations of ADPKD: the original polycystic kidney disease and phenocopies. *Pediatr Nephrol*. 2015;30:15–30.

35. Dumba M, Jawad N, McHugh K. Neuroblastoma and nephroblastoma: a radiological review. *Cancer Imaging*. 2015;15:5.

36. Szychot E, Apps J, Pritchard-Jones K. Wilms' tumor: biology, diagnosis and treatment. *Transl Pediatr*. 2014;3:12–24.

37. Capolicchio JP, Braga LH, Szymanski KM. Canadian Urological Association/Pediatric Urologists of Canada guideline on the investigation and management of antenatally detected hydronephrosis. *Can Urol Assoc J*. 2018;12:85.

38. Babu R, Venkatachalapathy E, Sai V. Hydronephrosis severity score: an objective assessment of hydronephrosis severity in children—a preliminary report. *J Pediatric Urol*. 2019;15:68–e1.

39. National Institute for Health and Care Excellence CG54. *Urinary tract infection in children: diagnosis, treatment and long term management*. London: National Institute for Health and Care Excellence; 2007.

40. Larcombe J. Urinary tract infection in children: recurrent infections. *BMJ Clin Evidence*. 2015;2015.

41. Tullus K. Vesicoureteric reflux in children. *Lancet*. 2015;385:371–379.

42. Chao HC, Kong MS, Chen JY, Lin SJ, Lin JN. Sonographic features related to volvulus in neonatal intestinal malrotation. *J Ultrasound Med*. 2000;19:371–376.

43. Zhang W, Sun H, Luo F. The efficiency of sonography in diagnosing volvulus in neonates with suspected intestinal malrotation. *Medicine (Baltimore)*. 2017;96.

44. Daneman A. Malrotation: the balance of evidence. *Pediatr Radiol*. 2009;39:164.

45. Gómiz EB, Ayats AT, Feliubadaló CD, Martínez CM, Tarragó AC. Intestinal malrotation–volvulus: imaging findings. *Radiología*. 2015;57:9–21.

46. Niedzielski J, Kobielski A, Sokal J, Krakós M. Accuracy of sonographic criteria in the decision for surgical treatment in infantile hypertrophic pyloric stenosis. *Arch Med Sci*. 2011;7:508.

47. Dias SC, Swinson S, Torrão H, et al. Hypertrophic pyloric stenosis: tips and tricks for ultrasound diagnosis. *Insights Imaging*. 2012;3:247–250.

48. Bradshaw CJ, Johnson PRV. Intussusception *Surg (Oxf)*. 2019;37:216–220.

49. Edwards EA, Pigg N, Courtier J, Zapala MA, MacKenzie JD, Phelps AS. Intussusception: past, present and future. *Pediatric Radiol*. 2017;47:1101–1108.

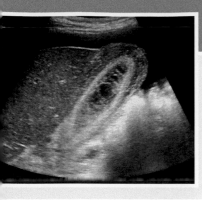

10

Ultrasound of the Acute Abdomen

Nicola J. Davidson

CHAPTER OUTLINE

Introduction, 321
Trauma, 322
  Focused Assessment of Sonography in Trauma (FAST), 322
  Performing Fast Scan, 323
    Scan 1. Right Upper Quadrant (RUQ), 323
    Scan 2. Left Upper Quadrant (LUQ), 324
    Scan 3. Pelvis, 324
    Scan 4. Pericardial Subcostal/Subxiphoid, 324
    Scan 5. Pleura, 324

  Free Fluid, 325
  Visceral Rupture, 327
Gastrointestinal Tract, 328
Hepatobiliary Emergencies, 328
The Acute Pancreas, 329
Renal Tract Emergencies, 330
Other Retroperitoneal Emergencies, 331
References, 331

INTRODUCTION

In many circumstances, ultrasound may be used as a first-line investigation assessing and triaging patients who attend with acute abdominal pain. Ultrasound examinations and scans should only be performed by those trained to do so, and operators should only perform scans that fall within their scope of practice. As ultrasound machines become more accessible, it can be tempting to pick up the probe and scan; however, this should be done with caution as in inexperienced hands vital "clues" can be missed, and there is a tendency for false negatives and positives which could delay management of the patient.

The introduction of smaller, portable, and hand-held ultrasound machines has greatly increased the accessibility of ultrasound. Over the last two decades, there has been an increase in clinicians using point-of-care ultrasound (POCUS) to help in the management of patients and in the emergency setting. There are now ultrasound

devices on the market that consist of a probe that contains all of the software required to be plugged into a mobile phone or tablet and provide scans of good quality. While the resolution may not be suitable for diagnosing small lesions within the liver or characterizing a renal cyst, they provide imaging that is more than sufficient for diagnosing hydronephrosis or pools of free fluid within the abdomen. There are also "portable" machines that are easily maneuvered to allow scans to be performed on wards and emergency departments. These machines are now of a high standard as the improvements in ultrasound technology are developing but tend to have fewer functions than the higher specification machines used within a radiology department.

Computed tomography (CT) has become increasingly accessible in most hospitals and many will place CT as an integral part of the diagnosis and management of the patient. This means that trauma victims with multiple injuries are often best served by immediate CT scanning, where a comprehensive report on all injuries related to the trauma can be provided. This allows the medical team to be aware of all potential injuries and will allow them to prioritize those which are most likely to impact the patients' well-being. While ultrasound may have a role in the triaging of patients where there are multiple casualties or monitoring of patients, there is now acceptance that ultrasound should not delay the transfer to CT for imaging. However, CT does incorporate the risk to the patient from the radiation dose, and this must be carefully balanced by the potential benefit of the investigation. In non-trauma cases, women with gynecological symptoms/pain, some pediatrics, and the acutely ill or unstable patients are likely to benefit from an ultrasound examination by a trained practitioner with good quality equipment.

Ultrasound examinations should always be performed by a trained practitioner. Whether it be as part of medical training, postgraduate course, or in-house, there should be the opportunity for an individual to gain competency in the area of ultrasound they are performing. In 2010, the Royal College of Emergency Medicine introduced POCUS as a mandatory component of emergency medicine training. This includes Focused Assessment of Sonography in Trauma (FAST), assessment of the abdominal aorta for suspected aneurysm, focused echocardiography in life support and training in ultrasound guided vascular access. General physics principles and the governance aspects surrounding performing POCUS are also included in the mandatory training. Following review by the National Patient Safety Agency requiring the use of ultrasound in pleural procedures, specific components were also included in the training of respiratory physicians several years later. The Royal College of Radiologists recognizes that other specialties are keen to undertake ultrasound as part of their clinical examination and have stated that all training should be conducted by an experienced individual. The minimum requirements for training would include that the examination needs to be performed safely and accurately. Trainees need to be able to recognize normal anatomy and pathology, diagnose the common abnormalities associated with the area being scanned, and recognize when a second opinion is required. The limited number of POCUS-trained individuals in the United Kingdom is largely due to the lack of trained supervisors/trainers.[1]

Due to the nature of ultrasound being a dynamic examination and the benefit of "real-time" imaging, it is extremely useful to the practitioner performing the scan. The ability to take a comprehensive clinical history from the patient, and the patient to interact with the scan, by directing the practitioner to the location of pain or site of palpable mass can often help build the clinical picture and context. A positive Murphy's sign in a patient with suspected cholecystitis or being able to scan at the point of maximum tenderness in suspected appendicitis can often help with confidence in the diagnosis or help the practitioner assess further if they feel the clinical question has not been answered.

TRAUMA

Internal organ injury resulting from trauma is extremely difficult to assess clinically, especially as many patients are admitted unconscious or in a highly unstable condition. Such trauma patients may require emergency laparotomy, and ultrasound may help in triaging these patients. CT has the advantage of being able to recognize other injuries which may be present, such as bony, spinal, or retroperitoneal trauma which may not be accessible to ultrasound investigation and is often the first choice for imaging in multiple injury trauma patients.

Focused Assessment of Sonography in Trauma (FAST)

FAST has become widely adopted in many trauma centers and is intended as a limited, directed examination designed to answer a specific clinical question, usually whether free fluid is present (Box 10.1). Indications for performing FAST examination include trauma in pregnancy, penetrating trauma, blunt trauma, and unexplained hypotension. Around 12% of blunt trauma will result in intraperitoneal hemorrhage,[2] and if left untreated, death due to hypovolemic shock is a possibility. Therefore, rapid access to diagnostic testing is important to detect signs early to prevent deterioration. Historically this would have been done by diagnostic peritoneal lavage where a needle is inserted into the abdomen between the umbilicus and symphysis pubis and aspiration performed to look for frank hemorrhage. If none is seen, saline is injected into the peritoneal cavity via a catheter, then re-drained several minutes later. This sample can then be sent for analysis to look for smaller quantities of blood. Since ultrasound machines have become more readily available and provide a quick result with no requirement for invasive technique, the use of ultrasound in trauma situations has increased.

The results are highly dependent on proper training, and a number of standardized training and accreditation programs have been devised. Scan protocols can ensure a repeatable technique that is reproducible between operators. FAST scanning involves a minimum four-view examination, principally to detect the presence of hemoperitoneum and hemopericardium, which may result from the rupture of internal organs. Numerous studies have demonstrated sensitivities between 85% to 96% and specificities exceeding 98%.[3] The four-view scan should include the right and left flanks (for hepatorenal space, perisplenic regions, and spaces above and below the

diaphragm), the subcostal region (to include the pericardial space), and the pelvis (retrovesical and retrouterine spaces) (Fig. 10.1).[4] An additional fifth view can be included to assess the pleura. In experienced hands, this scan can be performed in less than 5 min, making this an extremely quick and useful tool.

Performing FAST Scan

A standard curvilinear probe can be used to perform a FAST scan. A phased array probe may be useful in some cases as this has a smaller footprint, improving visualization intercostally. The patient needs to be in a supine position. This will ensure that any free fluid present will "pool" in the anatomical locations the user is trained to inspect. When starting to scan, ensure that a standard abdominal preset is selected. This will optimize the settings for assessing the abdomen. The depth, focus, and gain settings can then be manipulated by the operator to improve image quality.

Scan 1. Right Upper Quadrant (RUQ)

Place the probe in the right mid-axillary line and adjust until the probe sits parallel to the ribs roughly level with the xiphisternum (Fig. 10.1). The probe can be moved in a cephalic/caudal manner until the appropriate view is obtained.

On this view, the hepto-renal interface needs to be visualized. This is sometimes referred to as a Morrison's

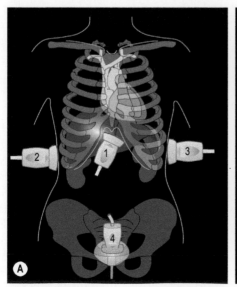
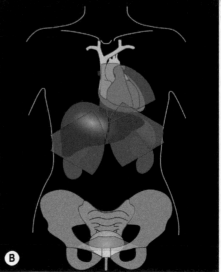

Fig. 10.1 The basic focused assessment of sonography in trauma scan: (A) subcostal (1), upper right quadrant (2), upper left quadrant (3), and pelvic (4). (B) The ultrasound planes. (Source: Critical Care Ultrasound Manual, 2013.)

pouch. Free fluid noted in this space would indicate a positive FAST scan in the presence of trauma. Once this view is obtained, slide the probe cephalically to assess the subphrenic space for free fluid. Then scan caudally to assess the lower pole of the kidney and paracolic gutter.

Scan 2. Left Upper Quadrant (LUQ)

Place the probe in the left mid-axillary line, level with the xiphisternum (Fig. 10.1). It will be positioned slightly higher than the right side, as the spleen is usually much smaller than the liver, resulting in the kidney being positioned slightly higher in the abdomen. Again, rotate the probe slightly until parallel with the ribs. If you are struggling with this view due to rib shadowing, the smaller footprint of a phased array probe can often be useful. Ensure that the entire spleen is visualized, looking specifically at the interfaces with the diaphragm, left kidney, and lower pole of the left kidney/paracolic gutter.

Scan 3. Pelvis

The probe is now moved to the pelvis, which must be assessed in both transverse and longitudinal planes. First, place the probe with the heel against the symphysis pubis in the midline to obtain a longitudinal view (Fig. 10.1). Identify the bladder; this should be thin-walled and anechoic when full. Place the focus posteriorly to the bladder and, where appropriate, look for the uterus; once visualized look posteriorly to the uterus for free fluid (pouch of Douglas). This can sometimes be difficult when the uterus is retroverted. It is important to remember that a small amount of free fluid in the pelvis in a young person may be a normal finding as part of ovulation. It is important to question patients about their menstrual cycle and the possibility of being pregnant to rule out a false positive scan including in transgender patients where ovaries and uterus may remain in situ. In a male patient, the prostate will often be visualized at the bladder base. Scan into both iliac fossa to assess for free fluid and then return to the midline and turn the probe 90 degrees, so that the probe is now in a transverse position; repeat assessment of the pouch of Douglas if applicable and also both iliac fossae. If there is a possible gynecological concern, a transvaginal scan should be requested to assess the uterus and ovaries in more detail.

> **TIP BOX**
>
> If the pelvic organs are obscured by the bowel, then fill the patient's bladder. This will push the bowel laterally and give an acoustic window to improve visualization.

Scan 4. Pericardial Subcostal/Subxiphoid

Position the probe at the xiphisternum and place downward pressure onto the probe, then angle cephalically under the xiphisternum toward the heart (Fig. 10.1). Assess for free fluid in the pericardial cavity and also watch the cardiac rhythm. In a normal case, a small amount of free fluid can be seen in the pericardium. A depth measurement of 5 mm or less measured anteriorly to the right ventricle equates to 15–50 mL of free fluid and would be considered a normal finding. A moderate effusion would measure 5–10 mm, and a large effusion measures >10 mm anteriorly to the right ventricle and extends to the left atrium.

> **TIP BOX**
>
> If the images obtained are limited, the patient, if conscious, can be asked to breathe in and suspend respiration. The lungs will push the heart caudally and improve visualization as the heart is moved closer to the ultrasound probe.

Cardiac tamponade results when a large pericardial effusion affects the rhythm of the heart due to pressure of the fluid within the pericardium. This results in the heart wall motion becoming unsynchronized, and this can be seen with the right ventricular wall bowing inwards during diastole.

Scan 5. Pleura

The probe is now placed longitudinally on the upper anterior chest wall at the level of the clavicle in the mid-clavicular line. A high-frequency linear probe is often useful in assessing this area as the structures are fairly superficially positioned. The focus must also be moved up into the near field of the image to improve image resolution. Scan systematically, progressively moving caudally, pausing at each intercostal space. The purpose is to visualize the pleural edge, which should be seen as a smooth surface that can be seen sliding back and forth (sliding sign) with an echobright artifact known as "twinkle" artifact seen arising from the pleural edge as the patient breathes in and out. In the case of pneumothorax, a white line will be seen at the interface of the lung and trapped air; no sliding sign or twinkle artifact will be seen.

Free Fluid

Free fluid is associated with numerous types of injury, including rupture of the liver, spleen, kidney, pancreas, or bowel (Fig. 10.2). Free fluid in the pelvis may be difficult to detect (due to overlying bowel and underfilled bladder). Ultrasound is more successful in detecting free fluid than detecting organ injury directly. One study reported a 74% sensitivity for detection of fluid, with a specificity of 95%.[5] Ultrasound has several limitations. It is only 85% sensitive, requiring more than 150 cc to 200 cc of intraperitoneal fluid to be detected.[6] False positives include ascites, ruptured ovarian cyst, or ectopic pregnancy. Older hemorrhage can also have a more solid, mixed echogenicity appearance rather than the anechoic appearance of fresh fluid, which can often be confusing to less experienced operators. It must also be acknowledged that scans can be limited by patient habitus, bowel gas, and also is poor at assessing retroperitoneal structures.[7]

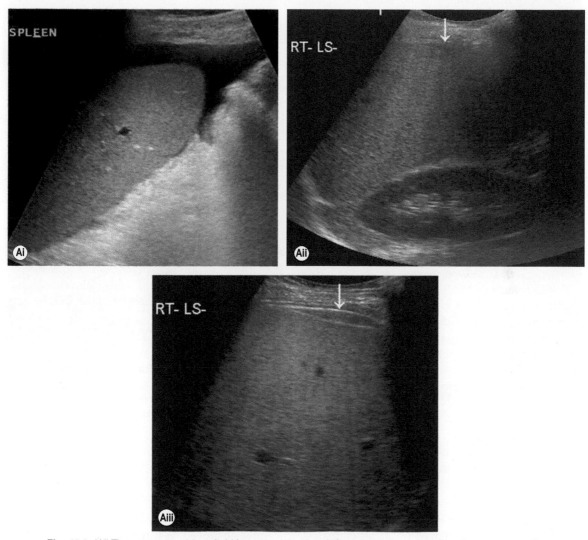

Fig. 10.2 (Ai) The presence of free fluid in a trauma patient infers organ injury. (Aii) Free fluid may be difficult to detect immediately following trauma. This patient has a trace of free fluid following blunt trauma (arrow), which is more clearly demonstrated (Aiii) when the focal zone is placed in the near field.

Continued

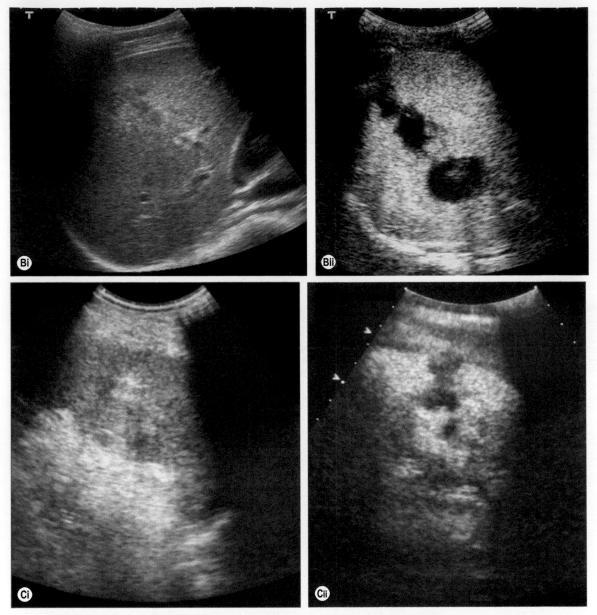

Fig. 10.2, cont'd (Bi) A patient with a right upper quadrant injury following trauma has altered echotexture in the liver but no frank hemoperitoneum at this stage. (Bii) Contrast-enhanced ultrasound (CEUS) clearly demonstrates the extent of the injury in the sinusoidal phase as a non-vascular rupture. (Ci) Laceration of the spleen immediately following a road traffic accident demonstrates hardly any free fluid. (Cii) CEUS confirms a splenic laceration which was managed conservatively.

Continued

The published studies have concentrated only on the presence or absence of free fluid rather than a comprehensive assessment of the abdomen by suitably qualified sonographers. There is a clear case for the latter, especially if the patient is unstable and cannot be moved, as ultrasound is able to offer valuable information about the viscera, which can direct management quickly and appropriately.

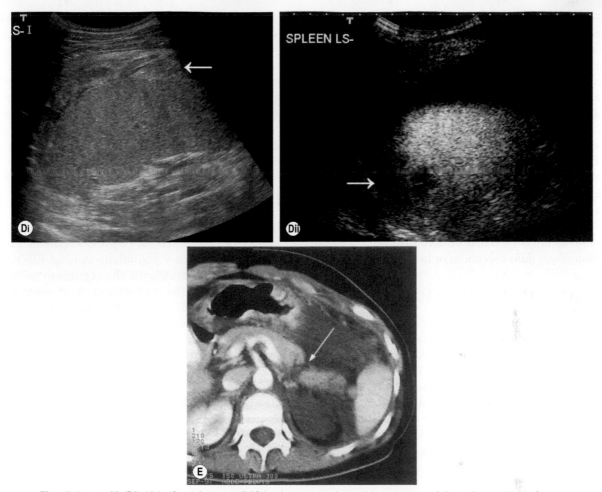

Fig. 10.2, cont'd (Di) 48 h after injury, a solidifying hematoma (arrow) is seen around the spleen with no free abdominal fluid. (Dii) CEUS demonstrates the injury at the dome of the spleen (arrow). (E) Computed tomography (CT) demonstrating pancreatic fracture (arrow) in the tail of pancreas following a road traffic accident. Ultrasound could not demonstrate the fracture but did demonstrate free fluid following the accident and diagnosed devascularization of the left kidney (no Doppler flow within the kidney) following a severed left renal artery, also confirmed on CT.

Visceral Rupture

Direct visualization of organ rupture by ultrasound is difficult unless a hematoma or other collection is seen. Laceration or contusion may be demonstrated in the liver, kidneys, or spleen, but less easily in the pancreas and very infrequently in the bowel. A subtle change in texture may be observed by the experienced operator, or a fine, high reflectivity linear band representing an organ tear (Fig. 10.2B–D). The use of contrast-enhanced ultrasound (CEUS) is particularly helpful in assessing liver and spleen damage, especially in the absence of hematoma or before a hemoperitoneum is established. CEUS is not routinely performed, possibly due to the cost of contrast, the procedure being highly operator dependent, and the difficulty in getting adequate images in deeper structures. However, it may be considered in the pediatric setting due to the lack of ionizing radiation.[8,9]

Small visceral lacerations not visible on ultrasound may become apparent when imaged with CT. In particular, pancreatic damage (often due to the sudden pressure of a seat belt across the abdomen during road accidents) may not be obvious immediately post-trauma on either ultrasound or CT.[10] Damage to the pancreatic duct

(Fig. 10.2E) causes leakage of pancreatic fluid into the abdominal cavity, resulting in pancreatitis and possible pseudocyst formation or peritonitis. Free fluid may be present because of a vessel rather than organ rupture. A reduction or loss of blood flow to all or part of the relevant organ, for example, the kidney, may be demonstrated using color and power Doppler ultrasound or CEUS.

The finding of free fluid in a patient with female reproductive organs should prompt a detailed scan of the pelvis where possible. Gynecological masses may rupture or hemorrhage, presenting acutely, and in those of childbearing age, ectopic pregnancy should be included in the list of differential diagnoses.

When visceral trauma is treated conservatively, a follow-up ultrasound may be used to monitor the resolution of any fluid collections or hematoma.

GASTROINTESTINAL TRACT

Most acute presentations of gastrointestinal tract pathology are due to obstruction or inflammation (see Chapter 8). Appendicitis and its possible complications are one of the most common reasons for referral. Ultrasound has a high sensitivity for acute appendicitis, particularly in children (see Chapter 9). Although the detailed assessment of the primary gastrointestinal pathology usually requires evaluation by an experienced operator with a high-frequency linear probe, many useful indicators can be found with the basic curvilinear abdominal probe.

Dilated loops of fluid-filled bowel, which may also show "overactive" peristalsis, should alert the operator to the possibility of acute intestinal obstruction. Such segments frequently lie proximal to the obstructing lesion, and so the point at which they appear to end should be the subject of detailed examination. Ultrasound is highly accurate in demonstrating obstruction. However, it is less successful in finding its cause, and contrast CT or other bowel studies are usually undertaken when an obstruction is diagnosed.

HEPATOBILIARY EMERGENCIES

Ultrasound scanning is invariably the first-line investigation for suspected biliary tract emergencies. These include inflammatory conditions causing RUQ and epigastric pain, mostly acute cholecystitis or gallstone pancreatitis, and the various causes of obstructive jaundice (Fig. 10.3). If possible, interventional treatment should be delayed until a detailed imaging assessment of the cause of biliary obstruction has been made since the presence of a biliary stent can compromise subsequent imaging by CT, MRI, or endoscopic ultrasound (EUS). Similarly, biliary stents frequently cause bile duct wall thickening and may introduce gas into the biliary tree. These will prevent the diagnosis of cholangitis or ductal calculi with ultrasound and may impede detailed Doppler investigation of, for example, the portal vein.

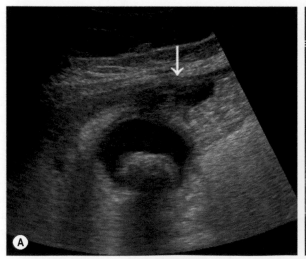
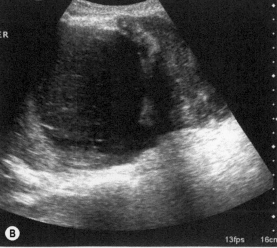

Fig. 10.3 (A) An acutely tender, inflamed gallbladder containing a large stone has a small anterior inflammatory collection (arrow). (B) A large subphrenic collection associated with gallbladder empyema.

Continued

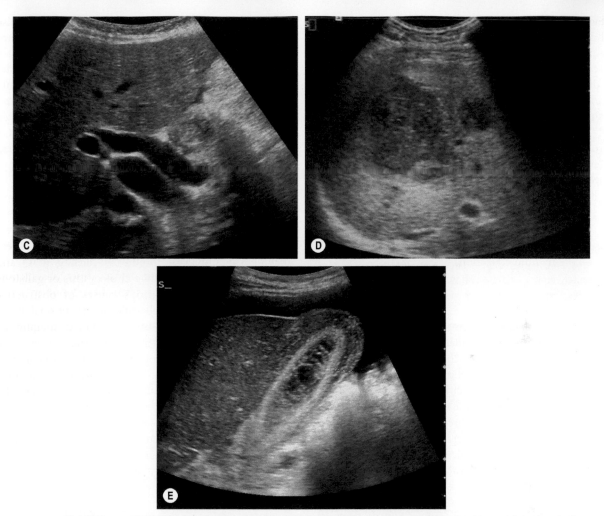

Fig. 10.3, cont'd (C) Obstructive jaundice; a stent that had been placed to palliate carcinoma of the head of the pancreas has become blocked. (D) Large liver abscess in an acutely ill patient. (E) Acute, acalculous cholecystitis in a patient on intensive care. The gallbladder wall is grossly edematous and tender.

There is an increasing trend toward less invasive diagnostic and therapeutic procedures, which has improved the mortality rate from biliary emergencies. The use of magnetic resonance cholangiopancreatography (MRCP) and EUS can avoid a diagnostic endoscopic retrograde cholangiopancreatography (ERCP).[11] If urgent biliary drainage is required, particularly when the bile is infected, this can quickly be achieved by endoscopic stent placement or sphincterotomy.[12]

The management of liver abscesses is determined by their size, number, and cause. Ultrasound is used to guide diagnostic aspiration and drainage procedures, and most types of hepatic abscesses can be treated successfully using these techniques combined with appropriate antibiotics therapy.

THE ACUTE PANCREAS (see also Chapter 4)

Most cases of acute pancreatitis are suspected clinically, with raised amylase levels and often a history of recurrent epigastric pain pointing to the diagnosis of acute pancreatitis (Fig. 10.4). Although pancreatitis may be due to abdominal trauma, it is more frequently due to gallstone obstruction or alcohol abuse. The pancreas often

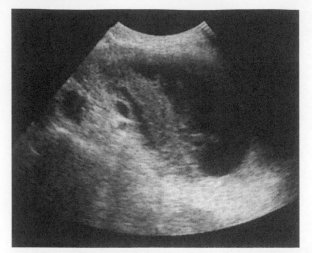

Fig. 10.4 Pancreatitis with a large pseudocyst. The patient was acutely tender, and the cyst was drained under ultrasound guidance.

appears normal even when acutely inflamed, so ultrasound examination should focus on the possible causes (such as gallstones, biliary dilatation, or evidence of alcoholic liver disease) and complications (pseudocysts, portal, or splenic vein thrombosis). EUS offers an accurate and less-invasive diagnosis than ERCP, with a complication rate of around 0.03% compared to 5%–10%.[13] Many pancreatic pseudocysts are now managed successfully by endoscopic ultrasound-guided transgastric drainage.[14]

RENAL TRACT EMERGENCIES (see also Chapter 6)

Ultrasound is the first-line investigation in the assessment of acute loin pain, which in the absence of trauma is commonly due to acute urinary tract obstruction and/or renal infection (Fig. 10.5). Less common acute

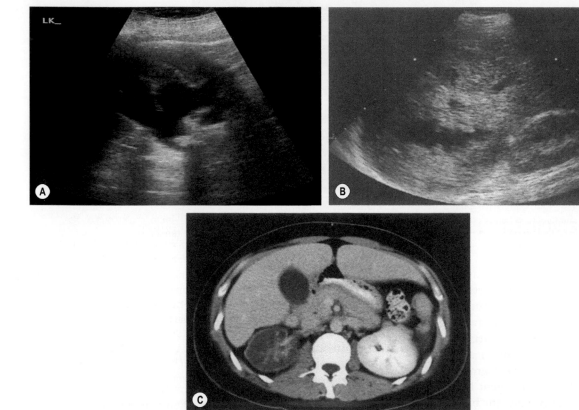

Fig. 10.5 (A) Obstructed kidney with pelvicalyceal system dilatation and a stone at the pelviureteric junction. (B) Severe laceration to the liver following a road traffic accident. (C) The same patient's CT scan confirms the liver injury and demonstrates an avascular right kidney (compared with the normal left kidney) due to laceration of the renal vessels.

presentations include renal vein thrombosis or spontaneous hemorrhage – usually from a renal tumor or cyst.

Ultrasound is also useful in assessing patients with acute renal colic due to suspected ureteric calculus and readily detects stones, obstruction, and other causes of pain (Fig. 10.5). Low-dose unenhanced multislice CT is increasingly the method of choice for locating ureteric calculi.[15,16]

The main limitation of ultrasound in acute ureteric obstruction is that obstruction may be present in the early stages without collecting system dilatation. Nevertheless, the minimally dilated renal pelvis, which would normally be dismissed as unremarkable in a patient with a full bladder, should raise the operator's suspicion in the patient with acute loin pain. Doppler ultrasound of the kidneys shows a higher resistance index in the obstructed kidney than in the normal side and can be a useful indicator.[17] Upper tract obstruction can be relieved via cystoscopy-guided ureteric stent placement. Ultrasound-guided percutaneous nephrostomy may be required if this is not practicable or there is evidence of infection.

Renal infection with parenchymal involvement (acute pyelonephritis) may be the cause of severe acute loin pain with fever, but ultrasound examination mostly shows no abnormality. Many patients will be particularly tender when scanning the affected kidney, a sign which should be included in the report. This, combined with ruling out potential other causes, can help support the diagnosis, which is usually based on clinical criteria but can be supported with CT if necessary.

OTHER RETROPERITONEAL EMERGENCIES (see also Chapter 8)

Ultrasound has an established role in identifying the presence of an abdominal aortic aneurysm (AAA) but should not be used to assess subacute leakage or rupture. However, where rupture is suspected and no previous imaging results are available, ultrasound can be a time-saving triage tool to exclude an aneurysm from the differential diagnosis of abdominal pain. Suitably trained emergency department clinical staff can perform this quickly and successfully, and as mentioned earlier, this is now included as part of the training of all high-level specialty trainees in emergency medicine. It is reported that ultrasound has a sensitivity of 99% and specificity of 98% for AAA detection (Fig. 10.6).[18] Rupture of an

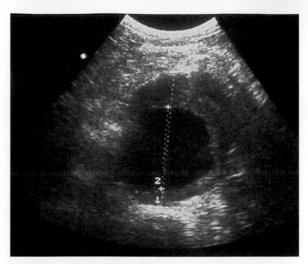

Fig. 10.6 Abdominal ultrasound showing a transverse section through a large abdominal aortic aneurysm. Measurement 1 shows the front to back (AP) diameter of the AAA from wall to wall while measurement 2 shows the diameter of the lumen through the thrombus lining the aneurysmal sac. (Source: Principles and Practice of Surgery: Adapted International Edition , Sixth Edition, 2012.)

aortic aneurysm is a catastrophic event, and although an urgent contrast-enhanced CT can be helpful, emergency surgery based on clinical findings should not be delayed by imaging investigations.

REFERENCES

1. Smallwood N, Dachsel M. Point of care ultrasound (POCUS): unnecessary gadgetry or evidence based medicine? *Clin Med*. 2018;1813:219–224.
2. Poletti PA, Mirvis SE, Shanmuganathan K, et al. Blunt abdominal trauma patients: can organ injury be excluded without performing computed tomography? *J Trauma*. 2004;57:1072–1081.
3. Pearl WS, Todd KH. Ultrasonography for the initial evaluation of blunt abdominal trauma: a review of prospective trials. *Ann Emerg Med*. 1996;27:353–361.
4. Scalea TM, Rodriguez A, Chiu WC, et al. Focused assessment with sonography for trauma (FAST): results from an international consensus conference. *J Trauma*. 1999;46:466–472.
5. Stengel D, Leisterer J, Ferrada P, Ekkernkamp A, Mutze S, Hoenning A. Point-of-care ultrasonography for diagnosing thoracoabdominal injuries in patients with blunt trauma. *Cochrane Database Syst Rev*. 2018;12, CD012669.

6. Von Kuenssberg Jehle D, Stiller G, Wagner D. Sensitivity in detecting free intraperitoneal fluid with the pelvic views of the FAST exam. *Am J Emerg Med.* 2003;21:476–478.

7. Bloom BA, Gibbons RC. *Focused assessment with sonography for trauma (FAST)*; 2019. Available at: https://www.ncbi.nlm.nih.gov/books/NBK470479/.

8. Miele V, Piccolo CL, Galluzzo M, Ianniello S, Sessa B, Trinci M. Contrast-enhanced ultrasound (CEUS) in blunt abdominal trauma Br. *J Radiol.* 2016;89, 20150823.

9. Trinci M, Piccolo CL, Ferrari R, et al. Contrast-enhanced ultrasound (CEUS) in pediatric blunt abdominal trauma. *J Ultrasound.* 2019;22:27–40.

10. Gupta A, Stuhlfaut JW, Fleming KW, et al. Blunt trauma of the pancreas and biliary tract: a multimodality imaging approach to diagnosis. *Radiographics.* 2004;24:1381–1395.

11. Lee YT, Chan FK, Leung WK, et al. Comparison of EUS and ERCP in the investigation with suspected biliary obstruction caused by choledocholithiasis: a randomized study. *Gastrointest Endosc.* 2008;67:660–668.

12. Sawas T, Arwani N, Al Halabi S, Vargo J. Sphincterotomy with endoscopic biliary drainage for severe acute cholangitis: a meta-analysis. *Endosc Int Open.* 2017;5:E103–E110.

13. Jenssen C, von Lampe B, Kahl S. Endoscopic ultrasound in acute pancreatitis. *Video J Encycl GI Endosc.* 2013;1:554–559.

14. Agalianos C, Passas I, Sideris I, Davides D, Dervenis C. Review of management options for pancreatic pseudocysts. *Transl Gastroenterol Hepatol.* 2018;3:18.

15. Drake T, Jain N, Bryant T, Wilson I, Somani BK. Should low-dose computed tomography kidneys, ureter and bladder be the new investigation of choice in suspected renal colic?: a systematic review. *Indian J Urol.* 2014;30:137–143.

16. The National Institute for Health and Care Excellence. Renal and ureteric stones: assessment and management. Imaging for diagnosis. NICE guideline NG118. Diagnostic evidence review (B), 2019.

17. Nuraj P, Hyseni N. The diagnosis of obstructive hydronephrosis with color doppler ultrasound. *Acta Informatica Medica.* 2017;25:178.

18. Rubano E, Mehta N, Caputo W, Paladino L, Sinert R. Systematic review: emergency department bedside ultrasonography for diagnosing suspected abdominal aortic aneurysm. *Academ Emerg Med.* 2013;20:128–138.

11

Interventional Techniques

Sidi H. Rashid

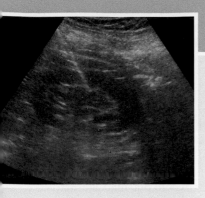

CHAPTER OUTLINE

Introduction, 333
Ultrasound-Guided Biopsy, 333
   General Considerations, 333
Methods of Ultrasound Guidance, 335
   Guided Biopsy, 335
   Freehand Biopsy, 335
Equipment and Needles, 335
   Non-Coaxial Technique, 336
   Coaxial Technique, 337
     Fine Needle Biopsy, 337
   Fine Needle Aspiration Cytology, 337
Specific Organ Ultrasound-Guided Biopsy
   Procedures, 337
   Liver Biopsy, 337
   Native Kidney Biopsy, 338

Renal Transplant Biopsy, 339
Complications of Ultrasound-Guided Biopsy, 340
Ultrasound-Guided Drainage, 341
   Paracentesis, 341
Pleural Drainage and Aspiration, 342
Abscess Drainage, 342
   Gallbladder Drainage, 343
Nephrostomy, 343
Cyst Drainage, 344
Ultrasound-Guided Vascular Access, 344
Tumor Ablation, 344
References, 345
Recommended Further Reading, 345

INTRODUCTION

The use of ultrasound-guided procedures, including diagnostic biopsy, therapeutic drainage, and treatment techniques, is an accepted and essential practice in the management of many conditions. These minimally invasive methods are responsible for improvements in inpatient mortality and morbidity compared to more invasive options, together with increased patient acceptability and cost-effectiveness.

The relative speed and ease with which these procedures can be carried out have resulted in a significant reduction of the diagnostic laparotomy or laparoscopy and more prompt and appropriate patient treatment. While ultrasound and computed tomography (CT) may

be suitable for many of these procedures, in general, ultrasound is often the first-line method. It is effective in most cases, generally more accessible, and does not carry a radiation risk. Also, ultrasound has the advantage of "real-time" placement, avoiding structures that could otherwise be damaged and effecting accurate and safe placement of the needle or drain.

ULTRASOUND-GUIDED BIOPSY

General Considerations

Percutaneous biopsy of solid organs, masses, or focal visceral lesions is an integral part of the diagnostic process for many patients.[1] Although changes on ultrasound may confirm the clinical suspicion (i.e., a hyperechoic liver may indicate fatty change, a nodular liver may indicate cirrhosis, or enlarged hyperechoic kidneys suggest glomerulonephritis), imaging alone is insufficient and frequently non-specific, so a definitive histological diagnosis is required.

The advantages of using ultrasound to guide such procedures are numerous:

- The needle tip is directed, in real-time, along the biopsy path and visualized within the lesion.
- Greater precision is obtained; needle guidance is essential for all small lesions and lesions at depth.
- Fewer needle passes are required to obtain the desired result, so post-procedure complications are minimized.
- The best route can be utilized and vital structures, such as blood vessels, avoided.
- Confidence in the biopsy result – particularly a negative one – is increased because of direct visualization of the needle tip in the lesion.
- All the advantages of ultrasound over other imaging methods apply (quick, direct vision, no radiation hazard, low cost). The limitations because of bone and air-filled structures also apply.
- The capability to perform bedside procedures for critically ill patients and to use in conjunction with other imaging techniques, for example, fluoroscopy, is advantageous.
- New image fusion technology allowing the fusion of CT, magnetic resonance imaging (MRI), or positron emission tomography images with real-time ultrasound (US) visualization is now another added benefit.

With ultrasound, the biopsy procedure is quick, safe, accurate, and usually acceptable to the patient. There are several accepted methods of performing a guided biopsy, but certain general rules are common to the procedure, regardless of the organ under investigation:

- A written or electronic request from a medical practitioner with the results of any previous investigations should be available. The reason for the biopsy should be appropriate.
- Assessment of blood clotting status should occur within at least seven days:
- Activated partial thromboplastin time ratio <1.2
- Platelet count >75,000/mL
- International normalized ratio <1.5.
- Anti-platelet agents (e.g., clopidogrel and aspirin) should be withheld five days before.

- Novel oral anticoagulants (should be withheld for at least seven days). The results of any previous investigations should be available.
- Identification of possible contraindications to biopsy. Contraindications are relative and include an unsuitable biopsy pathway, an uncooperative patient, and uncorrectable coagulation. These should be assessed on an individual patient basis, in conjunction with the patient's medical practitioner.
- Careful explanation of the procedure to the patient, including risks, benefits, and potential alternatives.
- Informed consent for the procedure should be obtained directly by the operator who will carry out the procedure.[2]
- Patients should be fasted for 4–6 h prior to the procedure, in particular when sedation is needed.
- The procedure should be performed in a quiet and clean environment. Infection control measures should be observed, and steps taken to preserve pre-, peri-, and post-procedure sterility.
- Before undertaking the procedure, any relevant cross-sectional imaging (usually CT or MRI) should be reviewed.
- A pre-biopsy scan is performed to identify a suitable biopsy route avoiding vital structures.
- Satisfactory care of the patient is required both during and after the biopsy procedure with relevant observations of vital signs. A pulse oximeter and appropriate nurse cover are recommended.
- Appropriate preparation of the specimen.
- Analgesia.

For most biopsy procedures, a local anesthetic is administered following the localization of the biopsy site with ultrasound. Lidocaine (1% or 2%) is commonly used; the volume will depend on patient build, depth of the lesion, and patient anxiety, but weight-dependent maximum doses should not be exceeded. It is also useful to inject the anesthesia under ultrasound guidance, so that lidocaine (or other local anesthetic agents) can be targeted exactly to the biopsy route, enabling effective pain relief throughout the procedure. A useful tip is initially creating a subdermal bleb with about 1–2 mL of local anesthetic followed by deeper infiltration to the organ capsule, pleura, or peritoneum, depending on the nature of the intervention. This has the benefit of making the procedure more tolerable and creating a hypoechoic tract to enable better needle visualization for the biopsy needle.

Usually, a short period, commonly 3–4 minutes depending on the nature of anesthetic, can work, after which a small scalpel incision is made in the skin to facilitate the biopsy. This has the benefit of making the procedure more tolerable, but local anesthetic may be unnecessary with a 22G needle or smaller.

Particularly apprehensive patients may require pre-procedure medication with a sedative such as Diazepam or a similar anxiolytic agent. However, this is uncommon. Peripheral venous access (18–20G) should be obtained before the procedure, to ensure immediate intravenous access in case medications or transfusions are required, except for very superficial biopsies (e.g., thyroid FNAB), depending on the operator's preference. Occasionally, intravenous analgesia and/or sedation may be required during the procedure.

The use of general anesthesia for children is common practice to enable the procedure to be carried out quickly and accurately while the child remains still.

METHODS OF ULTRASOUND GUIDANCE

There are various ways of performing ultrasound-guided procedures, i.e., guided or freehand. The choice of method depends on the procedure in question, equipment, and the experience and skill of the operator.

Guided Biopsy

Most manufacturers provide a biopsy guide that fits snugly onto the transducer head and provides a rigid pathway for the needle (Fig. 11.1). These are now common and widely accepted methods of biopsy. The fixed biopsy guide contains a groove for a series of plastic inserts ranging from 14G to 22G size, depending upon the size of the biopsy needle. It is usual to use one size greater than the needle (i.e., a 16G insert for an 18G needle), as the needle tends to move more freely. The guide is fitted onto the transducer over a sterile sheath. The needle pathway is displayed on the ultrasound monitor electronically – as a line or narrow sector - through which the needle passes. The operator then scans to align the electronic pathway along the chosen route, the needle is inserted, and the biopsy is taken. These attachments should be tested regularly to ensure the needle follows the correct path (Fig. 11.2).

Freehand Biopsy

A freehand approach, in which the operator scans with one hand and introduces the needle near the transducer with the other, is the most commonly used technique for most experienced operators. This technique can be used for any lesion and is typically used for drainages. The needle is inserted from one end of the probe. The technique allows for a greater degree of operator control and flexibility than the needle guide platform.

EQUIPMENT AND NEEDLES

The core of tissue for histological analysis is obtained with a specially designed needle consisting of an inner needle with a chamber or recess for the tissue sample

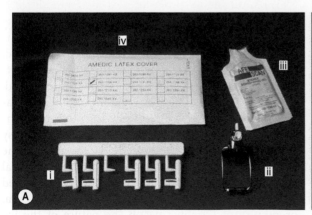
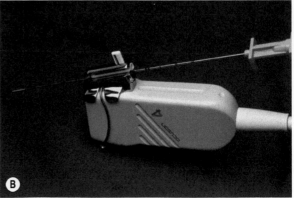

Fig. 11.1 (A) Necessary component parts to perform an ultrasound-guided biopsy procedure. A series of plastic inserts (Ai) range in size from 14G to 22G. The appropriate insert is inserted into a fixed biopsy guide (Aii). The procedure is performed with sterile jelly (Aiii) and a sterile probe cover (Aiv) if required. (B) The assembled biopsy guide.

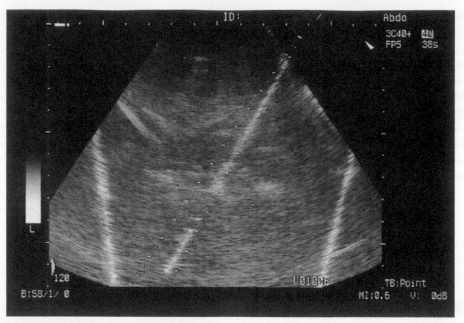

Fig. 11.2 Testing the alignment of the biopsy guide. The electronic pathway is activated on the image, and the needle is scanned as it is passed into a jug of water.

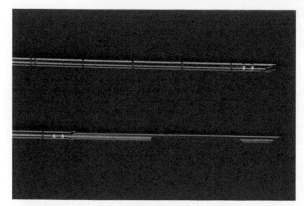

Fig. 11.3 Biopsy needle closed (top) and open (bottom).

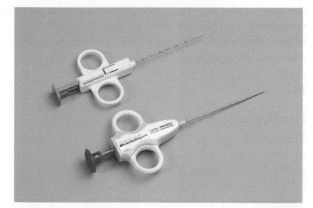

Fig. 11.4 Examples of semi-automatic core biopsy instruments. These allow placement of the central notch at the exact position required with the cutting sheath subsequently fired over the stylet. (Source: Grainger & Allison's Diagnostic Radiology: Interventional Radiology, Sixth Edition, 2016).

and an outer, cutting needle which moves over it, i.e., the Tru-cut needle. The biopsy is obtained in two stages with a specially designed needle into the tissue. Then the outer cutting sheath is advanced over it, and the needle is withdrawn, containing the required tissue core (Fig. 11.3). The use of a spring-loaded needle in two stages with a special design can be viewed in Fig. 11.4. It is designed to enable the operation of the needle with one hand (while holding the probe with the other) and has the advantage of being sterile and disposable.

Non-Coaxial Technique

The whole needle is advanced into the tissue, just in front of the area to be biopsied. By pressing the spring-loaded control, the inner part is quickly advanced into the lesion, followed rapidly by the cutting sheath over it. Needles can be obtained in various sizes, generally 14,

16, 18, or 20G. Most focal lesions are biopsied with a standard 16G or 18G needle. The needle advances approximately 1.5–2.0 cm during a biopsy, so it is advisable to position the needle tip on the edge of a lesion to obtain a good histological sample. Most lesion necrosis tends to be centrally located, which might compromise the result if sampled. Because the gun enables the operator to scan with one hand and biopsy with the other, the needle can be observed within the lesion, yielding a high rate of diagnosis with a single-pass technique[1] and minimizing post-biopsy complications.

Coaxial Technique

In the coaxial technique, a guide needle, larger than the biopsy needle (typically 12–19G), is advanced under image guidance, reaching the edge of the target. The inner stylet is removed, with the operator's finger placed over the lumen to prevent air aspiration. A biopsy needle is then introduced into the guide needle coaxially. This technique allows the collection of multiple specimens in a single puncture and may prevent possible tumor cells from seeding along the needle tract by re-inserting the inner stylet of the coaxial needle before removal. Compared to the non-coaxial method, the coaxial technique does not increase the rate of complications. Moreover, it also allows the injection of embolic agents (such as gel foam slurry or plugs) across the biopsy tract, thus reducing the risk of post-biopsy hemorrhage.[1]

Fine Needle Biopsy

Fine needle histology, involving the use of needles of 21G or less, reduces even further the possibility of post-procedure complications. These are rarely used because of the small tissue yield and the tendency of these needles to bend, making them difficult to retain within the plane of the scan. Biopsy of deep lesions with these needles is, therefore, almost impossible.

Fine Needle Aspiration Cytology

Cytology is the analysis of individual cells rather than a core of tissue such as that obtained for histology. This is generally more difficult to interpret pathologically, as the characteristic architecture and intercellular relationships seen in a histological sample are absent. Therefore, it requires a highly trained and specialized cytopathologist to interpret the samples (whereas all trained pathologists can view histological specimens) – a major disadvantage. However,

it has the advantage of allowing a finer needle to be used, which can be passed through structures, e.g., the stomach, blood vessels, en route to the site of interest, with no adverse effects. For many conditions, histological diagnosis is required, although cytology remains a useful tool in the diagnosis of breast and thyroid pathologic conditions.

Fine needles for cytology are of size 21G or smaller. They are of a simple design with a beveled, hollow core and no cutting mechanism. The needle is introduced under ultrasound guidance to the required position. Fragments of tissue are removed into the needle by applying negative (sucking) pressure with a syringe to the needle while moving the needle to and fro to loosen the tissue. These can then be expelled onto a microscope slide and smeared.

SPECIFIC ORGAN ULTRASOUND-GUIDED BIOPSY PROCEDURES

Liver Biopsy

The most common indication for an ultrasound-guided biopsy is focal lesion characterization. The liver is one of the most frequent sites for metastases, and histology may be required to confirm this diagnosis or, more usually, to identify the origin of an unknown primary lesion (Figs. 11.5–11.7). In contrast, a biopsy of suspected hepatocellular carcinomas (HCCs) is generally avoided, as it is associated with a poorer treatment outcome, and there is a small risk of tumor seeding. Instead, contrast-enhanced and diffusion-weighted MRI can now characterize many of these lesions. That said, focal lesion liver biopsy is generally safe and yields reliable tissue for histological analysis, with minimal complications. In general, an accuracy of 96%–98% should be achievable.[3]

A liver biopsy can also provide tissue to assess for the presence and severity of parenchymal liver disease. It may also identify the cause of the disease process. This is often performed in patients with abnormal liver function tests with no evidence of biliary obstruction. While the clinical history and serological analysis can help determine the cause, a biopsy is often required. This is usually performed with a 14G or 16G Tru-cut needle. A biopsy may also be performed for patients with suspected rejection following hepatic transplantation.

Care should be taken to assess and correct any coagulopathy in patients undergoing liver biopsy. Where coagulation profiles are not correctable (and most

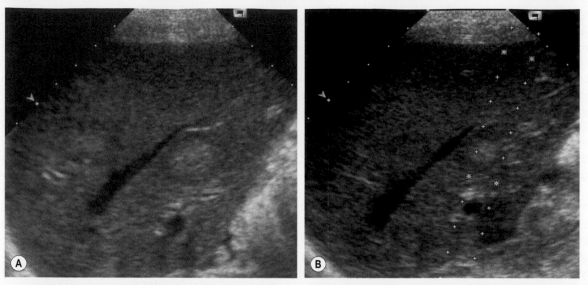

Fig. 11.5 (A) A liver lesion is identified in the right lobe prior to biopsy. (B) A route is chosen avoiding the adjacent hepatic vein.

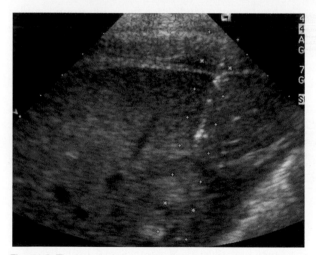

Fig. 11.6 The needle is introduced into the liver, just in front of the lesion under ultrasound guidance.

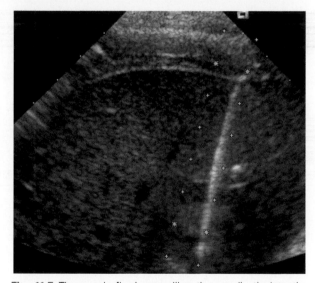

Fig. 11.7 The gun is fired, propelling the needle tip into the lesion. This visually confirms that the biopsy has been taken from the correct area.

generally are), liver biopsy can be performed using a "plugged" technique or, alternatively, by the transjugular route (Fig. 11.8).

Native Kidney Biopsy

Histology is frequently required to direct the management of diffuse renal disease. Biopsy of a solid renal mass is rarely performed as the diagnosis of renal cell or transitional cell carcinoma is usually clear from imaging. However, confirmatory biopsies are still performed

before chemotherapy or new therapeutic regimens in patients who are not having surgery.

Biopsy of the native kidney is performed in most centers under ultrasound guidance. Contraindications to biopsy include hydronephrosis (more appropriately treated with retrograde ureteric stenting or nephrostomy) or small kidneys measuring <8 cm in length

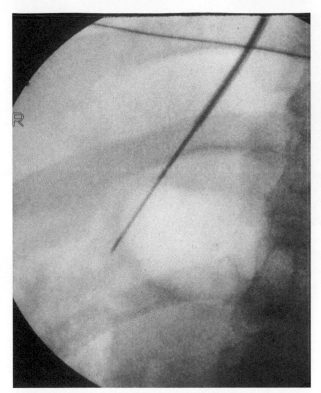

Fig. 11.8 Transjugular biopsy of the liver. Access is via the right internal jugular vein, through the SVC, and into the inferior vena cava and hepatic veins. Once the catheter is wedged in the hepatic vein, the cutting needle is released, and a biopsy is taken.

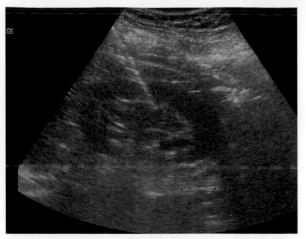

Fig. 11.9 Ultrasound-guided biopsy of the native left kidney. The tip of the needle is positioned on the outer aspect of the kidney. When the biopsy gun is fired, the cutting needle progresses forward into the kidney, acquiring a tissue sample.

(indicative of chronic renal impairment). Kidneys >9 cm in length can potentially be biopsied. However, other factors, including cortical thickness, age, clinical history, and the requirement for a definitive diagnosis, will all have a bearing on whether a biopsy is performed or not. Hydronephrosis and kidney size are easily assessed with a pre-biopsy scan.

In most cases, the biopsy is performed with the patient prone over a small bolster to maximize access to the kidney. The shortest route, avoiding adjacent structures, is selected subcostally, traversing the cortex of the lower pole and avoiding the collecting system and major vessels. For diffuse disease, either kidney may be chosen, and accessibility will vary between patients. The depth of penetration and angle of approach are carefully assessed. The biopsy is normally performed with a 16G needle.

The patient's cooperation is required in suspending respiration at the crucial moment. This avoids undue damage to the kidney as the needle is introduced through the capsule. The needle should be positioned just within the capsule before biopsy so that the maximum amount of cortical tissue is obtained for analysis as the throw of the needle may be up to 2 cm (Fig. 11.9).

RENAL TRANSPLANT BIOPSY

Biopsy is a valuable tool in the postoperative management of a transplant recipient (Chapter 6), enabling the cause of graft dysfunction to be identified, and in particular, differentiating acute tubular necrosis from acute rejection. Ultrasound guidance is essential to reduce complications such as hematoma, vascular damage (which may result in an arteriovenous [AV] fistula or pseudoaneurysm formation), and laceration of the renal collecting system.

A single-pass technique, using the spring-loaded biopsy gun with an 18G needle, is usually sufficient for histological purposes. However, two passes may be required so that electron microscopy and immunofluorescence can also be performed. The procedure is well tolerated by the patient, and the complication rate is low at about 5%.[4]

A full scan of the kidney is first performed to highlight potential problems (e.g., perirenal fluid collections) and establish the safest and most effective route. The transplanted kidney lies in an extraperitoneal position,

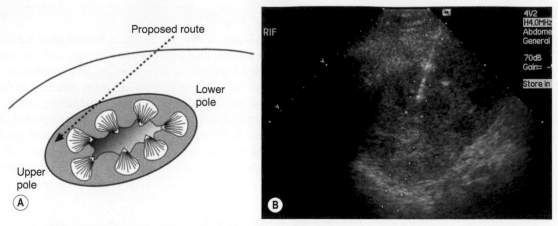

Fig. 11.10 (A) The transplanted kidney lies in the iliac fossa and is biopsied with the patient in a supine position. (B) The needle is seen entering the cortex of a transplanted kidney.

and the chosen route should avoid puncturing the peritoneum to minimize the risk of infection. Unlike the native kidney, the upper pole of the transplanted kidney is usually chosen to avoid major blood vessels and the ureter, both of which pass close to the lower pole.

The biopsy aims to harvest glomeruli, and the chosen route should, therefore, target the renal cortex. Identifying the renal capsule before the biopsy to avoid puncture into the medulla is the most important element to prevent complications.[4] An angle is chosen to include the maximum thickness of the cortex and, where possible, avoid the renal hilum (Fig. 11.10).

COMPLICATIONS OF ULTRASOUND-GUIDED BIOPSY

Post-procedure complications such as hematoma, requiring blood transfusion, and trauma to adjacent viscera occur very infrequently when ultrasound guidance is used. As expected, the risk of complications is less in fine needle biopsy than with larger needles. However, there is no significant difference in the complication rate between a standard 18G Tru-cut needle and a 22G Chiba needle.[1]

A biopsy is usually considered a minimally invasive and safe procedure, with a procedure-related mortality rate lower than 0.05%. The mortality rate for liver biopsy, in particular, is <0.1%.[5] The Society of Interventional Radiology quality improvement guidelines suggest a 2% quality improvement threshold for the overall incidence of major complications.[6]

The risk of hemorrhage is increased in patients with coexistent cirrhosis and is more likely to occur with malignant than benign lesions.[6] As with any procedure of this nature, there is a very small risk of infection, which can be minimized by using an aseptic technique.

Significant bleeding is a rare complication of liver biopsy. In a single-center, retrospective review of over 15,000 biopsies, Atwell et al. reported 0.5% of cases of significant hemorrhage within three months, varying according to biopsy site from 0.7% for the kidney to 0.1% in pancreatic biopsy.[7]

Tumor seeding occurs when malignant cells are deposited along the needle path. The best-known tumors for this are mesothelioma and hepatocellular carcinoma. It is a rare yet catastrophic complication, particularly when it occurs in otherwise potentially curable oncologic patients, such as surgical candidates. The risk of seeding varies according to the tumor type and location. The risk is negligible after biopsy of renal tumors (<0.01%), while it increases in liver biopsies.[1] The reported overall risk of needle tract seeding following biopsy of hepatocellular carcinoma is around 2.3–2.7%[8] but can be as high as 16–19% in colorectal liver metastases.[9]

Complications following abdominal biopsy are increased with multiple passes and are at least in part related to the skill and experience of the operator. If the biopsy result is negative or unexpected, several scenarios should be considered, including sampling error, poor histological specimen, sonographic or pathological misinterpretation, or a true negative finding. A repeat biopsy is sometimes justified.

ULTRASOUND-GUIDED DRAINAGE

While many fluid collections result from surgical intervention, others, such as pleural effusions and ascites, occur because of the natural disease process. Diagnostic aspiration may sometimes be used to establish the exact nature of a post-surgical collection, which may include hematoma, lymphocele, urinoma, biloma, pseudocysts, and others.

Postoperative hematomas are usually treated conservatively and tend to resolve spontaneously. Insertion of a drain into such a collection is at high risk of converting the collection into an abscess.

Paracentesis

Drainage of abdominal ascites is most often carried out in terminally ill patients or patients with decompensated liver failure, in whom the accumulation of fluid has become uncomfortable, often affecting breathing and mobility, or preceding chemotherapy and/or liver biopsy. Patients with refractory and/or infected ascites also benefit from paracentesis. Ultrasound guidance has the advantage of being able to assess the volume of fluid, selecting a suitable site and a route avoiding bowel and omental deposits (Fig. 11.11A). There is a growing

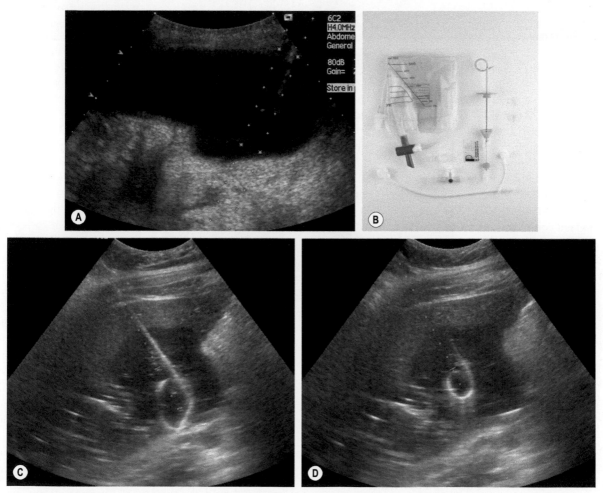

Fig. 11.11 Ultrasound-guided drainage. (A) Paracentesis under ultrasound guidance. Such procedures are often repeated regularly in the terminally ill, and ultrasound guidance facilitates an acceptable, pain-free procedure, focusing the area of local anesthetic injection and avoiding omental deposits. (B) Perkustay drain kit. (C) Postoperative subhepatic collection. This has been accessed with an 18G needle and guidewire inserted. (D) Guidewire has been withdrawn, and an 8Fr pigtail catheter is seen within the collection.

Continued

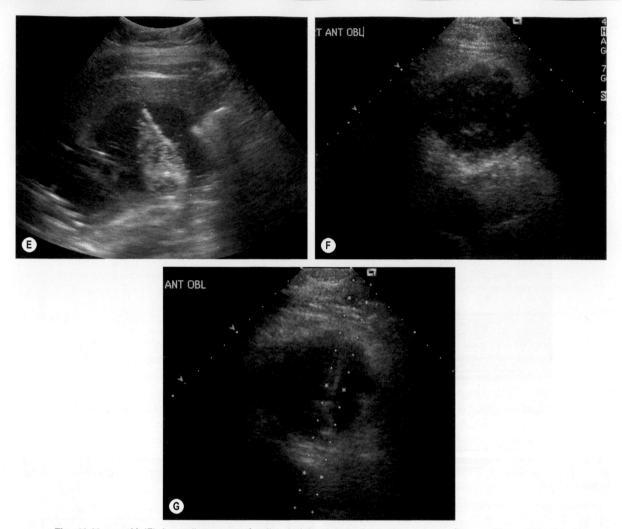

Fig. 11.11, cont'd (E) A small amount of saline is injected via the catheter to confirm position within the collection. A renal abscess (F) undergoing ultrasound-guided drainage (G).

trend to place tunneled catheters, such as the Pleurx drain (usually with the help of fluoroscopy) or dedicated low profile, long-term catheters, such as the Perkustay (Fig. 11.11B), which allow patients to mobilize freely and continue their paracentesis at home without the need for repeated drain insertions.

PLEURAL DRAINAGE AND ASPIRATION

The British Thoracic Society (BTS) strongly recommends thoracic ultrasound guidance for all pleural procedures for pleural fluid. Overall, ultrasound-guided pleural aspiration has been shown to increase the yield and reduce the risk of complications, particularly pneumothoraces and inadvertent organ puncture.[10] It is even more important when aspirating small or loculated pleural effusions, where there is a near or completely radio-opaque hemithorax.

ABSCESS DRAINAGE

Ultrasound-guided drainage of abscesses is the preferred treatment when the collection can be visualized on ultrasound, and a safe route is chosen. Abscesses may result from postoperative infection, inflammatory bowel conditions, such as Crohn's disease, appendicitis,

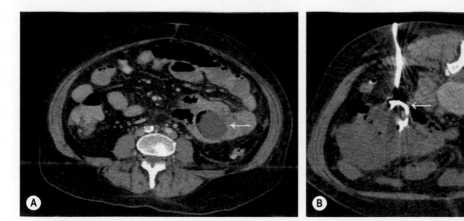

Fig. 11.12 (A) CT scan through the lower abdomen and upper pelvis. This shows an abscess cavity (arrows) which has tracked superiorly almost certainly from a perforated diverticulum more inferiorly. (B) This would almost certainly not be drainable with ultrasound. The surrounding small bowel loops mean that a posterior approach is required, so CT is the modality of choice. The abscess cavity was accessed with an 18G needle and an 8Fr drain (arrow) left *in situ*.

or other sources of infection, particularly in immuno-suppressed patients. Drains come in different sizes, and generally, the more viscous the pus, the larger the bore of drain required. While aspiration is initially performed to confirm the nature of the collection and provide microbiology samples, often a drain is left *in situ*, which, together with targeted antibiotic therapy, is usually effective. At the very least, it can improve the overall clinical condition to allow definitive treatment and, at best, can be definitive in itself.

Ultrasound is particularly useful in cases of hepatic and renal abscesses, postoperative abdominal wall seromas, and lymphoceles and in draining the subphrenic, pericolic, and subhepatic areas (Fig. 11.11C–G). Superficial collections, usually associated with wound sites, are also readily accessible to ultrasound. Collections obscured by bowel gas are better drained under CT guidance (Fig. 11.12).

Gallbladder Drainage

Gallbladder drainage under ultrasound control is a temporary procedure that tends to be reserved for particularly ill patients with acute cholecystitis and sepsis refractory to antibiotic therapy to stabilize their condition prior to surgery. The drainage of a gallbladder empyema buys valuable time and reduces the risk of perforation and subsequent bilious peritonitis. The portable nature of ultrasound allows a bedside procedure

to be performed, particularly useful in patients under intensive therapy who cannot be moved. However, this procedure carries a high risk of mortality and morbidity to the patient, and therefore full anesthesia, nursing, and medical support are required regardless of the physical location of the procedure (see Chapter 3, Fig. 3.31). There is evidence that percutaneous cholecystostomy may be the preferred first treatment option for patients with acute acalculous cholecystitis, except in perforation or gallbladder gangrene cases.[11]

NEPHROSTOMY

Renal obstruction, in which the pelvicalyceal system is dilated, can be decompressed by the percutaneous introduction of a nephrostomy tube under ultrasound guidance. This procedure relieves pressure in the renal collecting system and avoids potential, irreversible damage to the renal parenchyma (Fig. 11.13), thus preserving renal function. In cases of superadded infection to an obstructed renal tract, nephrostomy permits drainage of the system, protection/preservation of the renal parenchyma (from the insults of infection and pressure), and collection of microbiology samples, and is critical in reversing sepsis. Although the procedure may be carried out completely under ultrasound control, it is more common for the procedure to be performed in combination with fluoroscopy.[12]

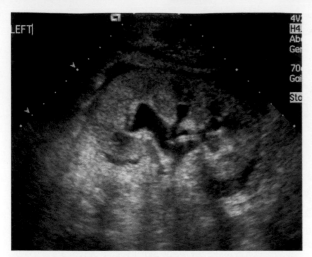

Fig. 11.13 Longitudinal ultrasound scan of the left kidney immediately following nephrostomy. A small rim of fluid, probably urinoma, surrounds the previously obstructed kidney.

CYST DRAINAGE

The percutaneous treatment of renal and hepatic cysts, by simple aspiration, may afford only temporary relief as they frequently recur. A more permanent result may be achieved by injecting a sclerosant, for example, absolute alcohol or tetracycline, into the cyst. In addition, percutaneous treatment of hydatid liver disease has been successfully performed by the injection of 95% ethanol solution or hypertonic saline solution.[13] Recently, the injection of sclerosing agents (sterile talc powder, tetracyclines, polidocanol solution or foam) following cyst aspiration has been found to be an effective and safe treatment in the management of postoperative seromas.[14]

ULTRASOUND-GUIDED VASCULAR ACCESS

Ultrasound-guided vascular access is a technique that can increase safety, as well as technical and procedural success when performing a wide range of invasive cardiovascular procedures.[15,16] The National Institute for Health and Care Excellence (NICE) recommends ultrasound-guided venepuncture as the preferred method for insertion of central venous catheters into the internal jugular vein in adults and children in elective situations.[17]

The probe most conducive to vascular access is a linear-array high-frequency (12–18MHz) probe. Once a site has been chosen, it should be evaluated with ultrasound to identify both the artery and the vein.

Arteries appear thick-walled, more circular, and pulsatile on ultrasound. Arteries do not compress with light pressure. Veins are more irregular in shape, sometimes appearing triangular rather than round, and compress with light pressure. Either a transverse or longitudinal approach is possible, depending on the scenario and expertise of the operator. Pressure over this area with a blunt object, such as a fingertip, can confirm the correct location. The needle should then be inserted at a 45-degree angle to the skin at a distance from the probe equal to the depth of the target vessel. Immediately after entering the skin, the needle tip should be identified on the screen. It will appear as hyperechoic within the subcutaneous tissue. The needle tip should be followed with the transducer as it advances toward the vessel. As the needle tip reaches the vessel, the wall of the vessel will be seen to deform. A flash of blood confirms that the needle has entered the vessel (arterial punctures typically result in pulsatile flow). A wire is then usually placed through the needle to enable subsequent access and a range of procedures. This is the basis of the Seldinger technique.[18]

TUMOR ABLATION

Ultrasound-guided (in combination with CT and/or MRI) percutaneous radiofrequency (RF) or microwave ablation has become one of the most promising local cancer therapies for both resectable and non-resectable hepatic tumors. Currently, RF ablation is recognized as a curative modality for early-stage HCC, the outcomes of which are comparable with those of surgical resection. Ablation for liver tumors is widely performed because of its ease of use, relatively low cost, short hospitalization time, and minimal invasiveness. Furthermore, major complications of hepatic ablation have been reported as rarely occurring, ranging between 2% and 3%. Complication rates do vary with pathologic conditions: a complication rate of 1.8% was seen in cases of HCC compared to 5.8% in the treatment of metastases.[19]

Although treatment algorithms differ worldwide, ablation is generally recommended for patients with three or fewer HCCs (diameter ≤3 cm) and who have contraindications for surgery.[19] Current NICE guidelines also support the use of radiofrequency (RF) ablation for colorectal liver metastases in patients unfit or otherwise unsuitable for hepatic resection or in those who have previously had hepatic resection.[20]

Ablation therapy has been developed for the treatment of small renal tumors to provide a less invasive, nephron-sparing treatment for patients that cannot or do not wish to undergo surgery. The advantage of ultrasound is that it provides real-time imaging for needle placement and deployment. However, the exact anatomical relationship with the surrounding organs (particularly the bowel loops) cannot be easily delineated with ultrasound. Furthermore, post-ablation bleeding cannot always be assessed because of the ablation acoustic shadow. For these reasons, US without concomitant real-time cross-sectional imaging (usually CT) is not recommended as the first-line guidance modality unless it is performed in selected patients by a very experienced operator in both b-mode and contrast-enhanced ultrasound.[21]

REFERENCES

1. Veltri A, Bargellini I, Giorgi L, Almeida PAMS, Akhan O. CIRSE guidelines on percutaneous needle biopsy (PNB). *Cardiovasc Intervent Radiol.* 2017;40:1501–1513.
2. Decision making and consent. https://www.gmc-uk.org/ethical-guidance/ethical-guidance-for-doctors/decision-making-and-consent.
3. Howlett DC, Drinkwater KJ, Lawrence D, et al. Findings of the UK national audit evaluating image-guided or image-assisted liver biopsy. Part I. Procedural aspects, diagnostic adequacy, and accuracy radiology. *Health Policy Prac.* 2012;265(12).
4. Tsai SF, Chen CH, Shu KH, et al. Current safety of renal allograft biopsy with indication in adult recipients: an observational study. *Medicine (Baltimore).* 2016;95(6):e2816.
5. Howlett DC, Drinkwater KJ, Lawrence D, et al. Findings of the UK national audit evaluating image-guided or image-assisted liver biopsy. Part II. Minor and major complications and procedure-related mortality. *Radiology.* 2013;266.
6. Gupta S, Wallace MJ, Cardella JF, Kundu S, Miller DL, Rose SC. Society of Interventional Radiology Standards of Practice Committee. Quality improvement guidelines for percutaneous needle biopsy. *J Vasc Interv Radiol.* 2010;21:969–975.
7. Atwell TD, Smith RL, Hesley GK, et al. Incidence of bleeding after 15,181 percutaneous biopsies and the role of aspirin. *Am J Roentgenol.* 2010;194:784–789.
8. Silva MA, Hegab B, Hyde C, Guo B, Buckels JA, Mirza DF. Needle track seeding following biopsy of liver lesions in the diagnosis of hepatocellular cancer: a systematic review and metaanalysis. *Gut.* 2008;57:1592–1596.
9. Jones O, Rees M, John T, et al. Biopsy of resectable colorectal liver metastases causes tumour dissemination and adversely affects survival after liver resection. *Br J Surg.* 2005;92. 1165Bi.
10. Havelock T, Teoh R, Laws D, Gleeson F. BTS Pleural Disease Guideline Group. Pleural procedures and thoracic ultrasound: British Thoracic Society pleural disease guideline 2010. *Thorax.* 2010;65. ii61–76.
11. Soria Aledo V, Galindo Iñíguez L, Flores Funes D, Carrasco Prats M, Aguayo Albasini JL. Is cholecystectomy the treatment of choice for acute acalculous cholecystitis? A systematic review of the literature. *Rev Esp Enferm Dig.* 2017;109:708–718.
12. Pabon-Ramos WM. Quality improvement guidelines for percutaneous nephrostomy clinical practice guidelines. *J Vasc Interv Radiol.* 2016;27:410.
13. Botezatu C, Mastalier B, Patrascu T. Hepatic hydatid cyst—diagnose and treatment algorithm. *J Med Life.* 2018;11(3):203–209.
14. Sood A, Kotamarti VS, Therattil PJ, Lee ES. Sclerotherapy for the management of seromas: a systematic review. *Eplasty.* 2017;28(17):e25.
15. Egan G, Healy D, O'Neill H, Clarke-Moloney M, Grace PA, Walsh SR. Ultrasound guidance for difficult peripheral venous access: systematic review and meta-analysis. *Emerg Med J.* 2013;30:521–526.
16. Mustapha JA, Diaz-Sandoval LJ, Jaff MR, et al. Ultrasound-guided arterial access: outcomes among patients with peripheral artery disease and critical limb ischemia undergoing peripheral interventions. *Invasive Cardiol.* 2016;28:259–264.
17. Guidance on the use of ultrasound locating devices for placing central venous catheters. Technology Appraisal Guidance [TA49], NICE; 2002. https://www.nice.org.uk/guidance/ta49.
18. Seldinger SI. Catheter replacement of the needle in percutaneous arteriography: a new technique. *Acta Radiologica.* 1953;39:368–376.
19. Kim JW, Shin SS, Heo SH, et al. Ultrasound-guided percutaneous radiofrequency ablation of liver tumors: how we do it safely and completely. *Korean J Radiol.* 2015;16(6):1226–1239. doi:10.3348/kjr.2015.16.6.1226.
20. Radiofrequency ablation for colorectal liver metastases. Interventional Procedures Guidance [IPG327], NICE; 2009. https://www.nice.org.uk/guidance/ipg327.
21. Krokidis ME, Orsi F, Katsanos K, Helmberger T, Adam A. CIRSE guidelines on percutaneous ablation of small renal cell carcinoma. *Cardiovasc Intervent Radiol.* 2017;40:177–191.

RECOMMENDED FURTHER READING

Kaufman JA, Lee MJ. Vascular and interventional radiology: the requisites. In: *The Core Requisites.* 2nd ed. Elsevier; 2013.
Mauro MA, Murphy Kieran PJ, Thomson KR, Venbrux AC, Morgan RA. Image-guided interventions. In: *Expert Radiology Series.* 3rd ed. Elsevier; 2020.

INDEX

Note: Page numbers followed by *f* indicate figures, *t* indicate tables, and *b* indicate boxes.

As the subject of this book is ultrasound and its variants, subentries under these terms relate to the theory and techniques of these methods. All other references can be found under specific anatomical features or individual diseases/disorders.

To save space in the index, the following abbreviations have been used:

CEUS–contrast enhanced ultrasound

CT–computed tomography

MRCP–magnetic resonance cholangiopancreatography

A

Abdominal aorta, 266–270, 266–267*f*
Abdominal aortic aneurysm (AAA), 268–270, 269–270*f*, 331, 331*f*
  CEUS, 268, 269–270*f*
  complications, 268–270
  diameter measurement, 266–267*f*, 268
  dissection, 268
  leakage, 268–270, 269–270*f*
  rupture, 268
  screening, 268
  surgery, 268
Abdominal wall layers, 285*f*
Abnormal liver function tests, 101
Abscesses
  post-operative liver transplants, 84, 85*f*
  renal transplants, 223
  ultrasound-guided drainage, 341–343*f*, 342–343
Acalculous cholecystitis, 118–119, 119*f*
  biliary sludge, 118–119, 119*f*
Acceleration index (AI), renal artery stenosis, 216*f*
Acceleration time (AT)
  renal artery stenosis, 216*f*
  liver transplants, 76, 77*f*
Acquired cystic disease, 195
Acute cholecystitis, 101*t*, 116–117, 117*f*
Acute fatty liver, pregnancy, 74
Acute idiopathic pancreatitis (AIP), 151, 152–153*f*
Acute kidney injury (AKI), 214
Acute lymphoblastic leukemia (ALL), 251–252, 253*f*

Acute pyelonephritis, 211
Acute scrotal pain, 240–242
Acute tubular necrosis (ATN), renal transplants, 226–227
Adenocarcinoma, 251
Adenomas
  benign focal liver lesions, 46, 46*f*
  renal tract, 196
Adenomatoid tumor, epididymis, 243–244, 244*f*
  Adenomyomatosis, gallbladder, 112–116
ADPKD *see* Autosomal dominant polycystic kidney disease (ADPKD)
Adrenal glands, 274, 274–275*f*
  adenoma, 274, 275*f*
  metastases, 274, 275*f*
  myelolipomas, 275*f*
Adrenal rest tumors, 248–249, 249*f*
Air enema, intussusception, 317*f*
Alcohol abuse
  acute pancreatitis, 151*t*
  cirrhosis, 61
  hepatitis, 70
Alpha-fetoprotein (AFP)
  cirrhosis, 61
  hepatocellular carcinoma, 52–53
Amoebic abscesses, liver, 40
Amyloid disease, renal tract, 215–216
Aneurysms
  abdominal aorta *see* Abdominal aortic aneurysm (AAA)
  splenic artery, 179
Angiomyolipoma (AML)
  renal tract *see* Renal tract
  tuberose sclerosis, 195

Appendicitis, 278–279, 278*f*, 328
  acute, 279*f*
  perforation, 278, 279*f*
Appendix epididymis, 234
Appendix testis, 234, 234*f*
Ascaris, biliary colic, 133–134, 134*f*
Ascending cholangitis, 107–108
Ascites
  acute cholecystitis, 116–117, 117*f*
  Budd–Chiari syndrome, 71–73
  portal vein thrombosis *vs.*, 64–66
Aspiration *see* Drainage, ultrasound-guided
Autosomal dominant polycystic kidney disease (ADPKD), 194, 195*f*, 308, 308*f*
  family history, 194
Autosomal recessive polycystic kidney disease (ARPCKD), 293, 308, 308*f*

B

Bacterial cholangitis, 128
Balanced flow, portal hypertension, 63, 64–65*f*
Bell-clapper deformity, 232, 233*f*
Benign focal lesions
  liver *see* Liver lesions, benign focal
  pancreas, 160–162, 162*f*
  renal tract, 196
Benign prostatic hypertrophy (BPH), 258–259, 259*f*
Bile crystals, 134–135
Bile duct(s), 30*f*, 97–99, 98–99*f*
  measurements, 98–99
    previous cholecystectomy, 99, 99*f*

Bile duct dilatation, 123–129
  causes, 124t
  obstructive jaundice, 123–128
Bile duct obstruction, 129
  choledochal cysts, 128, 128f
  duct wall fibrosis, 129
  intrahepatic tumors, 127–128
  treatment, 126–127
    malignancies, 126, 127f
  see also Obstructive jaundice
Bile, echogenic, 134–136
Biliary atresia
  cystic, 292
  diagnosis, 291–292, 292f
  pediatric ultrasound, 291
Biliary reflux
  choledocholithiasis, 107–108
  cystic duct insertion, 108, 109f
Biliary sludge, 134, 134f
  acalculous cholecystitis, 118–119,
    119f
Biliary stasis, 134–135
  acalculous cholecystitis, 118
  cholelithiasis, 134–135, 135f
  obstructive causes, 135
Biliary tree, 93–141
  malignant disease, 136–139
  parasites, 133–134
  see also Bile duct(s); Gallbladder;
    specific diseases/disorders
Bilirubin, 99–100
Biochemical analysis
  liver transplants, 79
  pancreas, 146–147
Biological effects (of ultrasound), 15–16
  mechanical effects, 16
  thermal effects, 15–16
Biopsy, ultrasound-guided, 333–335
  advantages, 334
  blood clotting assessment, 334
  coaxial technique, 337
  complications, 340
    hematoma, 340
    tumor seeding, 340
  contraindications, 334
  environment, 334
  equipment and needles, 335–337,
    336f
  fine needle, 337
    aspiration cytology, 337
  kidney, 338–339, 339f
    contraindications, 338–339

Biopsy, ultrasound-guided (Continued)
  liver, 337–338, 338–339f
  liver metastases, 49–52
  non-coaxial technique, 336–337
  renal transplant, 339–340, 340f
Bladder, 186, 189
  chronic wall thickening, 211, 212–213f
  diverticula, 212, 212–213f
  focal wall thickening, 212–213,
    212–213f
  pediatrics, 301–303
  transitional cell carcinoma see
    Transitional cell carcinoma
    (TCC)
  ureteric jets, 188
  volume measurement, 189
Bosniak classification, renal cysts, 194,
    194t
Bowel carcinoma, 282f
Bowel scanning technique, 277f
Budd–Chiari syndrome, 71–73, 72f
  ascites, 71–73

C

Calcification
  chronic pancreatitis, 154–156, 155f
  renal cysts, 194
  spleen, 175f, 176
Calcium renal tract stones, 207
Candidiasis, liver abscesses, 40
Caroli's disease, 132–133, 133f
  cholangiocarcinoma, 132–133
  choledochal cysts, 132, 133f
Cavernous transformation, portal
    hypertension, 63, 66–67f
Chemoembolization
  cirrhosis, 63
  liver metastases, 52
Chemotherapy
  spleen leukemia, 173
  spleen lymphoproliferative disorders,
    171
Cholangiocarcinomas, 124–126,
    137–138, 137f
  Caroli's disease, 132–133
  contrast-enhanced ultrasound, 132f, 137
  malignant focal liver lesions, 56, 58t
  management, 137–138
  multifocal, 137, 138f
  primary sclerosing cholangitis,
    130–131, 132f
  see also Klatskin tumors

Cholangitis, 128, 129f
  bacterial, 128
Cholecystitis, 115–123
  acalculous see Acalculous
    cholecystitis
  acute, 116–117, 117f
  acute on chronic, 119, 119f
  chronic, 117, 118f
    cholelithiasis, 117, 118f
  complications, 119–123
  emphysemous, 120, 121f
    pneumobilia, 136
  gangrenous, 119, 120f
Choledochal cysts
  bile duct obstruction, 128, 128f
  Caroli's disease, 132, 133f
  pediatrics, 293, 294f
Choledocholithiasis, 105–108
  biliary reflux, 107–108
  common bile duct, 105, 106–107f
  complications, 107, 108f
  management, 108
Cholelithiasis, 101–104, 102–103f
  acute, 101t
  acute pancreatitis, 151t
  associated conditions, 101
  biliary stasis, 134–135, 135f
  causes, 101t
  chronic cholecystitis, 117, 118f
  clinical features, 101, 101b
  contracted gallbladder, 111–112
  extracorporeal shock wave lithotripsy,
    108
  floating gallstones, 103f
  impaction, 104, 106f
  mobility, 102f, 104, 105f
  pigment stones, 101
  reflectivity, 104
  shadowing, 101, 104f
  stone size, 103, 103f
Cholesterol gallbladder polyps, 113–115
Cholesterolosis, 115–116, 116f
Chronic active hepatitis, 70
Chronic cholecystitis see Cholecystitis
Chronic kidney injury, 214
Chronic persistent hepatitis, 70
Chronic pyelonephritis, 211, 212–213f
Cirrhosis, 57–70
  alcohol abuse, 61
  alpha-fetoprotein, 61
  biopsy, 63
  clinical features, 62–63

Cirrhosis *(Continued)*
  congenital forms, 62
  cryptogenic, 62
  drug-induced, 62
  elastography, 63
  hemodynamics, 61
  hepatic fibrosis, 57–70, 59*f*
  hepatitis, 61
  hepatitis B, 61
  hepatitis C, 61
  hepatocellular carcinoma, 52–53,
    54–56*f*, 61
  liver size, 58
  macronodular, 58, 60*f*
  management, 62–63
  micronodular, 58, 60*f*
  nodules, 58–61
  primary biliary cirrhosis, 60*f*, 61–62
  secondary biliary cirrhosis, 62
  ultrasound appearances in, 58, 62*t*
Coeliac axis, 26*f*, 90*f*
Color Doppler ultrasound, 6, 6*f*
Common bile duct (CBD), 28*f*, 90*f*, 92*f*
  choledocholithiasis, 105, 106–107*f*
  diameter, 99
  dilatation, 123
    post-surgical, 128–129, 130*f*
    post-operative liver transplants, 79
Complex cysts, liver, 37
Compound imaging, 10
Congenital abnormalities
  pancreas, 147–148
  see also specific diseases/disorders
Congenital cirrhosis, 62
Congenital intrahepatic biliary
    dilatation *see* Caroli's disease
Congestive cardiac disease, liver disease,
  73
Conjugated bilirubin, 99–100
Contracted gallbladder *see* Gallbladder
Contrast angiography, portal vein
    thrombosis, 63–64
Contrast-enhanced ultrasound (CEUS),
  36
  benign focal liver lesions, 46
  focal nodular hyperplasia, 43–46
  liver hemangioma, 43
  liver metastases, 49, 50–51*f*
  male urogenital tract, 230–231
Cortex, kidneys, 186–187
Courvoisier's law, bile duct stones, 126
Creatinine, renal function assessment, 189

Crohn's disease, 279–280, 280*f*
Crossed fused renal ectopia, 192
Crossed renal ectopia, 192
Cryptogenic cirrhosis, 62
Cryptorchidism, 235–236
Cystadenoma, liver, 37, 38*f*
Cystic biliary atresia, 292
Cystic duct insertion, bile reflux, 108,
  109*f*
Cystic fibrosis, 73, 73*f*
  pediatric patients, 293–295
    gallbladder, 293–295
    liver fibrosis, 293
  pancreatic cysts, 161–162
Cystinuria, renal tract stones, 207
Cystitis, 211
Cysts
  pancreas, 160–162
  as prostate gland diseases, 259, 260*f*
  renal *see* Renal cysts
  spleen, 174–175
  ultrasound-guided drainage, 344
  see also specific types
Cytomegalovirus, hepatitis, 70

D
Diabetes mellitus
  focal pyelonephritis, 212–213
  pancreatic transplantation, 162
  pyogenic liver abscesses, 39
Dimercaptosuccinic acid (DMSA) scan
  multicystic dysplastic kidney, 308
  renal agenesis, 303
  renal function assessment, 303
Dissection, abdominal aortic aneurysm,
  268
Diverticulitis, 281, 281*f*
Doppler ultrasound, 6–8
  flow velocities, 8, 8*f*
  liver transplants, 76–78, 76*b*
  pulse repetition frequency, 8
  sensitivity, 8, 9*f*
  techniques, 8
Drainage, ultrasound-guided
  abscess drainage, 341–343*f*, 342–343
  complex liver cysts, 37
  cyst, 344
  gallbladder, 343
  liver abscesses, 40
  nephrostomy, 343, 344*f*
  paracentesis, 341–342, 341–342*f*
  pleural, 342

Drug-induced acute pancreatitis, 151*t*
Drug-induced cirrhosis, 62
Duodenum, 92*f*
  gallbladder mimic, 95, 97*f*
Duplex kidneys, 189–192, 191–192*f*,
  304–306, 304*f*
  partially duplication, 305
Duplication, inferior vena cava, 271

E
Echinococcus granulosus, 39
Ectopic kidneys, 192
Elastography, 11
  cirrhosis, 63
Electrical safety, 16
Emphysemous cholecystitis *see*
  Cholecystitis
Empyema, gallbladder, 120–123, 122*f*
Endoscopic retrograde
    cholangiopancreatography
    (ERCP)
  cholelithiasis management, 108
  Mirizzi's syndrome, 111
  obstructive jaundice, 124–126
  pancreas, 148
  pancreatic adenocarcinoma,
    156–158*f*, 160
Endoscopic ultrasound (EUS)
  common bile duct stones, 126
  common biliary duct obstruction
    management, 126
  gallbladder polyps, 113–115
Epidermoid cysts, 248, 248*f*
Epididymal torsion, 240, 240*f*
Epididymis, 240–241, 241–242*f*
  acute, 241*f*
  adenomatoid tumor, 243–244, 244*f*
  chronic, 243
  cysts, 243, 243–244*f*
  sperm granulomas, 243, 244*f*
Epigastric hernia, 286, 286*f*
Equipment, 12–14
  biopsy attachments, 13
  capabilities and functions, 13
  cost, 12
  dimensions, 14
  ergonomics, 14
  image quality, 13
  keyboard design, 14
  knowledge, image optimization, 2, 2*b*
  maintenance, 14
  portability, 14, 321

Equipment (*Continued*)
  probes, 13, 13*f*
  tests, quality assurance, 18
  upgradeability, 14
ERCP *see* Endoscopic retrograde
      cholangiopancreatography
      (ERCP)
Erythrocyte sedimentation rate (ESR),
      liver abscesses, 40
Esophageal carcinoma, 278*f*
Esophagus, 68, 276*f*, 277–278, 278*f*
  EUS, 277–278
EUS *see* Endoscopic ultrasound (EUS)
External renal pelvis, pelvicalyceal system
      dilatation, 191–192*f*, 201
Extracorporeal shock wave lithotripsy
      (ESWL), cholelithiasis
      management, 108
Extrarenal pelvis, kidneys, 191–192*f*,
      192

F

Falciform ligaments, liver, 23–24
Fetal lobulations, kidney development,
      187, 188*f*
Fibrosis
  bile duct obstruction, 129
  chronic pancreatitis, 154
  liver *see* Liver
Fine needle aspiration (FNA) cytology,
      337
Floating gallstones, 103*f*
Flow velocities
  Doppler ultrasound, 8, 8*f*
  portal hypertension, 63
Fluid collections
  liver transplants, 85–86, 86*f*
  renal transplants, 221–223
Fluid content, pancreatic malignancies,
      160
Focal fatty changes, benign focal liver
      lesions, 46
Focal fatty sparing
  benign focal liver lesions, 48
  pancreas, 160–161, 161*f*
Focal nodular hyperplasia, benign focal
      liver lesions, 43–46, 45*f*
Focal orchitis, 249
Focal pyelonephritis, 212–213, 212–213*f*
Focal zones, image optimization, 2, 3*f*
Focused assessment with sonography
      for trauma (FAST), 322–323

Focused assessment with sonography for
      trauma (FAST) (*Continued*)
  free fluid, 325–326, 325–327*f*
  purpose of, 323*b*
  scan, 323–325
    left upper quadrant, 323*f*, 324
    pelvis, 323*f*, 324
    pericardial subcostal/subxiphoid,
        323*f*, 324
      cardiac tamponade, 324
    pleura, 324–325
    right upper quadrant, 323–324,
        323*f*
Folded gallbladder, 95, 96*f*, 97
Fournier's gangrene, 241–242
Fulminant hepatitis, 70

G

Gallbladder, 28*f*, 89*f*, 92*f*, 94–101, 94*f*
  adenomyomatosis, 112–116
  cholesterolosis, 115–116, 116*f*
  cholesterol polyps, 113–115
  contracted (small), 111–112
    pathological causes, 105*f*, 111–112,
        111*f*
    post-prandial, 111, 111*f*
  dilatation, 106*f*, 123
  duplication, 95, 97*f*
  empyema, 120–123, 122*f*
  enlargement, 108–111, 110*f*
  folded, 95, 96*f*, 97
  inflammatory disease (cholecystitis)
      see Cholecystitis; *specific
      diseases/disorders*
  metastases, 138–139, 139*f*
  mucocoele, 106–107*f*, 110
  normal variants, 95–97
  pediatric cystic fibrosis, 293–295
  pathology, *see also specific diseases/
      disorders*, 93–141
  polyps, 113–115, 114*f*
    cholecystectomy, 113–115, 114*f*
  porcelain *see* Porcelain gallbladder
  post-fasting appearance, 94–101
  primary carcinoma, 136–137, 136*f*
  scanning pitfalls, 95–97
    duodenum mimic, 95, 97*f*
    missing, 95–97
    previous surgery, 95
  ultrasound-guided drainage, 343
  wall hyperplasia, *see also specific
      diseases/disorders*, 112–116

Gallbladder (*Continued*)
  wall varices, portal vein thrombosis,
      68
  see also Bile duct(s)
Gallstone ileus, 108*f*
Gallstones *see* Cholelithiasis
Gangrenous cholecystitis, 119, 120*f*
Gastric varices, portal vein thrombosis,
      68
Gastrinomas, pancreas, 160
Gastroduodenal artery, 90*f*, 92*f*
Gastrointestinal tract, 265–287
  acute abdomen, 328
  anatomy, 276, 276–277*f*
  congenital abnormalities, 313–314
  inflammatory conditions, 278–281
  intestinal malrotation and volvulus,
      313–314, 314*f*
  malignant tumors, 281
  obstruction, 282, 283*f*, 328
  pediatrics, 313–314
  techniques, 276–277
  see also specific anatomical features
Glomerulonephritis, 214
Glycogen storage diseases
  cirrhosis, 62
  liver adenoma, 46
Granuloma, benign focal liver lesions,
      48, 48*f*

H

Haemobilia, 135
HCC *see* Hepatocellular carcinoma
      (HCC)
HELLP syndrome, pregnancy, 74–75,
      74*t*, 75*f*
Hemangiomas
  benign focal liver lesions, 42–43, 44*f*
  complications, 296
  congenital hepatic, 295–296
  infantile hepatic, 295–296
  pediatrics, 295–296
  pancreas, 162, 162*f*
Hematomas, ultrasound-guided
      biopsy, 340
Hematuria, 189, 210–211
Hemochromatosis, 46
  cirrhosis, 62
Hemodynamics
  cirrhosis, 61
  inferior vena cava, 271
  liver, 31

Hemolytic anemia, 176, 177f
Hemoperitoneum, 162
Hemorrhages
  pancreatic malignancies, 160
Hepatic artery (HA), 25f, 29, 31–32f,
    33–34, 90–91f
  portal vein thrombosis, 68, 68f
  post-operative liver transplants, 79
  pseudoaneurysms, 80–81, 82f
  stenosis, post-operative liver
      transplants, 80
  thrombosis, 80, 81f
Hepatic vein (HV), 27f, 29–31, 32f, 89f
  color Doppler, 6f
  and IVC complication, 83–84
  post-operative liver transplants, 79
Hepatitis, 70, 71f
  acute cholecystitis, 116–117, 117f
  alcoholic, 70
  cirrhosis, 61
  clinical features, 70
  cytomegalovirus, 70
  herpes virus, 70
  infectious mononucleosis, 70
  inflammation, 70, 71f
  viral see Viral hepatitis; specific types
Hepatitis A, 70
Hepatitis B, 61
Hepatitis C, 61, 70
Hepatitis E, 70
Hepatobiliary iminodiacetic acid
    (HIDA), 293
Hepatobiliary emergencies see Acute
    abdomen
Hepatobiliary scintigraphy
  bile duct stones, 126
Hepatobiliary system, 21–92
  common diseases/disorders, see also
      specific diseases/disorders,
      99–101
  see also Bile duct(s); Biliary tree;
      Gallbladder; Liver
Hepatoblastoma, 296, 297f
Hepatocellular carcinoma (HCC),
    52–56, 296–298, 298–299f
  alpha-fetoprotein, 52–53
  CEUS, 53, 54–56f
  cirrhosis, 52–53, 54–56f, 61
  high intensity focused ultrasound,
      53–56
  transcatheter arterial
      chemoembolization, 53–56

Hepatomegaly, fatty infiltration
    (steatosis), 56–57
Hepatopetal flow, portal hypertension,
    33f, 63
Hernia, 283–286
  anatomy, 283, 285f
  epigastric, 286, 286f
  incisional, 286, 286f
  paraumbilical, 286
  spigelian, 286
  technique, 283–286
  umbilical, 286
Herpes virus, hepatitis, 70
High intensity focused ultrasound (HIFU)
  hepatocellular carcinoma, 53–56
HIV infection/AIDS, liver disease,
    73–74
Hodgkin's lymphoma, 199
  renal tract, 199
Horseshoe kidneys, 191–192f, 192
Human chorionic gonadotropin (β
    HCG), 251
Hydatid cysts
  benign focal liver lesions, 39
  ultrasound-guided drainage, 344
Hydatids of Morgagni, 240
Hydrocele, 245–246, 246f
Hyperparathyroidism, 209–210
  primary, 209
  secondary, 209–210
Hypertrophic pyloric stenosis (HPS),
    pediatrics, 315–316f
Hypertrophied column of Bertin, 189,
    191–192f, 192

I
Iatrogenic splenic trauma, 179
Image optimization, 2–6
  equipment knowledge, 2, 2b
  essential controls of, 2
  focal zones, 2, 3f
  frequency changes, 3, 4f
  fundamentals of ultrasound, 2
  line density, 5, 5f
  time gain compensation (TGC), 4–5
Image quality, equipment, 13
Image recording, 14–15, 23
  digital imaging networks, 15
  patient records, 14–15
Immunocompromised individuals,
    spleen lymphoproliferative
    disorders, 173

Incisional hernia, 286, 286f
Infantile hepatic hemangioma, 295–296,
    297f
Infantile hypertrophic pyloric stenosis
    (IHPS), 314–315
Infarction, spleen, 176–179, 178f
Infectious mononucleosis, hepatitis, 70
Inferior vena cava (IVC), 25–28f, 89f,
    91f, 271–274
  compression, 271, 273f
  duplication, 271
  hemodynamics, 271
  pathology, 271–274
  stenosis, post-operative liver
      transplants, 84, 84f
  thrombi, 271
  tumors, 274
    thrombi, 271, 272–273f
Infertility as prostate gland diseases,
    260, 260f
Inflammatory bowel conditions,
    278–281
  bowel scanning technique, 277f
  see also specific diseases/disorders
Inflammatory bowel disease (IBD), 279
Insulinomas, pancreas, 160
Interventional techniques, see also
      specific techniques, 333–345
Intestinal malrotation, gastrointestinal
    tract, 313–314, 314f
Intratesticular masses, 246–250
  adrenal rest tumors, 248–249, 249f
  benign, 247
  epidermoid cysts, 248, 248f
  intratesticular cysts, 248, 248f
  microlithiasis, 247
Intussusception, pediatrics, 316–317,
    317f

J
Jaundice, 99–100
  causes, 52t, 58t, 100f
  liver metastases, 49–52
  non-obstructive, 100
  obstructive see Obstructive jaundice

K
Keyboard design, equipment, 14
Kidneys, 6f, 186–189
  agnesis, 303
  cortex, 186–187
    thickness, 187f, 189

Kidneys (Continued)
    development, 187
    duplex, 189–192, 191–192f, 304–306,
        304f
    ectopic, 192
    extrarenal pelvis, 191–192f, 192
    fetal lobulations, 187, 188f, 302f, 303
    fusion, 303–304, 303f
    horseshoe, 191–192f, 192, 303
    measurements, 188–189
    medullary pyramids, 186–187, 187f
    pediatric, 302–303, 302–303f
    renal artery stenosis, 216
    renal cortex, 302–303
    renal cystic disease, 307–308
    renal sinus, 187
    renal size, 302
    transplant see Renal transplants
    trauma, 216
    ultrasound-guided biopsy, 338–339,
        339f
Kidney stones see Renal tract stones
Klatskin tumors, 137, 138f

L
Lactate dehydrogenase (LDH), 251
Laparoscopic cholecystectomy,
        cholelithiasis management, 108
Laparoscopic fenestration, complex liver
        cysts, 37
Laparoscopic ultrasound
    biliary duct obstruction management,
        126
    cholelithiasis management, 108, 110f
Laparotomy, abdominal trauma, 322
Laser ablation, liver metastases, 52
Left hepatic vein (LHV), 27f, 29–31, 33f,
        89f, 91f
Left lobe, liver, 25–29f
Left renal artery (LRA), 92f
Left renal vein (LRV), 90f, 92f, 189
Leukemia, spleen see Spleen
Ligamentum teres, 23–24, 26f, 28f, 91–92f
Ligamentum venosum, 23–24, 25f, 89f
    Line density, image optimization, 5, 5f
Liver, 23–34, 25–29f
    benign lesions see Liver lesions,
        benign focal
    calcification, 48–49
        metastases, 48–49
        parasitic infestations, 48–49, 48f
    capsule, 23, 24f

caudate lobe, 25f, 27f, 89–90f
cystadenoma, 37, 38f
diffuse conditions, see also specific
        diseases/disorders, 56–75, 57t
fatty infiltration (steatosis), 46f,
        56–57, 59f
    CEUS, 53, 59f
fibrosis
    cirrhosis, 57–70, 59f
    pediatric cystic fibrosis, 293–295, 295f
focal lesions, 36
    mass effect, 36
hemodynamics, 31
left lobe, 25–29f
malignant lesions see Liver lesions,
        malignant focal
normal appearance, 23–29
Reidel's lobe, 24–29, 29f
right lobe, 24f, 27f, 89f
segments, 29
size determination, 24–29, 24f
tumor ablation, 344
ultrasound-guided biopsy, 337–338,
        338–339f
vasculature, 29–31
Liver function tests, abnormal, 101
Liver lesions, benign focal, 36–49
    abscesses, 39–40, 41–43f
    adenoma, 46, 46f
    complex cysts, 37, 37f
    focal fatty infiltration, 46
    focal fatty sparing, 48
    focal nodular hyperplasia, 43–46, 45f
    granuloma, 48, 48f
    haemangioma, 42–43
    hematoma, 40–42, 44f
    hepatocellular carcinoma see
        Hepatocellular carcinoma
        (HCC)
    hydatid (echinococcal) cysts, 39, 39f
    lipomas, 48
    polycystic liver, 39
    simple cysts, 36
Liver lesions, malignant focal, 49–56
    cholangiocarcinoma, 56, 58t
    metastases, 49–52, 50–51f
        ascites, 49–52
        clinical features, 49–52
        intraoperative ultrasound, 53f
        lymphadenopathy, 49
        prognosis, 52
        staging, 49–52

Liver transplants, 75–86
    acceleration times (ms), 76, 77f
    complications, 79t, 80–81
    Doppler principles, 76–78, 76b
    fluid collections, 85–86, 86f
    indications, 78t
    intraoperative ultrasound, 79
    model of end-stage liver
        disease, 78
    operative procedure, 79
    post-operative assessment, 79–80,
        79t, 80f
        abscesses, 84, 85f
        biochemical monitoring, 79
        focal lesions, 84
        hepatic artery pseudoaneurysms,
            80–81, 82f
        hepatic artery stenosis, 80
        hepatic artery thrombosis, 80, 81f
        hepatic artery assessment, 80, 81f
        hepatic veins, 83–86
        IVC, 83–86
        IVC stenosis, 84, 84f
        portal vein assessment, 81–83, 83f
        renal dysfunction, 79
    post-transplantation malignancy,
        84–85, 85f
    preoperative assessment, 78–79
    rejection, 86
    resistive index values, 77–78, 77f
    waveform interpretation, 76, 77f
Lymphadenopathy, 179, 180–182f
    liver metastases, 49–52
    pancreatic adenocarcinoma, 160
    spleen lymphoproliferative disorders,
        173
Lymphangioma, 182–183, 182f
Lymphatic system, 179–182, 180–182f
Lymph nodes, 182
Lymphocoele, renal transplants see
        Renal transplants
Lymphoma
    renal tract, 199, 200f
    spleen, 171, 172–173f
Lymphoproliferative disorders, spleen
        see Spleen

M
Magnetic resonance
        cholangiopancreatography
        (MRCP)
    acute pancreatitis, 154

Magnetic resonance cholangiopancreatography (MRCP) *(Continued)*
biliary duct obstruction management, 125–126*f*, 126
choledocholithiasis, 107–108
cholelithiasis, 108
chronic pancreatitis, 154
obstructive jaundice, 124, 125–126*f*
pancreas, 148
pediatric biliary atresia, 292
primary sclerosing cholangitis, 130–131
Main portal vein (MPV), 27*f*, 29, 30*f*, 33*f*, 90–91*f*
color Doppler, 30*f*
Main renal artery, duplication, 192
Main renal vein, duplication, 192
Male urogenital tract, 230–232
adenocarcinoma, 251
atrophy, 250
benign penile mass, 255
epididymis, 240–241, 241–242*f*
acute, 241*f*
hydrocele, 245–246, 246*f*
intratesticular masses, 246–250
adrenal rest tumors, 248–249, 249*f*
epidermoid cysts, 248, 248*f*
focal orchitis, 249
intratesticular cysts, 248, 248*f*
malignant, 250–253
microlithiasis, 247
sarcoidosis, 249, 249*f*
small, 249, 249*f*
malignant penile mass, 255, 256*f*
orchitis, 241, 242*f*
Fournier's gangrene, 241–242, 243*f*
mumps, 241
perfusion assessment, 241, 242*f*
palpable scrotal masses, 242–246
penis, 230–232, 230*f*
anatomy, 253–254, 254*f*
CEUS, 230–231
color Doppler, 230–231
examination of, 232
patient dignity, 232
shear wave elastographic techniques, 231, 231*f*
ultrasound elastography, 231
prostate gland, 255–261
scrotal pearls, 245, 246*f*
scrotum, 232–253

Male urogenital tract *(Continued)*
anatomy, 232–234, 233*f*
appendix epididymis, 234, 234*f*
appendix testis, 234, 234*f*
bell-clapper deformity, 232, 233*f*
cystic ectasia, 232–233, 234*f*
testicular volume measurement, 234–235, 235*f*
tunica albuginea, 232–233
tunica vaginalis, 232
tunica vasculosa, 234
sex-cord stromal tumors, 251
testicular appendix, 240, 240*f*
testicular lymphoma, 251–252, 253*f*
testicular torsion, 237–239, 238*f*
missed torsion, 239, 240*f*
spectral Doppler, 238
undiagnosed torsion, 238–239, 239*f*
testicular tumors, 251
secondary, 252–253, 253*f*
trauma, 236–237
CEUS, 237
TWIST score, 237–238
tumor mimicking abnormalities, 249, 250*f*
undescended testes, 235–236
clinical examination, 236, 237*f*
MRI, 236, 237*f*
orchidopexy, 236
urethral carcinoma, 256*f*
varicoceles, 235
color Doppler, 235
diagnosis, 235, 236*f*
retractile testis, 236
spectral Doppler, 235, 236*f*
Malignant disease *see* Tumors
Malignant intratesticular masses, 250–253
primary malignant lesions, 251–252, 252*f*
non-seminoma, 251
seminoma, 251, 252*f*
MCDK *see* Multicystic dysplastic kidney (MCDK)
Mechanical effects (of ultrasound), 16
Mechanical index (MI), 16
Medicolegal issues, 17
Medullary pyramids, kidneys, 186–187, 187*f*
Medullary sponge kidney, 209, 214–215

MELD (model of end-stage liver disease), liver transplants, 78
Metastases
adrenal glands *see* Adrenal glands
gallbladder, 138–139, 139*f*
hepatic calcification, 48–49
liver, 50–51*f*
pancreas, 160
pancreatic carcinoma, 156
renal tract, 199
spleen, 173–174, 174*f*
Microgallbladder, cystic fibrosis, 112, 112*f*
Microlithiasis, 134–135
testicular, 247, 247*f*
Middle hepatic vein (MHV), 29–31
Mirizzi's syndrome, 110–111, 110*f*
endoscopic retrograde cholangiopancreatography, 111
Mitral valve disease, 73, 74*f*
Model of end-stage liver disease (MELD), liver transplants, 78
Monophasic waveform, portal vein, 32
Morrison's pouch, 24*f*
Mucocoele, gallbladder, 106–107*f*, 110
Multicystic dysplastic kidney (MCDK), 196, 308, 309*f*
Multifocal cholangiocarcinoma, 137, 138*f*
Mumps orchitis, 241
Myelolipomas, adrenal glands, 275*f*

N
Needle visualization, 12, 12*f*
Nephroblastoma, 309–311, 310*f*
Nephrocalcinosis, 209, 210*f*
Nephrostomy, ultrasound-guided drainage, 343, 344*f*
Nephrotic syndrome, 215–216
Neuroblastomas, 309–311, 311*f*
Neuroendocrine tumors, pancreas, 160
Nodules, cirrhosis, 58–61
Non-alcoholic steatohepatitis (NASH), 57, 59*f*
Non-Hodgkin's lymphoma
adrenal gland metastases, 274
renal tract, 199
Non-obstructive hydronephrosis, 207
post-obstructive dilatation, 207
reflux, 207
Non-obstructive jaundice, 100
Non-obstructive uropathy, 311, 312*f*

O

Obstruction, gastrointestinal tract, 282, 283f
Obstructive jaundice, 100, 328, 328–329f
  biliary duct dilation, 123–128
  diagnosis/assessment, 106–107f, 124–126, 124t, 125–126f
  early ductal obstruction, 107f, 123
  endoscopic retrograde cholangiopancreatography (ERCP), 124–126
  management, 126–127
Operator safety, 17
Oral contraceptives, liver adenoma, 46
Orchidopexy, 236
Orchitis
  focal, 249
  Fournier's gangrene, 241–242
  male urogenital tract, 241, 242f
  mumps, 241
  perfusion assessment, 241, 242f

P

Pediatric ultrasound, 289–319
  abdomen and pelvis ultrasound technique, 290
  congenital anomalies, 303–307
  equipment, 290
  general tips, 290
  hepatobiliary pathologic conditions, 290–295
    biliary atresia, 291
    choledochal cysts, 293, 294f
    focal liver lesions, 295–298, 296t
    hepatoblastoma, 296, 297f
    hepatocellular carcinoma, 296–298, 298–299f
    normal pediatric US appearances, 290, 291t
    "starry night" liver, 291, 291t
  liver haemangioma, 43
  posterior urethral valves, 306–307, 306f
  renal ultrasound technique, 301–303, 302f
  spleen, 298
Pancreas, 143–165, 144f
  adenocarcinoma, 156–158f, 159
    color Doppler ultrasound, 159–160
    ERCP, 156–158f, 160
    gallbladder dilatation, 160
    liver metastases, 160

Pancreas (Continued)
    lymphadenopathy, 160
    secondary findings, 160
  age-related changes, 146, 147f
  benign cysts, 161–162, 162f
  benign focal lesions, see also specific diseases/disorders, 160–162
  biochemical analysis, 146–147
  carcinoma, 156–160, 156–158f
    clinical features, 156–159
    CT, 156–159
    differential diagnosis, 159, 159t
    endosonography-guided aspiration, 159
    management, 156–159
    metastases, 156, 156–158f
    surgery, 159
  congenital abnormalities, 147–148
  duct, dilatation, 123
  endoscopic ultrasound, 148, 155f
  focal fatty sparing, 160–161, 162f
  focal pancreatitis, 161, 161f
  gastrinomas, 160
  hemangiomas, 162, 162f
  insulinomas, 160
  malignant disease, 156–160
  metastases, 160
  MRCP, 148
  neuroendocrine tumors, 160
  pediatrics, 299, 300–301f
  pseudocysts
    benign focal liver lesions, 37
  scanning pitfalls, 146
  texture, 146
  trauma, 162
  visualization techniques, 143–146
Pancreas anulare, 147–148
Pancreas divisum, 147–148
Pancreatic transplantation, 162–163
  color Doppler, 163, 163f
  contrast CT, 163
  with kidney transplant, 163
  postoperative complications, 163
Pancreatitis, 150–156
  focal, 161, 161f
Pancreatitis, acute, 150–154, 152–153f, 329–330, 330f
  causes, 151t
  clinical features, 150
  CT, 151–154
  Doppler ultrasound, 154
  focal occurrence, 154

Pancreatitis, acute (Continued)
    management, 154
    MRCP, 154
    pseudocysts, 151
    recurrent chronic vs., 154–156
Pancreatitis, chronic, 154–156, 155f
  calcification, 154–156, 155f
  duct obstruction, 156
  fibrosis, 154
  MRCP, 154
  recurrent acute vs., 154–156
  serum enzymes, 154
Paracentesis, ultrasound-guided drainage, 341–342, 341–342f
Parapelvic renal cysts, 193
Parasitic infections
  biliary tree, 133–134
  hepatic calcification, 48–49, 48f
  see also specific infections
Paraumbilical hernia, 286
Partial pancreaticoduodenectomy, pancreatic carcinoma, 159
Parvus tardus pattern, renal artery stenosis, 216f
Pelvicalyceal system dilatation, renal transplants, 217
Penile mass
  benign, 255
  malignant, 255, 256f
  palpable, 254
Penis
  anatomy, 253–254, 254f
  CEUS, 230–231
  color Doppler, 230–231
  examination of, 232
  general considerations, 230–231, 230–231f
  patient dignity, 232
  scanning technique, 232
  shear wave elastographic techniques, 231, 231f
Peraumbilical varices, portal vein thrombosis, 66–67f, 68
Percutaneous nephrostomy, renal tract obstruction, 203–205f
Phaeochromocytoma, adrenal glands see Adrenal glands
Peyronie's disease, 254, 255f
Physiological dilatation, renal tract, 191–192f, 201
Pigment stones, cholelithiasis, 101

Pneumobilia, 135–136, 135*f*
  emphysemous cholecystitis, 136
Polycystic liver, 39, 39*f*
Polyps, gallbladder, 113–115, 114*f*
Porcelain gallbladder, 105*f*, 112, 112*f*
Porta hepatis varices, portal vein
      thrombosis, 68
Portal hypertension, 62*t*, 63
  balanced flow, 63, 64–65*f*
  cavernous transformation, 63, 66–67*f*
  color Doppler, 63
  damping, 63
  flow velocity, 63
  hepatopetal flow, 63
  liver transplants, 78
  portal vein signs, 63–68
  reversed flow, 63, 64–67*f*
  spectral Doppler, 63
  thrombosed, 63, 64–65*f*
Portal vein (PV), 23–24, 27*f*, 31–32*f*
  complications, 81–83, 83*f*
  diameter, 32
  Doppler ultrasound, 63–64
  monophasic waveform, 32
  post-operative liver transplants,
      81–83, 83*f*
  stenosis, post-operative liver
      transplants, 82–83
  thrombosis, 63–64, 66*t*, 83
    liver transplants, 78
    management, 68–70
  velocity, 32
Positron emission tomography (PET)
  adenomyomatosis, 112–113
  spleen lymphoproliferative disorders,
      171
Posterior urethral valves, pediatrics,
      306–307, 306*f*
Post-obstructive dilatation, non-
      obstructive hydronephrosis,
      207
Post-transplantation malignancy, liver
      transplants, 84–85, 85*f*
Post-transplant lymphoproliferative
      disorder (PTLD), 171,
      172–173*f*
Power Doppler ultrasound, 6–7
Pregnancy
  acute fatty liver, 74
  HELLP syndrome, 74–75, 74*t*, 75*f*
  liver disease, 74–75
  pelvicalyceal system dilatation, 201

Primary biliary cirrhosis (PBC), 132
  biliary stasis, 135
  cirrhosis, 60*f*, 61–62
Primary carcinoma, gallbladder,
      136–137, 136*f*
Primary hyperparathyroidism, 209
Primary sclerosing cholangitis (PSC),
      71, 129–131, 130–132*f*
  biliary stasis, 135
  cholangiocarcinoma, 129–130, 132*f*
  clinical features, 129–130
Probes, 13, 13*f*
Processing, image optimization, 6
Prostate cancer, 260–261, 261*f*
Prostate gland, 188*f*
  anatomy, 255–257, 257*f*
  benign prostatic hypertrophy,
      258–259, 259*f*
  diseases
    cysts, 259, 260*f*
    infection and prostatitis, 259–260,
        260*f*
    infertility, 260, 260*f*
    prostate cancer, 260–261, 261*f*
    ultrasound-guided biopsy, 261,
        261*f*
  measurements, 257–258, 258*f*
  zonal anatomy, 256, 257*f*
Prostatitis, 259–260, 260*f*
Pseudoaneurysms, 225–226
  color Doppler, 225–226, 226*f*
  renal transplants, 225–226, 226*f*
  spleen, 179
Pseudocysts, acute pancreatitis, 151
Pulsed Doppler ultrasound, 7, 8*f*
  thermal effects, 15–16
Pulse repetition frequency (PRF), 8
Pyelonephritis, 211–214
  acute, 211, 331
  bladder diverticula, 212, 212–213*f*
  pyonephrosis, 202–207, 206*f*,
      212–213*f*
  renal abscess, 212–213*f*, 213
  xanthogranulomatous, 213–214, 214*f*
Pyloric stenosis, 315, 315–316*f*
Pylorus, 314, 315*t*
  ultrasound examination, 315
Pyonephrosis, 202–207, 206*f*, 212–213*f*

Q
Quadratus lumborum, 24*f*, 89*f*, 92*f*
Quality assurance, 18

Quality assurance (*Continued*)
  equipment tests, 18
  testing regimens, 18, 19*f*

R
Radiofrequency microwave ablation
  liver metastases, 52
RCC *see* Renal cell carcinoma (RCC)
Rectum, malignant tumors, 281
Reflux
  non-obstructive hydronephrosis, 207
  urinary tract infections, 207
Reidel's lobe, 24–29, 29*f*
Rejection, liver transplants, 86
Renal abscesses, pyelonephritis,
      212–213*f*, 213
Renal artery stenosis, 216
  acceleration index, 216*f*
  acceleration time, 216*f*
  Doppler ultrasound, 223
  parvus tardus pattern, 216*f*,
      223–224
  renal transplants, 223–224
Renal cell carcinoma (RCC), 197,
      198–199*f*
Renal cystic disease, 307–308
  ADPKD, 308, 308*f*
  MCDK, 308, 309*f*
Renal cysts, 193–196
  acquired disease, 195, 195*f*
  benign *vs.* malignant, 193*f*, 194, 194*t*
  Bosniak classification, 194, 194*t*
  calcification, 194
  CEUS, 194, 199, 199*f*
  CT, 194
  simple, 307–308
Renal dilatation, 311
Renal pelvis dilatation, 301, 302*f*
  non-obstructive uropathy, 311, 312*f*
  obstructive uropathy, 311
  postnatal renal dilatation, 311
Renal ectopia, 303–304
Renal failure, 214–216
  acute, 214
  chronic, 214
Renal function assessment, 189
  serum creatinine, 189
  serum urea, 189
Renal humps, 192–193
Renal measurements, 188–189
Renal sinus, 187
Renal size, pediatrics, 302

Renal tract, 185–228
  acute renal colic, 330f, 331
  adenomas, 196
  amyloid disease, 215–216
  anatomical variants, *see also specific
      variants*, 189–193
  angiomyolipoma, 195f, 196
    CT, 196
  benign focal tumors, *see also specific
      tumors*, 196
  calcification, *see also* Renal tract
      stones, 207–211
  diffuse disease, 214–216
  hemodynamics, 189
    color Doppler, 189, 190–191f
    see also specific blood vessels
  infections, 211–214, 331
  inflammation, 211–214
  lymphoma, 199, 200f
  malignancies, 196–201
  metastases, 199
  non-Hodgkin's lymphoma, 199
  obstruction *see* Renal tract
      obstruction
  physiological dilatation, 191–192f
  renal failure *see* Renal failure
  trauma, 216
  ureteric calculi, 331
  vascular pathology, 216
  von Hippel–Lindau disease, 201
  see also Kidneys
Renal tract obstruction, 201–202,
      203–205f
  causes, 201–202, 201–202t
  CT, 201–202
  non-dilated, 204–206, 206f, 207t
  percutaneous nephrostomy, 203–205f
  vesicoureteric junction, 203–205f, 207
    color Doppler, 188f, 207
Renal tract stones, 206f, 207–211, 208–209f
  calcium stones, 207
  CT, 209
  cystine stones, 207
  cystinuria, 207
  Doppler ultrasound, 207–211,
      208–209f
  staghorn calculi, 207, 208–209f, 209
  struvite (triple phosphate) stones, 207
  uric acid stones, 207
Renal transplants, 217–227
  abscesses, 223
  acute tubular necrosis, 226–227
  ciclosporin nephrotoxicity, 227

Doppler ultrasound correlation, 227
  hematoma, 222
  infections, 226, 226f
  lymphocoele, 221–222
    spectral Doppler, 221–222, 223f
  with pancreatic transplantation, 163
  postoperative complications, 217–219
  posttransplant monitoring, 217,
      218–219f
    morphological appearance, 217
    pelvicalyceal system dilatation, 217
    perirenal fluid, 217
  rejection, 219–223, 222f
    acute, 219
    chronic, 221, 223t
  ultrasound-guided biopsy, 339–340,
      340f
  urinoma, 222–223
  vascular anatomy, 217, 218–219f
  vascular complications, 223–226
    graft nephrectomy, 223
    pseudoaneurysms, 225–226, 226f
    renal artery stenosis, 223–224
    renal vein thrombosis, 224–225
    vascular occlusion, 223, 224f
Renal vein thrombosis, 219, 220f,
      224–225
  Doppler spectrum, 224, 225f
  renal transplants, 224–225
Resistive index values, liver transplants,
      77–78, 77f
Retroperitoneum, 265–287, 266f
Reversed flow, portal hypertension, 63,
      64–65f
Right hepatic vein (RHV), 24f, 27f,
      29–31, 33f, 91f
Right lobe, liver, 24–25f, 27f, 89f
Right portal vein (RPV), 27f, 91f
  color Doppler, 30f
Right renal artery (RRA), 25f, 89f
Rokitansky–Aschoff sinuses,
      adenomyomatosis, 112, 113f

S

Safe practice (of ultrasound), 17, 17b
Safety indices, 16
Sarcoidosis, 249, 249f
Sarcoidosis, liver granuloma, 48
Scintigraphy, hepatobiliary *see*
      Hepatobiliary scintigraphy
Scrotum, 232–253
  anatomy, 232–234, 233f
  appendix epididymis, 234, 234f

Scrotum *(Continued)*
  appendix testis, 234, 234f
  bell-clapper deformity, 232, 233f
  cystic ectasia, 232–233, 234f
  testicular volume measurement,
      234–235, 235f
  tunica albuginea, 232–233
  tunica vaginalis, 232
  tunica vasculosa, 234
Scrotal pearls, 245, 246f
Secondary biliary cirrhosis, 62
Secondary hyperparathyroidism, 209–210
Serum creatinine, renal function
      assessment, 189
Serum tumor markers, 251
Serum urea, renal function assessment,
      189
Sex-cord stromal tumors, 251
Sinus fat, renal tract stones *vs.*, 209
Soft tissue thermal index (TIS), 16
Sperm granulomas, 243
Sphincterotomy, biliary duct obstruction
      management, 126
Spigelian hernia, 286
Spleen, 91f, 167–171
  abscesses, 175–176, 175f
    immunosuppressed individuals, 175
  anatomical variants, 168
  benign conditions, *see also specific
      diseases/disorders*, 174–176
  calcification, 175f, 176
  cysts, 174–175
  ectopic, 168
  hemolytic anemia, 176, 177f
  leukemia, 173
    chemotherapy, 173
    immunocompromised individuals,
        173
    lymphadenopathy, 173
    metastases, 173–174, 174f
  lymphoproliferative disorders, 171,
      172–173f
    chemotherapy, 171
    diagnosis, 171
    focal lesions, 171
    lymphoma, 171, 172–173f
    positron emission tomography, 171
  malignant disease, *see also specific
      diseases/disorders*, 171–174
  pediatrics, 298
  pseudoaneurysms, 179
  scanning pitfalls, 171
  size, 168

Spleen *(Continued)*
  splenic infarction, 176–179, 178*f*
  splenunculi, 168–171, 170*f*
  trauma, 179
  vascular abnormalities, 176–183
Splenic artery (SA), 25*f*, 28*f*, 90–91*f*,
      168, 169*f*
  aneurysm, 179
Splenic vein, 26*f*, 33*f*, 90*f*, 92*f*, 143, 168,
      169*f*
  thrombosis, 178
Splenomegaly, 168, 169–170*f*, 170*b*
  portal vein thrombosis *vs.*, 66
Splenorenal varices, portal vein
      thrombosis, 66–67*f*, 68
Sporadic aniridia, Wilms tumor, 310
Staghorn calculi, 208–209*f*, 209
Steatosis *see* Liver, fatty infiltration
      (steatosis)
Stomach, 26*f*, 28*f*, 90–92*f*, 277*f*
  EUS, 277–278
Strawberry gallbladder *see*
      Cholesterolosis
Struvite (triple phosphate) stones, renal
      tract stones, 207
Subcostal scanning, ultrasound
      technique, 23
Superior mesenteric artery (SMA), 26*f*,
      28*f*, 90*f*, 92*f*, 144*f*, 146, 189,
      190–191*f*
Superior mesenteric vein (SMV), 89*f*

T
Technique (of ultrasound), 1–2, 23
  image optimization, 2–6
Testicular appendix, 240, 240*f*
  Doppler assessment, 240–241
Testicular lymphoma, 251–252, 253*f*
Testicular microlithiasis, 247, 247*f*
Testicular seminoma, 251, 252*f*
Testicular torsion, 237–239, 238*f*
Testicular tumors, 237
Testing regimens, quality assurance,
      18, 19*f*
Thermal index (TI), 16
Thrombi, inferior vena cava, 271
Thrombosed flow, portal hypertension,
      63, 64–65*f*
Thrombosis, splenic vein, 178
Time gain compensation (TGC), 4–5
TIPSS (transjugular intrahepatic
      portosystemic shunt), portal
      vein thrombosis, 68, 69*f*

Tissue harmonics, 8–10
  image optimization, 5, 10*f*
Torsion
  missed, 239, 240*f*
  spermatic cord, 238, 239*f*
  testicular, 237–239, 238*f*
    extravaginal torsion, 238
    supravaginal torsion, 238
  undiagnosed, 238–239, 239*f*
Transcatheter arterial
      chemoembolization,
      hepatocellular carcinoma,
      53–56
Transitional cell carcinoma (TCC), 197,
      200*f*
Transplantation
  kidney *see* Renal transplants
  liver *see* Liver transplants
  pancreas *see* Pancreatic
      transplantation
Trauma
  acute abdomen *see* Acute abdomen
  acute pancreatitis, 151*t*
  male urogenital tract, 236–237
  pancreas, 162
  spleen, 179
Tru-cut needles, 335–336, 336*f*
Tuberculosis
  liver granuloma, 48
Tuberose sclerosis, 195, 195*f*
Tubular necrosis, acute *see* Acute
      tubular necrosis (ATN)
Tumors
  ablation, 344–345
  biliary tree, 136–139
  inferior vena cava, 274
  liver lesions *see* Liver lesions,
      malignant focal
  pancreas *see* Pancreas
  rectum, 281
  retroperitoneum, 283, 284–285*f*
  seeding, ultrasound-guided biopsy,
      340
  testicular tumors, 251
Tunica albuginea, 232–233
Tunica vaginalis, 232

U
Ulcerative colitis (UC), 281
Ultrasound elastography, 231
Ultrasound-guided vascular access, 344
Umbilical hernia, 286
Unconjugated bilirubin, 99–100

Undescended testes, 235–236
  clinical examination, 236, 237*f*
  MRI, 236, 237*f*
  orchidopexy, 236
Upgradeability, equipment, 14
Urachal remnant, 306
Urea, renal function assessment, 189
Ureteric jets, 188
Ureteric orifices, bladder, 188
Ureterocele, renal tract obstruction, 207
Urethral carcinoma, 256*f*
Uric acid stones, 207
Urinary tract infections (UTIs), 211
  reflux, 207
Urinoma, 222–223

V
Varices, portal vein thrombosis *vs.*, 66,
      66–67*f*
Varicoceles, 235
  diagnosis, 235, 236*f*
  Doppler, 235
VATER syndrome, renal agnesis, 303
Vesicoureteric reflux, 311–312,
      312–313*f*, 313*b*
Viral hepatitis, 70
  chronic active, 70
  chronic persistent, 70
  fulminant, 70
  see also specific types
Visceral rupture, abdominal trauma,
      325–327*f*, 327–328
Volvulus, 313–314, 314*f*
Von Hippel–Lindau disease, 194–195
  pancreatic cysts, 161–162
  renal tract, 201

W
Waveform interpretation, 76, 77*f*
Whipple procedure, pancreatic
      carcinoma, 159
Wilms tumor, 309–311, 310*f*
  CT, 310
  magnetic resonance imaging, 310
Wilson's disease, cirrhosis, 62
Wolffian duct, 240
Work-related musculoskeletal disorders
      (WRMSDs), 14

X
Xanthogranulomatous pyelonephritis,
      213–214, 214*f*